In-Services for Long-Term Care

Education for Frontline Staff

Kelly Smith Papa, MSN, RN

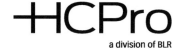

HCPro

a division of BLR

In-Services for Long-Term Care: Education for Frontline Staff is published by HCPro, a division of BLR

Copyright © 2015 HCPro, a division of BLR

All rights reserved. Printed in the United States of America.   5   4   3   2   1

Download the additional materials of this book at www.hcpro.com/downloads/12360

ISBN: 978-1-55645-285-7

HCPro provides information resources for the healthcare industry.

HCPro is not affiliated in any way with The Joint Commission, which owns the JCAHO and Joint Commission trademarks.

Kelly Smith Papa, MSN, RN, Author
Olivia MacDonald, Managing Editor
Adrienne Trivers, Product Manager
Erin Callahan, Senior Director, Product
Elizabeth Petersen, Vice President
Matt Sharpe, Production Supervisor
Vincent Skyers, Design Manager
Vicki McMahan, Sr. Graphic Designer
Diane Uhls, Layout/Graphic Design
Tyson Davis, Cover Designer

Advice given is general. Readers should consult professional counsel for specific legal, ethical, or clinical questions.

Arrangements can be made for quantity discounts. For more information, contact:

HCPro
75 Sylvan Street, Suite A-101
Danvers, MA 01923
Telephone: 800-650-6787 or 781-639-1872
Fax: 800-639-8511
Email: *customerservice@hcpro.com*

Visit HCPro online at *www.hcpro.com* and *www.hcmarketplace.com*

Contents

Introduction

Every day we are surrounded by the opportunity for learning. Whether it is learning a new policy, enhancing skills, reflecting on actions, or meeting a new person, in long-term care we have countless opportunities to learn and grow. I often find myself thinking about Michelangelo, who at the age of 87 wrote the inscription "*Ancora Imparo*" (*I am still learning*) in one of his sketches. The painter and sculptor, who had created magnificent works of art his entire life, was still learning.

I believe in lifelong learning; I don't think any person can ever feel they're done learning, growing, and becoming. Healthcare is an ever-changing world with constant challenges and new expectations of those we serve. The more we know about our jobs and those we serve, the more we know we need to learn.

If you are reading this book, you are inspired to bring new learning to your team. Your approach, in bringing enlightened learning to your team, is an essential factor in the building of skills. Quality clinical outcomes are the results of a talented team of staff with high clinical competence and empathy for those they are entrusted to care for. In this book you will find 40 essential in-services. Each chapter offers tools to help you create connections with your team as you help them deepen their awareness and skills in a variety of important long-term care topics. While using the materials in this book, keep in the mind the additional information your team will need to know regarding your facility's specific policies and procedures.

I believe we learn the most from authentic educators who are passionate about learning and developing. Educators who are excited about the topics that they are teaching and who also have a deep respect for their students have the biggest impact. As an educator, take the extra time to learn about how adults learn and infuse your classes with many types of communication and approaches to be sure that students are able to feel educated about the topic at hand. Use training time to build relationships to help with less formal learning that occurs in those unscheduled teachable moments.

1

Alzheimer's Disease

Teaching Plan

To use this lesson for self-study, the learner should read the material, do the activity, and take the test. For group study, the leader may give each learner a copy of the learning guide and follow this teaching plan to conduct the lesson. Certificates may be copied for everyone who completes the lesson.

Learning objectives

After this lesson, participants should be able to:

- Recognize signs of Alzheimer's disease (AD)

- Apply suggestions that may make caring for the person with AD easier

- Use techniques for handling distress in a compassionate way

Lesson activities

1. Ask participants to remember a time when they faced an unfamiliar situation. The first day of a new job, for example, usually requires talking to strangers, figuring out unfamiliar routines and tasks, and getting around in a strange building. Encourage the learners to tell you how they feel in such situations. Some natural feelings include confusion, puzzlement, nervousness, insecurity, or even fear. Explain to participants that a person with AD feels this way all the time. The world is more puzzling to them every day. Everyone seems to be a stranger, nothing seems familiar, and abilities they used to have are gone. When we try to see situations from the point of view of the person with AD, it is easy to understand why they are sometimes anxious, irritable, or upset.

2. Distribute index cards or paper. Ask each learner to take two cards and on one card write down a question about caring for people with AD and on the other card write down a joy found caring for people affected by AD. Have the learners fold the papers or cards that have the questions on them and place them in a box or basket you provide. Ask them to hold onto the card that has the joy on it. These can be shared later in the lesson when you

feel ready. Hand out copies of the learning guide. Have each learner draw a card from the basket. Instruct the learners to read the learning guide and try to find an answer to the question. Allow enough time for all learners to find their answer, and then ask them to read their question aloud to the group and explain the answer they found. If there is no answer for the question in the learning guide, have learners brainstorm possible approaches or ideas based on the principles in the lesson.

The lesson

Review the material in the lesson with participants. Allow for discussion.

Conclusion

Have participants take the test. Review the answers together. Award certificates to those who answer 70% of the test questions correctly.

Test answers

1. c	2. False	3. e	4. True	5. b, c, e
6. True	7. True	8. True	9. c	10. False

Alzheimer's Disease

Learning Guide

Contents:

- Understanding Alzheimer's Disease
    - Causes
    - Complications
    - Treatment
    - Prevention and research
- Caring for the Person With AD
    - Suggested approaches to caring for the person with AD
- Approaches for supporting the person with AD who is in distress

Understanding Alzheimer's Disease

Alzheimer's disease (AD) is the most common form of dementia. More than 4 million Americans have AD. The disease is characterized by memory loss, language deterioration, poor judgment, and inability to care for personal needs.

AD is a form of dementia that affects a person's ability to carry out daily activities. It involves the parts of the brain that control short- and long-term memory, speaking and understanding language, concentration, and the ability to perform complex tasks. Healthy brain tissue dies or deteriorates, causing a steady decline in memory and mental abilities.[1]

AD is not the only form of dementia. Doctors diagnose AD by doing tests to eliminate all the other possible reasons for the person's symptoms. People can suffer from more than one form of dementia at a time. This is why treatment approaches that are person-centered and based on the person's strengths are the most successful.

AD causes progressive degeneration of the brain. It may start with slight memory loss and confusion but eventually leads to severe, irreversible mental impairment that destroys a person's ability to care for him or herself without assistance. Usually, family members notice gradual—not sudden—changes in a person with AD.

As AD progresses, symptoms become serious, and family members usually seek medical help. Progression from simple forgetfulness to severe dementia might take 5–10 years or longer.

People with mild AD may live alone and function fairly well. People with moderate AD may need some type of assistance. People with advanced AD generally require assistance with all areas of their personal care.

Causes

Think of the way electricity travels along wires from a power source to the point of use. Messages travel through the brain in a similar way, but they are carried by chemicals instead of wires. Information travels through the nerve cells in the brain so we can remember, communicate, think, and perform activities.

Researchers have found that people with AD have lower levels of the chemicals that carry these important messages from one brain cell to another. In addition, people with AD have many damaged or dead nerve cells in areas of the brain that are vital to memory and other mental abilities. Although the person's mind still contains memories and knowledge, it may be impossible to find and use the information in the brain because of AD.

Abnormal structures in the brain called plaques and tangles are another characteristic of AD:

- **Plaques**

    – It is believed that plaque deposits form between brain cells early in the disease process.

- **Tangles**

    – This refers to the way that brain cells become twisted, causing damage and nerve cell death.

These structures block the movement of messages through the brain, causing memory loss, confusion, and personality changes.

People with AD may experience distress when they feel overwhelmed, confused, or misunderstood. As they lose the ability to communicate verbally, they may share their distress with physical signals. Always remember that all actions are forms of communication of a need. Use empathy to seek to understand what the person with dementia is feeling, then use validation to support their needs.

Complications

As people advance into late stages of AD, they may lose the ability to do normal activities and care for their own needs. They may have difficulty eating, going to the bathroom, or taking care of their personal hygiene. People with AD may suffer from poor safety awareness, and they might get lost or become injured. They may develop complicating health problems such as pneumonia, infections, falls, and fractures.

Treatment

There is no cure. Medications are available that may lessen the symptoms, but they are unable to stop or reverse the disease. These include tacrine (Cognex), donepezil (Aricept), rivastigamine (Exelon), and galantamine (Reminyl).

Medications are sometimes ordered to help with symptoms such as sleeplessness, pain, wandering, anxiety, agitation, and depression.

Prevention and research

There is no known way to prevent AD. Researchers continue to look for ways to reduce the risk of this disease. It is believed that a lifelong heart-healthy lifestyle with mental exercise and learning may create more connections between nerve cells and delay the onset of dementia. People should be encouraged to learn new things and stay mentally active as long as possible.

Caring for the Person With AD

AD progresses at a different rate with each person. It is important to focus on things that the person with AD can still do and enjoy.

All persons with AD need empathy and constant reassurance, no matter what stage of the disease they are in.

You will recognize the following signs in many people with AD:

- Increasing and persistent forgetfulness
- Difficulty finding the right word
- Loss of judgment
- Difficulty performing familiar activities such as brushing teeth or bathing

- Personality changes such as irritability, anxiety, pacing, and restlessness
- Depression, which may show itself in some of the following ways:
  - Wandering
  - Anxiety—this can be caused by noise, feeling rushed, and large groups
  - Weight loss
  - Sleep disturbance
- Pacing and agitation
  - Agitation often is a symptom of underlying illness or pain. Medication can also cause agitation, as can changes in the environment.
- Cursing or threatening language
- Distress related to pain, disorientation, delusions, or hallucinations
  - A person with hallucinations sees, hears, or feels things that are not there. A person with delusions believes strongly in something that is not true, such as believing that he or she has been captured by enemies. Symptoms of pain can look like agitation, aggression, or depression.
- Difficulties with abstract thinking or complex tasks
  - Balancing a checkbook, recognizing and understanding numbers, or reading may be impossible

The following suggestions will help you care for a person with AD

Learn their life story

Many times we ask people affected by AD questions that have only one correct answer, such as "What town are you from?" "How many kids do you have?" or "What type of job did you have?" These questions require the person with AD to come up with one correct answer. The ability to access this factual information may be hard for them to do as their brains change during the disease process. A person with AD may feel a sense of distress or sadness if they are frequently asked questions to which they can not think of the answers. Instead of asking these types of questions, ask them or their family members questions that seek to learn the richness of the person's life—the cool stuff! Ask about the interesting stories that convey the person's passions or give you clues into who they were when they were healthier. Ask questions such as "Can you tell me about your favorite things to do in the summer?" "Can you tell me about your first car?" or "What would your dream vacation be?" If the person has AD, give them time to think about their answers to your questions and share with you. It may feel like it is taking a long time, but the changes in their brain are what is causing the delay. Be careful not to ask multiple questions rapidly; instead, give the person time to process and share.

Work with the care team to find meaningful questions to ask family members to learn more about the person's life legacy. Rather than asking the typical "bio" form topics, create questions that build relationships. You can find countless conversation starter-type questions online. These questions seek more to learn about the person instead of quiz their ability to recall. Having engaging conversations about the things a person enjoyed doing in the summer months can help you to get to know them much better than simply knowing the town that they are from.

Provide structure

Serenity and stability reduce feelings of distress. When a person with AD becomes upset, their ability to think clearly declines even more. Follow a regular daily routine. Plan the schedule to match the person's normal, preferred routine, and find the best time of day to do things, when the person is most capable. Be sure to keep familiar objects around.

Bathing

Some people with AD won't mind bathing. For others, it is a confusing, frightening experience. Plan the bath close to the same time every day. Be patient and calm. Allow the person to do as much of the bath as possible. Never leave the person alone in the bath or shower. A shower or bath may not be necessary every day—try a sponge or partial bath some days. If a person with AD experiences distress from a shower such as feeling cold or feelings of modesty, it is more important to keep them feeling safe and in control. Some care partners have found that washing different areas of the body at different times decreases the distress associated with bathing. For example, in the morning, wash the person's face, neck, arms, chest, and underarms. Then, later in the day, wash the person's peri area, legs, and feet. If the person is still distressed, break up the bathing of areas of their body even more.

Dressing

Allow extra time for dressing, so the person won't feel rushed. Encourage the person to do as much of the dressing as possible.

Eating

Some people will need encouragement to eat, while others will eat all the time. A quiet, calm atmosphere may help the person focus on the meal. Finger foods will help those who struggle with utensils. If the person needs assistance with the meal, use visual and verbal cues to keep them independent. If more assistance is needed, care partners have found that using a hand-over-hand or hand-under-hand approach keeps the person engaged. Calming music, meaningful conversation, or aromas are other methods to keep the person engaged during meals.

Personal care

Set a routine for taking the person to the bathroom, such as every three hours during the day. Don't wait for the person to ask. Many people with AD experience incontinence as the disease progresses. Be understanding when accidents happen.

Communication

When talking, stand where the person can see you. Use simple sentences and speak slowly. Focus attention with gentle touching if permitted.

Environment

Make the environment familiar, free of clutter, and safe. Create spaces in which the person with AD has meaningful things to do. It should be the goal to keep the person with AD involved in activities that they find meaningful, rewarding, and person centered, not juvenile. Use spaces that have access to the outdoors and that have areas to sit and relax.

Exercise

Exercise helps improve motor skills, functional abilities, energy, circulation, stamina, mood, sleep, and elimination. Avoid pushing the person to exercise, but provide encouragement. Give simple instructions. Mild stretching exercises are good; some people enjoy chair stretching such as modified yoga moves. Demonstrate how to tense and release muscle groups in sequence, keeping the order the same each time. Exercise or walk at the same time each day. A daily walk may relieve discomfort and distress. Work with therapy and recreation to create plans for movement and exercise.

Evening routines

Evening routines are important to maximize the benefits of a good night's sleep. Distress is often worse at night. Create a routine that is calming. Soothing music is helpful for some. Leave a night-light on to reduce confusion and restlessness. Try to minimize disruptions at night to give the person more hours of sleep.

Approaches for Supporting the Person With AD Who Is in Distress

Sundown syndrome

Many patients with AD are more agitated, confused, or restless in the late afternoon or early evening. Some people with AD can experience these symptoms at any time of the day when they feel overwhelmed, misunderstood, in pain, or frustrated. The first key to understanding distress is to create environments in which all day-care partners are in tune with the person's reactions. Simply noticing when frustration begins and approaching with validation will help minimize the distress. Research shows the following things help:

- Learn the person's life story and past routines, and use empathy to seek to understand what the person with AD is communicating.

- Enjoy the outdoors.

- Provide more activity earlier in the day. This will use up energy, while reducing stress.

- Schedule essential activities and appointments early in the day.

- Encourage an afternoon nap every day. This reduces fatigue and agitation.

- Play classical music on a portable radio or music player through headphones or earpieces. This shuts out disturbing noises and may soothe the person.

- Give warm, relaxing baths, foot soaks, or massages. They may help.

- Reduce activity and distractions toward the end of the day.

- Discourage evening visits and outings.

- Avoid overstimulation. Turn off the television or radio before speaking to a person.

- Keep the person well-hydrated by offering plenty of water throughout the day.

- Assess for pain frequently.

Hiding, hoarding, and rummaging

These common actions can be disturbing to care partners and to others living with the person with AD. With the resident that struggles with hiding, hoarding, or rummaging, you can try the following strategies:

- Lock outside-going doors.

- If locking closets or drawers causes the person with AD more distress, remove items that might pose a safety risk.

- Watch for patterns. If a person keeps taking the same thing, provide one of his or her own.

- Leave things lying around in the open that are safe for the person who enjoys rummaging or hoarding; put things away that you would prefer the person not to use.

- Make duplicates of important items like family photos, keys, and eyeglasses.

- Designate an easily reached drawer as a rummage drawer. Fill it with interesting, harmless items like old keys on chains, trinkets, or plastic kitchen implements. Allow the patient to rummage freely in this drawer.

- Look through waste cans when something is lost and before emptying them.

- People with AD tend to have favorite hiding places for things. Look for patterns.

> All actions have meaning. Use empathy to seek to understand the reason for the action, and then respond in the most supportive way.

Repetition

A person with AD can become fixated on a task and repeat it over and over without stopping. Pacing, turning lights on and off, or washing hands repeatedly are examples of this. As long as the activity isn't dangerous, there is nothing wrong with letting the person continue doing it. When the time comes that the person must be asked to stop, try these tips:

- Touch the person gently.

- Lead the person by the arm away from the activity.

- Point out something distracting.

- Say things like "Thank you for folding all those towels. Now let's go to dinner."

Confusion

Enter the person's world through empathy. Ask questions to seek to understand what the person is seeing in his or her mind's eye. Use words that let the person know that he or she is safe with you and that you are a friend. Wait 20–90 seconds after asking the person with AD a question; this gives him or her time to understand what you have asked and to find the words to answer. Many times we rush people when it feels to us like we have given them enough time to respond. As their brain is changing, in order to keep them engaged, you should offer them the time to respond. Just like when you get caught in traffic, you still get to your destination, it just takes a bit longer. Ask questions with yes/no answers.

As stated previously, avoid asking questions that have one right answer or that could leave the person feeling like they should know the answer but can't come up with it. Recall how you felt when you were given a pop quiz in school. Our goal is to keep the person feeling positive, and when we ask questions the person does not know the answer to, it can cause him or her to feel emotions of distress.

- Make positive statements that let the person know what you want. For example, say "stand still" instead of "don't move."

- If there are many steps in a task, break them into very small steps so that there are things that the person can do to be successful. Instead of saying "Put on your shirt," break it into "Put your left arm in the sleeve," and then follow up with each additional small step.

- Give the person a limited number of choices.

- Lay out clothes in advance. Keep the wardrobe simple, and try the following things:

  - Avoid buttons and zippers if possible

  - Use Velcro fastenings and elastic waistbands

  - Limit the number of colors in the wardrobe

  - Eliminate accessories

- Use memory aids, such as posting a list of the daily routine or putting up a large calendar and clock. Other aids include:

  - Putting name tags on important objects.

  - Using pictures to communicate if the person doesn't understand words.

  - Making memory books with pictures of important people and places.

  - Posting reminders about chores or safety measures.

  - Painting the bathroom door a bright color, and putting a brightly colored seat cover on the toilet. These will remind the person where to go.

- Give simple, precise instructions. Reduce distractions during a task. Give only as much guidance as necessary.

- Say the person's name and make eye contact to get his or her attention before touching.

- Reassure the person if needed, but don't needlessly distract a patient who is doing a task.

- Each step of a process should be handled as a separate task. Instead of saying "It's time for your bath," say "Take off your shoes. That's good. Now take off your socks."

- Allow plenty of time for every task.

- If the person can't complete a task, praise him or her for what was accomplished and say "thank you" for helping you.

Wandering

We may call it wandering, but to the person with AD, this walking is purposeful. The person with AD who is walking around a lot may be looking for something that looks familiar, or it may feel good to them to stay active. Our goal is to keep our patient safe, positive, and engaged. Always remember that as their disease progresses, people with AD do not know they have dementia and, in some cases, may believe that they are in their twenties. When we use symbols that make them feel childlike or controlled, it will cause them distress or to not feel that those symbols are there for them. Things like STOP signs and painting over doorways are ineffective. The most effective thing to do is to be empathetic—enter the person's world and try to figure out what he or she is thinking or feeling. Then determine how to approach or create a person-centered intervention. For example, if there are glass windows on a door that exits their community, and people with AD are drawn to the door and want to go to the other side, consider that there is nothing engaging keeping them in the space where they are living. Try to determine what you can do to keep them engaged in a meaningful way. If the windowed door continues to be an area of interest for people, this could become a safety risk; you could consider putting tinting on the window so that to the person with AD, it looks like the lights are out on the other side of the door and there is nothing of interest to find there. When a person is constantly moving, find out if he or she needs something.

Look for patterns in the wandering and possible reasons, such as time of day, hunger, thirst, boredom, restlessness, need to go to the bathroom, medication side effect, overstimulation, or looking for a lost item. Perhaps the person is lost or has forgotten how to get somewhere. Help meet the need and keep the person safe by trying the following things:

- Remind the person to use the bathroom every two hours.

- Have healthy snacks and a pitcher of water readily available.

- Provide a quiet environment away from noise, distraction, and glaring light.

- Provide a purposeful activity such as folding clothes or dusting.

- Provide an outlet such as a walk, a social activity, a memory book, or classical music played through headphones.

- Offer a life-like baby doll to rock or hold. If the person enjoys the doll, be sure you also treat it like it is a real baby.

- Keep soft lights on at night.

- Remember that the use of alarms only upsets the person with AD. How would you feel if each time you had a need, an alarm went off and people came running to tell you to sit down? Instead, find creative ways to keep an eye on the person. Ask team members from other departments to help or use video monitors.

- When outside doors are not being monitored, they should have bells or alarms that sound when opened. Use child-resistant locks on doors and windows.

- Follow facility policies if you believe a person with AD has wandered away.

Distress manifesting as aggression and agitation

First, be sure that the person is not ill or in physical pain, such as from an infection or injury. Consider if your approach or anything in the environment is causing the person to feel out of control. Respond with empathy, showing the person that you understand and that he or she is safe. Try the following suggestions:

- Respond by validating the emotion that the person is expressing. Refrain from reality orienting; instead, seek to understand the meaning behind the person's words or behaviors. Ask yourself "What would I be feeling if I was reacting in that way?" Get to know the person's life story. Use this knowledge to help the person feel safe with you.

- Maintain a calm environment.

- Reduce triggers such as noise, glare, television, or too many tasks.

- Check for hunger, thirst, or a full bladder.

- Make calm, positive, reassuring statements. Use soothing words.

- Change the subject or redirect the person's attention.

- Give the person a choice between two options.

- Don't argue, raise your voice, restrain, criticize, demand, or make sudden movements.

- Don't take it personally if accused or insulted.

- Let the person know that he or she is safe. Encourage calming activities that have a purpose. Sorting and folding laundry, dusting, polishing, vacuuming, watering plants, and other quiet, repetitive tasks can be soothing.

Alzheimer's Disease

Test

Name _____ Date _____ Score _____

Directions: Circle the best answer. (Seven correct answers required.)

1. Which statement is not correct?

    a. AD is a form of dementia that makes a person unable to carry out daily activities.

    b. AD is a progressive, degenerative brain disease.

    c. AD symptoms usually begin suddenly.

    d. AD is characterized by memory loss, language deterioration, and poor judgment.

2. Medication will stop the progression of AD.   True or False

3. Benefits of exercise are that it _____.

    a. helps to retain motor skills

    b. improves circulation

    c. improves sleep

    d. aids in elimination

    e. All of the above

4. If the person is able to, a daily walk may reduce distress.   True or False

5. When you see a person is experiencing feelings of agitation, choose three things you can do that might help:

   a. Argue

   b. Offer choices between two options

   c. Make calm positive statements

   d. Restrain

   e. Create a calm environment

6. It is important to focus on things the AD person can still do and enjoy.   True or False

7. Serenity and stability reduces potential feeling of being out of control or distressed. True or False

8. Seek to understand the feeling or emotion behind the words or behaviors the person is exhibiting, then seek to validate them.   True or False

9. When a person exhibits behavior that shows that they are in distress, the first thing you should do is look for the _____.

   a. family

   b. nurse

   c. reason

   d. supervisor

10. People with AD never hide something in the same place twice.   True or False

CERTIFICATE OF COMPLETION

I hereby certify that

_____

has successfully completed the in-Service

Alzheimer's Disease

_____

Signature

2

Amputation: Understanding Barriers and Strategies for Quality of Life

Teaching Plan

To use this lesson for self-study, the learner should read the material, do the activity, and take the test. For group study, the leader may give each learner a copy of the learning guide and follow this teaching plan to conduct the lesson. Certificates may be copied for everyone who completes the lesson.

Learning objectives

After this lesson, participants should be able to:

- Understand the difficulties residents face after amputation

- Recognize ways to help alleviate these difficulties

- Identify ways to help improve an amputee resident's lifestyle

Lesson activities

After reviewing the lesson, have participants (as a group) list issues people who have undergone amputation might struggle with. Then, go through the list and brainstorm ways to help alleviate those issues.

Some issues to list might include:

1. Skin breakdown

2. Depression associated with a belief that independence won't improve

3. Pain at the area of amputation

4. Difficulty working with the prosthesis

5. Challenges associated with impaired mobility

Some solutions are:

1. Keep their skin clean, dry, and lubricated. Keep their bedding free of wrinkles.

2. Lifestyle is important. Ensure residents eat well and drink plenty of liquids and walk or exercise a few times daily in compliance with their plan of care. Therapy may create plans of care for residents who are in chairs most of the time to encourage them to stand, walk, or shift their weight every 15 minutes, do chair push-ups with their arms, and sit with their knees at the same level as their hips, with their thighs horizontal on the chair.

   For residents who are in bed most of the time, work with therapy and nursing to teach them how to use side rails and the trapeze to change position frequently, at least every two hours. Massage the skin when possible, but avoid massaging pressure points or irritated areas.

   For residents who use special chair cushions or mattress-overlay pads, staff should check to be sure that the pads are thick enough to do the job.

   For residents with pressure sores, keep weight and pressure off any reddened areas and wounds. Also, use pillows to elevate or separate body parts and keep pressure off an area, such as a pillow under the calf to raise the heel off the bed or a pillow between the legs to keep the knees from touching.

   When working on rehabilitation, divide tasks into simple steps for the resident. Follow the plan that physical therapy, occupational therapy, and nursing have written for your interventions. Minimize distractions. Try not to rush residents, and if possible given their conditions, do not hover over them while they perform tasks. Provide feedback and praise to encourage residents to continue the effort. It also helps to praise residents' efforts to their families. Keep in mind that in the process of rehabilitation, frequent ups and downs are to be expected. Be prepared to encourage residents and yourself through the difficult times and join with them in their happiness as they improve. Be sure to celebrate improvement.

3. Observe resident positioning to ensure proper positioning and elongation of the residual limb.

4. Document the pain, and tell appropriate care team members of the pain to ensure the prosthesis fits correctly and the resident is using it correctly.

5. Determine any environmental adaptations that can be used to accommodate the impaired mobility due to the amputation. Keep rooms, bathrooms, and hallways free of clutter for

ease of mobility. Keep the cane, walker, or other adaptive equipment within reach of the resident at all times. Observe resident positioning to ensure proper positioning and elongation of the residual limb.

Also, for any of these complaints, remember to do the following:

- Tell the nurse about any problems you observed and ask him or her to document according to facility policies. Tell a member of the therapy team a list of the problems you observed.

- Document your observations in the 24-hour report.

Conclusion

Have participants take the test. Review the answers together. Award certificates to those who answer 70% of the test questions correctly.

Test answers

1. d	2. c	3. a	4. b	5. True
6. True	7. c	8. d	9. True	10. a

Amputation: Understanding Barriers and Strategies for Recovery

Learning Guide

Contents:

- Introduction

- Amputee Care

    - Defining identification criteria

    - Interventions and plans of care

    - Preventing skin problems

    - Rehabilitation measures

    - Benefits to rehabilitation

    - Guidelines for rehabilitation

Introduction

Amputation and prosthetic care involve issues related to rehabilitation and recovery after the amputation of a limb. Residents with amputated limbs and/or prosthetics need extra care and attention.

It takes time and patience to assist an amputee or prosthetic resident to make even a partial recovery.

It is important to allot the amount of time that is needed in order to avoid potential complications with amputations or prosthetics in the future. Everyday processes, such as moving in and out of bed, become difficult for amputee and prosthetic residents. The residents often experience frustration and feelings of helplessness. Helping them realize that they can regain the ability to do things on their own and encouraging them to be independent is important. Different residents with amputations and prosthetics may be at a range of stages in the rehabilitation process. You can help improve the quality of life for these residents by supporting any progress that is made. There are many things to take into consideration with amputee and prosthetic residents.

Amputee Care

One of the more difficult aspects of caring for a person who is an amputee or who wears a prosthetic is learning about his or her personal care needs for quality of life.

Make sure you understand the criteria you should be looking for to see whether there is a decline in a resident's ability to manage his or her amputation. If you know what therapy can do to help a resident, you may be more likely to report changes or deficits to the nurse to help generate referrals.

Defining identification criteria

There are several triggers that may indicate that therapy services designed to address the deficits related to amputations or prosthetics are appropriate for a resident:

- The resident has had a recent amputation

- The resident had a past amputation and is now experiencing new deficits

- The resident has increased difficulty with ambulation or transfers due to use of a prosthesis

- The resident has increased difficulty with activities of daily living (ADL) due to use of a prosthesis

- The resident has poor posture/positioning in wheelchair or bed due to a residual limb or prosthesis

- There is noted shortening of muscle length around the knee, hip, shoulder, or elbow due to amputation

- The resident complains of muscle or joint stiffness near the amputation site

- Caregivers comment on increased difficulty with ADLs due to amputation

- The resident has impaired skin integrity of his or her residual limb

- The resident experiences increased falls due to ambulation problems with prosthesis

- The resident is expressing desire for increased independence

Interventions and plans of care

Therapy can include the following interventions and plans of care for assessing and treating a resident who has had an amputation or is having difficulty with a prosthesis:

- Notice range of motion (ROM) limitations compared to the normal values for passive and active ROM for the affected joint and contralateral side. Consider how the limitations in mobility due to the amputation affect functional activities.

- Determine any environmental adaptations that can be used to accommodate the impaired mobility due to the amputation. Work with occupational therapy on access to these interventions.

- Determine, in coordination with a prosthetist, whether a prosthesis is indicated to increase ROM for maximum function.

- Ensure muscle length is adequate for prosthesis fitting and gait training.

- Monitor the skin of the residual limb to see whether edema is present or whether skin breakdown is an issue. Report to the nurse if you see any changes.

- Monitor for changes in sensation of the extremity to determine protective responses and appropriate wearing schedule of the prosthesis.

- Work with therapy to utilize modalities to help facilitate increased ROM (hot packs, etc.).

- Develop positioning to ensure skin integrity and maintenance of the residual limb, and train staff members as appropriate.

- Understand the importance of residual-limb care and its effect on the resident's function.

- Use specialized stretching techniques, such as contract-relax techniques and prolonged positional stretching, to address any ROM deficits at the joints around the amputation site.

You can help residents who may be having trouble with amputations or prosthetic use in the following ways:

- Tell the nurse about the problems, concerns, or changes you observed and ask him or her to document them in the medical record

- Tell a member of the therapy team

- Document your observations per facility policy

What can therapy do to help these residents?

- Evaluate the residents to see what they are able to do

- Provide treatment to increase their safety and help them be as independent as possible

- Develop recommendations that can be integrated into a restorative program

- Use treatment to help the resident get stronger and increase flexibility, balance, and coordination to make him or her safer during functional mobility

You can also make recommendations regarding the environment to make it as safe as possible:

- Train the resident on how to use an assistive device

- Recognize when the resident may benefit from reminders of balance-compensation strategies (to help recover quickly when he or she loses balance)

- Assess the residual limb to determine the stage of recovery it is in, and recommend an active course of treatment

- Work with nursing and therapy to train the resident on donning and doffing the prosthesis

- Ask the resident if he or she has ideas about how to adjust the environment to help with independence and comfort

What can be done every day to help residents with use of prosthetics?

- Keep rooms, bathrooms, and hallways free of clutter for ease of mobility.

- Keep the cane, walker, or other adaptive equipment within reach of the resident at all times.

- Attend to the toileting needs of each resident at the appropriate time.

- If you see a resident who normally requires help moving without assistance, assist him or her immediately.

- Ensure rooms and hallways are well lit.

- Encourage residents who are able to walk by themselves to walk more to keep their strength up. If a resident walks with assistance and is on a restorative program, follow the instructions daily.

- Make sure residents lock their brakes when they stand up from wheelchairs.

- Observe resident positioning to ensure proper positioning and elongation of the residual limb.

- Be observant for signs of skin breakdown on the residual limb.

- If you notice that the person is resistive to wearing a prosthetic, ask why he or she may be feeling that way, and alert the nurse.

Preventing skin problems

Work with therapy and nursing to learn about measures and tips to prevent the deterioration of skin due to amputation or prosthetic use. Encourage and help residents to:

- Walk or exercise several times per day

- Keep their skin clean, dry, and lubricated

- Keep their bedding free of wrinkles

- Eat well and drink plenty of liquids

For residents who are in chairs most of the time, your role may be to:

- Encourage or help them to stand, walk, or shift their weight every 15 minutes.

- Teach them how to do chair push-ups with their arms.

- Teach them to sit with their knees at the same level as their hips, with their thighs horizontal on the chair. This will distribute their weight along their thighs and away from pressure points.

If a resident cannot do these things, he or she should return to bed after an hour in a chair.

For residents who are in bed most of the time:

- Teach them how to use side rails and the trapeze to change position frequently, at least every two hours. Be available to assist them if necessary. Even small shifts in body weight are helpful.

- When you are helping a resident to change position, move him or her carefully so you do not create friction and shearing between the skin and the bedding or clothes.

- The head of the bed should be raised as little as possible, no more than 30 degrees, to prevent sliding and pressure on the bony areas. If it must be raised higher for eating, it should be lowered an hour later.

- Massage the skin when possible, but avoid massaging pressure points or irritated areas.

For residents who use special chair cushions or mattress-overlay pads, check to be sure that the pads are thick enough to do the job. Place your hand under the pad while the resident is on top of it—if you can feel the resident's body through the cushion, the pad is too thin.

For residents with pressure sores, keep weight and pressure off any reddened areas and wounds. Also, use pillows to elevate or separate body parts and keep pressure off an area, such as a pillow under the calf to raise the heel off the bed, or a pillow between the legs to keep the knees from touching.

Rehabilitation measures

The term rehabilitation is most often used when trained professional therapists are involved in evaluating the resident and designing a plan of care. The term restorative may be used when the evaluation and care plan are performed by the nursing staff.

It is estimated that about one-third of disabled adults over the age of 65 would benefit from physical rehabilitation. These people can be divided into two groups. The first group is composed of those who have been disabled throughout their lives and who need continuous rehabilitation. The second group is made up of those people who have become disabled as the result of an accident or illness.

Most people with physical disabilities require rehabilitation due to amputation, as well as strokes, head injuries, spinal-cord injuries, and general debilitation.

There are several goals of rehabilitation for amputees. These goals include:

- Improving the level of functioning when possible

- Maintaining the current level of functioning if improvement is not possible

- Slowing deterioration when decline is inevitable

- Preventing the complications of inactivity

Benefits to rehabilitation

The higher the level of functioning that residents attain, the greater their ability to control their own lives and regain their independence. From the time we are children, we want to be independent, and we insist on it. As we grow older, we may begin to experience feelings of tiredness, illness, or discouragement.

Investing a little extra time in working with residents to increase their ability to perform their own ADLs will result in saving a significant amount of time in the long run. They may be reluctant to work on their own rehabilitation because they believe that no matter how hard they try, they will never be able to regain their independence. When they feel weak and tired, the required effort may seem too great. Losing a limb is often accompanied by depression, which makes any effort seem too difficult. Seek to understand how to best support each person with an individualized, person-centered approach. Work with the interdisciplinary team to create plans of care that encourage the resident to obtain the highest possible quality of life.

Guidelines for rehabilitation

There are certain techniques that will help make rehabilitation measures for a resident with a prosthetic more successful. These are:

- Divide tasks into simple steps for resident.

- Minimize distractions.

- Try not to rush the resident and, if possible given his or her condition, do not hover over the resident while he or she performs tasks.

- Provide feedback and praise to encourage the resident to continue the effort. It also helps to praise residents' efforts to their families.

- Report concerns, changes, or feedback to the therapists and nursing staff.

Monitor residents' progress and report and document their accomplishments. New goals may need to be established once a task has been mastered or if a task proves too difficult. Rehabilitation measures are necessary to produce positive results when caring for amputee residents. These measures can increase the resident's independence, prevent complications, or, at the very least, help slow deterioration.

Rehabilitation goals for many residents include a return to a previous lifestyle. For others, primarily the elderly, the goal may be independence in ADLs and restoration to an acceptable quality of life. Keep in mind that in the process of rehabilitation, frequent ups and downs are to be expected. Be prepared to encourage residents and yourself through the difficult times and join with them in their happiness as they improve.

Amputation: Understanding Barriers and Strategies for Quality of Life

Test

Name _____ Date _____ Score _____

Directions: Circle the best answer. (Seven correct answers required.)

1. What should you take note of when observing residents?

    a. Residents with residual limbs

    b. Residents with recent amputations

    c. Anyone experiencing skin breakdown

    d. All of the above

2. Assessing how limitations in mobility caused by an amputation affect functional activities is an example of _____.

    a. observation

    b. identification criteria

    c. interventions and plans of care

    d. none of the above

3. How can therapy help residents with amputations or residual limbs?

a. Provide treatment that promotes independence

b. Keep residents from becoming too active

c. Therapy isn't meant for issues that come with amputation

d. It doesn't—it's too challenging for elderly residents to undergo these types of therapy

4. What is one thing that can be done on a daily basis to help residents with amputations or prosthetics?

a. Let residents take care of their own needs

b. Keep areas clear of clutter to enhance mobility

c. Trust residents to check their skin for signs of breakdown

d. Help regardless of whether the resident seems to need assistance

5. For residents that are in bed most of the time, the care plan may instruct you to help encourage them to use side rails and the trapeze to change positions frequently and on their own. True or False

6. Keeping weight and pressure off of any reddened areas and wounds is beneficial for an amputee or prosthetic resident. True or False

7. Approximately how many disabled adults over the age of 65 would benefit from physical rehabilitation?

a. One-half

b. Three-fourths

c. One-third

d. Two-thirds

8. One of the goals to rehabilitation for amputees is _____.

a. to improve the level of functionality

b. to maintain the current level of functionality when improvement is not possible

c. to prevent complications of inactivity

d. all of the above

9. Investing a little extra time in working with residents to increase their ability to perform their own ADLs will result in saving a significant amount of time in the long run.   True or False

10. One way to make rehabilitation easier for a resident with a prosthetic is _____.

a. dividing tasks into simple steps

b. giving distractions and obstacles to overcome

c. rushing them to perform at a higher level

d. none of the above

CERTIFICATE OF COMPLETION

I hereby certify that

_____

has successfully completed the in-Service

Amputation

_____

_____
Signature

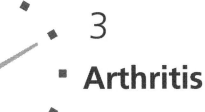

3

Arthritis

Teaching Plan

To use this lesson for self-study, the learner should read the material, do the activity, and take the test. For group study, the leader may give each learner a copy of the learning guide and follow this teaching plan to conduct the lesson. Certificates may be copied for everyone who completes the lesson.

Learning Objectives

After this lesson, participants should be able to:

- Name the symptoms of arthritis and be familiar with some different types of the disease

- State the things that can help prevent arthritis from occurring or getting worse

- Explain how to treat and care for people with arthritis

Objective 1: The symptoms and types of arthritis

1. If you have secured a speaker, ask him or her to address the group. If you did not find a speaker in advance, ask if anyone in your group has arthritis and is willing to talk about it. If someone responds, ask him or her to tell the group what kind of arthritis he or she has, what it feels like, and how it affects him or her.

2. Ask your learners to look at the picture of a normal joint in column two of the first page of the learning guide. Together, read and review the information in the sections "Who gets arthritis and why?" "What are the symptoms?" and "What happens in arthritis?" Try to find some photos on the Internet of people with arthritis to show during this lesson.

3. Discuss or lecture on the different types of arthritis as described in the learning guide section "Types of arthritis."

Objective 2: Things that might prevent arthritis from occurring or getting worse

1. Talk about the preventive measures as described in the learning guide section "Can you prevent arthritis?"

2. Tell your learners that research has shown that middle-aged and older women who lose 11 pounds or more over 10 years cut their risk of knee osteoporosis in half.

Objective 3: How to treat and care for people with arthritis

1. Go over the "Treatments that work" section of the learning guide in detail. Be sure your participants understand each of the six treatment methods. Review the case study learning activity and discuss the answers.

2. Emphasize how participants can assist residents with care and treatments. Depending on the plan of care and your policies, participants may be able to help with exercises, passive range of motion, medication assistance, heat and cold applications, pacing activities, and joint protection, and with encouraging self-care.

Lesson activities

Hand out the "Arthritis Case Study Learning Activity" to the participants before giving them the learning guide. Ask them to do the activity based on what they already know. Tell them they will learn the correct answers during the lesson. They should keep the activity for review during Objective 3.

Conclusion

Have participants take the test. Review the answers together. Award certificates to those who answer 70% of the test questions correctly.

Test answers

1. a, b, c, d	2. a	3. d	4. b	5. c
6. b	7. a, b, c, d, e, f	8. c	9. b	10. a

Arthritis

Learning Guide

Contents:

- Arthritis Case Study Learning Activity

- Arthritis Lesson Guide

    - Who gets arthritis and why?

    - What are the symptoms?

    - What happens in arthritis?

    - Types of arthritis

    - Can you prevent arthritis?

    - Treatments that work

- Arthritis Case Study Learning Activity Answers

Arthritis Case Study Learning Activity

Each of these case studies presents a situation that someone with arthritis and their caregivers might face. Based on what you already know, choose the best solution. After you have completed the activity, you will study the learning guide for answers.

1. Mrs. Jones has arthritis in both of her knees. She complains often about how much it hurts to walk. She has become inactive and gained weight in the past few years. What do you think might help Mrs. Jones? Circle all the answers that apply.

    a. Nothing will help her, because she is old and arthritis is part of growing old

    b. Losing weight would help

    c. Exercising would help

    d. She needs to rest more

    e. Using a walker would help

2. Warm compresses are applied to Mrs. Jones' knees several times per day. She says it doesn't help her knees feel better at all. What else might be tried for pain relief?

    a. Warm packs are the best treatment there is

    b. Cold compresses help some people and might help Mrs. Jones

    c. Probably neither heat nor cold will help

    d. She should keep warm compresses on the knees all day

3. Mrs. Jones doesn't like to take a bath early in the day because she usually wakes up feeling stiff, with pain in her joints. What should you do?

    a. Let her bathe later when she feels more flexible and less uncomfortable

    b. Tell her that she will feel better if she gets moving

    c. Bathe her in bed so she doesn't have to get up

4. Mrs. Jones likes to do needlework, and she will sit and work on her projects for long periods of time. She complains that her fingers hurt, but she doesn't want to give up her hobby. What might help her with this problem? Circle all that apply.

    a. She needs to stop doing needlework

    b. She should change to a different kind of hobby or craft that doesn't require repetitive finger movements

    c. She should alternate a period of needlework with a time of rest

    d. She should alternate needlework with something that doesn't use the fingers as much

Arthritis Lesson Guide

The term arthritis is taken from two Latin words:

- *arthro* means joint, or a part of the body where bones meet

- *itis* means inflammation; symptoms are redness, heat, swelling, and pain

Who gets arthritis and why?

People of all ages can have arthritis, but it occurs more often among older people. Nearly 43 million Americans are affected by this condition. We do not know the cause of most types of arthritis, but probably there are many different causes.

What are the symptoms?

There are six main signs of arthritis. They usually occur in or around a joint. Symptoms can include:

1. Pain

2. Stiffness

3. Swelling (sometimes)

4. Difficulty moving a joint

5. Redness around the joints

6. Decreased range of motion

Arthritis symptoms can vary widely among individuals. For example:

- Symptoms can develop suddenly or slowly

- Pain can be constant or can come and go

- Pain may occur when the person is moving or has been still for some time

- Pain may be felt in one spot or in many parts of the body

- Sometimes the skin over the joint may appear swollen and red and feel warm to the touch

- Some types of arthritis are associated with fatigue

- Often the pain and stiffness are more severe in the morning or after a period of inactivity

Arthritis is usually chronic, which means it lasts a long time and may never go away.

This condition can make it hard for people to do many of the daily tasks they used to do easily by themselves. This causes loss of independence and a need to rely on others for assistance.

What happens in arthritis?

Arthritis usually affects areas in or around joints. Joints are parts of the body where bones meet. The ends of the bones are covered by cartilage, which is a spongy material that works as a shock absorber to keep bones from rubbing together.

Joints are enclosed in a capsule, called the joint capsule. The joints are lined with tissue, called the synovium or synovial membrane. The synovial membrane releases a slippery fluid that lubricates the joint and helps it move smoothly and easily.

Muscles and tendons are connected to the bones. They support the joints and help with movement. Different types of arthritis can affect one or more different parts of a joint. When arthritis affects a joint, it can change the shape and alignment of the bones or the joints. Certain types of arthritis can also affect other parts of the body besides the joints, such as the skin and internal organs (Figure 3.1).

Figure 3.1 A Normal Joint

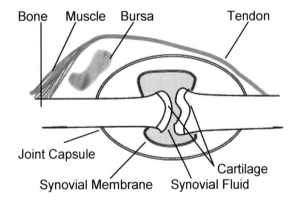

Types of arthritis

There are more than 100 different types of arthritis and related conditions. The following sections describe a few of the more common kinds.

Osteoarthritis (OA)

OA is the most common kind. It is also called degenerative arthritis or degenerative joint disease. OA affects many older people. It usually occurs after age 45 in both men and women.

With OA, the cartilage and bones begin to deteriorate or break down. This means the bones might rub together or not move smoothly within the capsule. The result is pain and stiffness. OA usually affects the fingers and the weight-bearing joints, such as the knees, feet, hips, and back.

Rheumatoid arthritis (RA)

RA is another common form. It occurs three times more often in women than in men, and usually begins in the young or middle adult years. Morning stiffness that usually lasts more than one hour is common with RA, and over time, joints may lose their range of motion and may become deformed.

With this type of arthritis, something goes wrong with the body's immune system. The immune system is usually the way the body defends itself against bacteria and viruses. When a person has RA, the immune system works improperly and attacks the body's own joints and organs. This problem causes warmth and swelling (inflammation) of the joint lining (synovium). This can cause damage to the cartilage, bone, and tendons of the joint. RA often affects the same joints on both sides of the body. If the right knee is swollen, then the left knee will probably be swollen also. The hands, wrists, feet, knees, ankles, shoulders, neck, jaw, and elbows are frequently affected.

Fibromyalgia

Fibromyalgia is a common condition that usually afflicts women. It affects muscles and the points where the muscles attach to bones. Fibromyalgia creates tender points in the body that are more sensitive to pain and touch. It also causes pain throughout the entire body. Fatigue and stiffness are associated with fibromyalgia, along with restless sleep and psychological distress.

Lupus

Lupus is a type of arthritis that causes inflammation of the skin, body tissues, and organs such as the kidneys, lungs, or heart. Lupus affects women 8–10 times more often than men and often first appears between the ages of 18 and 45. Arthritis in the joints can also be a symptom of lupus. Lupus can be fatal, but there are treatments that can help.

Gout

Gout causes severe pain and swelling in the big toes, ankles and knees. Gout results when the body produces or retains too much uric acid, which is a natural substance in the body. The excess uric acid forms needle-like crystals in the affected joint, causing pain. It is more common in men than women, because men more frequently have higher uric acid levels. Weight loss and limited alcohol intake help this condition, along with medication.

Can you prevent arthritis?

There are things we can do to reduce the risk of getting certain kinds of arthritis. These things also help reduce the level of disability in people who have arthritis and may keep the condition from getting worse. They are:

- Maintain recommended weight

    - People who are overweight have a higher frequency of OA, especially in the weight-bearing joints (knees and hips)

    - Women are especially at risk for developing OA from being overweight

    - In men, excess weight increases the risk of developing gout

- Guard against injury

    - Joint injuries caused by accidents or overuse increase the risk of OA

    - Keep the muscles around joints strong by exercising to reduce the risk of wear on the joint and to help prevent injury

    - Get adequate calcium and vitamin D to protect against bone fractures

Treatments that work

There are several things we can do to help most types of arthritis. First, anyone who has symptoms of arthritis should see a doctor for a correct diagnosis. Only a doctor can decide whether a person has arthritis and what kind it is. It is important to know the type of arthritis, because there are different treatments for different types.

Medication is important for reducing the pain and inflammation caused by arthritis. Doctors often prescribe the following:

- Aspirin-free pain relievers such as acetaminophen (Tylenol).

- Anti-inflammatory drugs such as aspirin, ibuprofen (Advil), and naproxyn (Aleve). These reduce the warmth and redness (inflammation) in the joints or skin and also relieve pain.

- Sleep aids.

If you are helping someone take medication, you should know the name of the medicine, how much the individual is supposed to take, how and when they should take it, how quickly it works, what it does, and what side effects to watch for. Anti-inflammatory drugs can cause stomach pain and bleeding and can also thin the blood so that a person bleeds excessively. Always report complaints of stomach pain.

Exercise is one of the best treatments for arthritis. There are different ways to exercise (Figure 3.2).

Figure 3.2 Exercises for Prevention

Type of Exercise	What It Does	How to Do It	How Often
Range of motion (ROM)	Reduces stiffness. Keeps joints flexible and moveable.	Gently move each joint through all the possible ways it can move. An assistant can do passive ROM, or someone with arthritis who is able to can do active ROM alone.	Daily
Strengthening	Builds muscle strength, which helps keep joints stable. Strong muscles make it easier to do things.	Lift light weights in sets of 8 to 10 repetitions. Start with weights no heavier than one to three pounds each.	Every other day
Endurance	Builds fitness. Keeps heart healthy. Helps control weight.	Walk or do something that raises the heart rate a little above normal for 20 to 30 minutes. Don't exercise so hard that it is difficult to talk.	Three times a week

Dementia and Arthritis: Be aware if you have residents who have dementia and also arthritis. They may not be able to self report pain. Be sure to recognize the symptoms of pain in a person with dementia and report your findings to the nurse for treatment plans.

Heat and cold applications can provide relief from some of the symptoms of arthritis. Heat relaxes aching muscles and can be applied with warm compresses and warm water soaks. Cold numbs the area and reduces pain and can be applied with ice or cold packs. Either heat or cold are fine to use, depending on the individual's preference. When using either type of application, it's important to remember the following:

- Never use heat with rubs or creams. The combination of heat and creams can burn the skin.

- It is helpful to use heat or cold before exercising to prepare the joints and muscles.

- Be safe! Don't leave a hot or cold treatment on the skin for more than 20 minutes at a time. Let the skin return to its normal temperature between treatments.

Pacing activities also saves energy, reduces fatigue, and protects joints from stress and injury. Keep the following in mind:

- Alternate heavy or repeated tasks with easy tasks

- Switch periods of activity with periods of rest

- Change tasks often so the joints don't stay in one position for a long time

Joint protection uses the joints in ways that avoid stress and can make it easier to do tasks. Pay attention to joint position and use the joints in the best way. Use larger or stronger joints to carry things, such as carrying a grocery bag with the forearms, not the hands. Use walking or assistive devices, such as canes, walkers, and reachers, to reduce stress on the joints and to make tasks easier. Use thick pens for writing, and only carry lightweight items.

Self-care skills means taking care of oneself by planning activities for the best times, when feeling more flexible or in less pain. The person should do enjoyable things and learn how to manage stress.

Arthritis Case Study Learning Activity Answers

The following are the answers to the case study problems.

1. Mrs. Jones has arthritis in both of her knees. She complains often about how much it hurts to walk. She has become inactive and gained weight in the past few years. What do you think might help Mrs. Jones? Circle all the answers that apply.

    a. Nothing will help her, because she is old and arthritis is part of growing old

    b. Losing weight would help

    c. Exercising would help

    d. She needs to rest more

    e. Using a walker would help

    Answers: b, c, and e. Weight loss will reduce the pressure on the knees. Exercise can strengthen the muscles around the knees and improve support to the joint. A walker can reduce pressure on the knees.

2. Warm compresses are applied to Mrs. Jones' knees several times per day. She says it doesn't help her knees feel better at all. What else might be tried for pain relief?

    a. Warm packs are the best thing there is

b. Cold compresses help some people and might help Mrs. Jones

c. Probably neither heat nor cold will help

d. She should keep warm compresses on the knees all day

Answer: b. Either warm or cold compresses are good, depending on what helps the individual the most. Neither heat nor cold should be left on for more than 20 minutes at a time.

3. Mrs. Jones doesn't like to take a bath early in the day because she usually wakes up feeling stiff, with pain in her joints. What should you do?

a. Let her bathe later when she feels more flexible and less uncomfortable

b. Tell her that she will feel better if she gets moving

c. Bathe her in bed so she doesn't have to get up

Answer: a. She should be allowed to schedule her bath for a time when she has more freedom of movement and less pain, a little later in the day.

4. Mrs. Jones likes to do needlework, and she will sit and work on her projects for long periods of time. She complains that her fingers hurt, but she doesn't want to give up her hobby. What might help her with this problem? Circle all that apply.

a. She needs to stop doing needlework

b. She should change to a different kind of hobby or craft that doesn't require repetitive finger movements

c. She should alternate a period of needlework with a time of rest

d. She should alternate needlework with something that doesn't use the fingers as much

Answers: c and d. Switching between a repetitive activity such as needlework and something that uses the joints less will help reduce the pain in Mrs. Jones' fingers. Periods of rest are also good.

Arthritis

Test

Name _____ Date _____ Score _____

Directions: Circle the best answer or fill in the blanks.

1. Write the four main symptoms of arthritis (four points):

    a. _____

    b. _____

    c. _____

    d. _____

2. What is the most common kind of arthritis?

    a. Osteoarthritis (degenerative arthritis)

    b. Rheumatoid arthritis

    c. Fibromyalgia

    d. Lupus

    e. Gout

3. What are the two main things that can help prevent arthritis or keep it from getting worse?

    a. Vitamins and vigorous exercise

    b. Daily meditation and at least eight hours of rest

    c. Avoiding alcohol and not smoking

    d. Maintaining recommended weight and guarding against injury

4. Which kind of exercise should people with arthritis do every day?

    a. Aerobic exercises for endurance

    b. Range-of-motion exercises

    c. Muscle strengthening exercises with weights

5. Two side effects of some arthritis medicines are:

    a. Confusion and dizziness

    b. Liver disease and jaundice

    c. Stomach upset and bleeding

    d. Kidney failure and gout

6. How should cold or warm compresses be used?

    a. Alternate heat with cold

    b. Apply either one for no more than 20 minutes at a time

    c. Use a muscle rub under a warm compress

    d. Keep them on continuously

7. There are six main treatments for arthritis. They are (fill in the blanks—two points):

    a. Medication

    b. Exercise

    c. Heat or cold

    d. Pacing activities

    e. _____

    f. _____

8. Self-care skills _____.

   a. are very selfish and self-centered

   b. are skills to wash one's own back

   c. means taking care of oneself by planning activities for the best times, when feeling more flexible or in less pain

   d. all of the above

9. Arthritis symptoms develop _____.

   a. rapidly

   b. rapidly or slowly, depending on the type and individual

   c. slowly

   d. because of a genetic disease

10. Fibromyalgia is _____.

    a. a condition that affects muscles and the points where they attach to bones, creating tender points in the body that are more sensitive to pain and touch; it causes body-wide pain, fatigue, stiffness, restless sleep, and psychological distress

    b. a type of arthritis that causes inflammation of the skin, body tissues, and organs such as the kidneys, lungs, or heart, often first appearing between the ages of 18 and 45, and which can be fatal

    c. a condition that causes severe pain and swelling in the big toes, ankles, and knees; it results when the body produces or retains too much uric acid, which forms needle-like crystals in the affected joint, causing pain

    d. is also called degenerative arthritis and causes the cartilage and bones to deteriorate or break down, allowing for the bones to rub together or not move smoothly within the capsule, resulting in pain and stiffness

CERTIFICATE OF COMPLETION

I hereby certify that

_____

has successfully completed the in-Service

Arthritis

_____
Signature

4
Assistive Devices

Teaching Plan

To use this lesson for self-study, the learner should read the material, do the activity, and take the test. For group study, the leader may give each learner a copy of the learning guide and follow this teaching plan to conduct the lesson. Certificates may be copied for everyone who completes the lesson.

Learning objectives

After this lesson, participants should be able to:

- Identify the role of assistive devices

- Recognize proper and improper uses, cleaning, and maintenance care for various assistive devices

- Understand the role of assistive devices for activities of daily living

Lesson activities

If you can, bring in some assistive devices, such as a wheelchair, a hearing aid, a reacher, or a walker. After participants review the lesson, have them use or clean the device in the manner indicated in this lesson. Ask another participant to point out what might be wrong or unsafe. Encourage participants to also point out if the devices are too big, too small, worn out, etc. You can also have the participants simply look at each device and discuss as a group whether anything looks like it should be fixed, such as the following:

- Resident is in wheelchair without footrests or with footrests not being used

- Resident is cleaning the hearing aid using a paper clip

- Resident is stooped over walker, which is far away from the resident's body

Conclusion

Have participants take the test. Review the answers together. Award certificates to those who answer 70% of the test questions correctly.

Test answers

1. True	2. d	3. b	4. True	5. c
6. c	7. d	8. d	9. b	10. b

Assistive Devices

Learning Guide

Contents:

- Introduction

- Mobility Aids

  - Wheelchair usage

  - Wheelchair etiquette

- Mobility Safety

- Hearing Aids

- Assistive Devices for ADLs

  - The role of the care partner

Introduction

An assistive device is anything that helps a resident with activities of daily living (ADL). Such a device may be something as simple as a walker to make moving around easier or a hearing aid to make sounds easier to hear (e.g., for talking on the telephone or watching television). These devices help a resident perform activities that might otherwise be difficult or impossible. Many people who use assistive devices have a disability, but assistive devices can also be used by residents who simply may not have the strength or agility to complete ADLs without help. These ADLs include ambulating, eating, bathing, grooming, and more. The person could also be using the device temporarily if they have recently suffered an injury.

Other examples of assistive devices include:

- A magnifying glass that helps someone who has poor vision read the newspaper

- A wheelchair that makes it possible to travel distances that are too far to walk

- A reacher device that makes it easier to grab out-of-reach objects

- A set of weighted utensils that helps a resident with a light grip or tremor grasp their fork, spoon, or knife

- A dressing stick that helps someone who has a hard time pulling their clothes on because of his or her limited reach

Safety in using these devices is paramount to their effectiveness for the resident. It is your responsibility to understand why your resident is using an assistive device, how it works, and how to ensure the resident is using it safely.

Mobility Aids

Mobility aids help residents ambulate from place to place if they are disabled or have an injury. Residents may need a walker or cane if they are at risk of falling. If they need to keep their body weight off a foot, ankle, or knee, they may need crutches. They may need a wheelchair or a scooter if an injury or disease has left them unable to walk.

Mobility aids include:

- Wheelchairs

- Scooters

- Walkers

- Canes

- Crutches

- Prosthetic devices

- Orthotic devices

- White cane and/or guide dog (for residents who are visually impaired or blind)

Choosing these devices takes time and research. Residents should be fitted for crutches, canes, and walkers by their therapist. Residents are also fitted for wheelchairs. If they fit, these devices give support; however, if they don't fit, they can be uncomfortable and unsafe. The person must learn how to use the device safely.

Wheelchair usage

There are many reasons for someone to use a wheelchair, and there is a wide range of physical abilities among those who do. This means that users may require different degrees of assistance (or no assistance at all). Some people do not use wheelchairs exclusively.

There are many different types of wheelchairs to meet residents' diverse needs. Some wheelchairs are moved manually, and others are motorized. They can also differ in size and shape. For example, a resident with hemiplegia (paralysis of the arm, leg, and trunk on the same side of the body) might have a lowered base of support and lowered seat to allow the resident to use the uninvolved foot to propel the wheelchair or a one-armed drive that enables maneuvering with one arm and hand.

Always make sure that the wheelchair fits the person and that it is in good repair with all parts working. This includes checking the footrests, as they are often missing. You should ensure that the person is positioned correctly and properly supported. Be sure to check the condition of the wheelchair cushion. This is important for comfort and to prevent skin breakdown. If you believe that the wheelchair is broken or not effective for the resident, you should report this to your supervisor.

Wheelchair etiquette

It's important to remember that a wheelchair is an extension of the person's body, and you must treat both with respect. The following are tips for proper wheelchair etiquette:

- When communicating with a resident who uses a wheelchair, you should accommodate the person. Remember to give the person a comfortable viewing angle of yourself. If the resident has to look straight up at you, it's probably not comfortable. If conversation lasts more than a few minutes, you may consider sitting down or kneeling to get yourself on the same level as the person using the wheelchair. Looking someone in the eyes is an important aspect of strong communication. Do not stand too close to the person in the wheelchair. Give the person the proper amount of personal space.

- Do not come up to someone who is using a wheelchair and start pushing them without asking—they may not want or need your assistance.

- It is a very common experience for people who use wheelchairs to be told that a place is accessible when it isn't. Listen carefully when anyone who uses a wheelchair tells you that an area that you thought was accessible is not. It may seem easy for you to navigate, but every wheelchair user has his or her own level of comfort.

- Inquire if the resident is comfortable in the chair. Are there things you can adjust so he or she is more comfortable, or should you ask your nursing supervisor or therapy for wheelchair modifications?

Mobility Safety

Many residents, regardless of their age, will find themselves in need of an assistive device for ambulating (getting from one place to another). Safety in using these devices is paramount to their effectiveness for the resident. The following are some safety tips for residents using an ambulation device:

- Always wear good supporting shoes

- Avoid wet surfaces when using a walker

- Use ramps with caution

- Stand tall and avoid walking bent over

- Keep the ambulation device close to the body to maintain balance

- Use caution on thick surfaces, such as shag carpet

- Check that the walker or cane's rubber tips are not worn; replace them when needed

- Remove any throw rugs or unnecessary objects on the floor

- Move all extension cords away from the walkways

Hearing Aids

Hearing loss is something that often occurs during the aging process, and many residents suffer from it. Hearing aids are assistive and sound-amplifying devices designed to aid people who have a hearing impairment.

Using hearing aids can be very frustrating for an older person during simple activities of daily living. Using an electric shaver or a hair dryer with hearing aids in the ears can be upsetting. The hearing aid amplifies the sound so it is almost painful. Many people talking at once can cause a garbled sound that is hard to understand. Background noise drowns out spoken words. New hearing-aid users will have to relearn how to ignore these background noises.

It can be hard for a person with memory problems to remember how to turn the volume down or what to do if the hearing aid squeals. Replacing the tiny batteries can be a problem if the person has arthritis. It can be hard to grip the batteries. A person with Parkinson's may drop the batteries and be unable to find them again, and trying to pick them up could cause a fall due to tremors and rigidity associated with the condition.

Hearing aids also need proper care to work well. Very hot or very cold temperatures can damage them, as can hair spray. The inside of the hearing aid is filled with delicate electronics that can be ruined by water. If sharp items such as a toothpick or paperclip are used to clean the hearing aid, they can break it. A special tool that is provided by the manufacturer is the only thing that should be used to clean the hearing aid.

Assistive Devices for ADLs

Assistive devices may not always be used as the result of a disability or injury. Many devices are used simply to make ADLs easier for the resident. These are often called adaptive devices because they aren't standalone devices, but attachments or simple adaptations that make everyday objects easier to use.

Residents are often elderly and may have lost some of their agility and strength. Residents may also live alone with no one to help them reach things, bathe, dress, or use the bathroom. Being able to feed or bathe yourself are things many may take for granted, but it can be very hard for residents when they can no longer do these things on their own. Assistive devices that enable these activities can help a resident live more independently.

The role of the care partner

Staff members have frequent interaction with residents and therefore play a key role in a number of areas related to assistive device usage and safety, such as:

- **Observing and reporting any improper use or lack of use:** If a staff member observes that the resident is not properly using his or her device or has decided to completely stop using it, this should be reported to a supervisor. Once the misusage is reported, a clinician can speak to the resident about properly using the device, discuss why the resident might not want to use it, and offer an alternative to provide quality care.

- **Ensuring safe practices when using assistive devices:** You play a key role in maintaining safety during ADLs regardless of whether the resident needs assistance, but when assistive devices are in the mix, you must pay even closer attention. Ensure that devices are working properly and that the resident is using them properly. If the resident gives pushback, explain why the device is important and how to properly use it. The home should be clean enough to make sure there are no hazards to get in the way.

- **Maintaining, cleaning, and caring for the assistive device:** Observe the condition of the resident's assistive devices and make sure they are clean and in good shape. This includes ensuring that walkers or canes are at the proper height, hearing aids have fresh batteries, wheelchairs are working properly, and the rubber tips of canes are intact.

Assistive Devices

Test

Name _____ Date _____ Score _____

Directions: Circle the best answer or fill in the blank.

1. Assistive devices are effective only for residents with long-term injuries or permanent disabilities. True or False

2. A _____ would NOT be considered an assistive device.

    a. reacher

    b. prosthetic device

    c. hearing aid

    d. hairbrush

3. What could be a reason that a resident would need to use a mobility aid?

    a. The resident is having a hard time hearing

    b. The resident is at risk of falling

    c. The resident needs help reaching things on high shelves

    d. The resident's eyesight is failing

4. If a mobility device isn't fitted properly, it can prove not only uncomfortable but also unsafe for a resident. True or False

5. A wheelchair that fits a resident well and is in good condition should _____.

    a. be a standard size and shape

    b. be motorized whenever possible

    c. have a supportive cushion

    d. not have footrests

6. A safe practice for residents who use ambulation devices is _____.

    a. for the resident to stoop over the device to maintain balance

    b. for the resident to walk on throw rugs rather than floored surfaces, as they provide more cushioning in the case of falls

    c. to replace a walker's or cane's rubber tips when they become worn to improve traction

    d. to line walkways with extension cords, which can double as cordons for dangerous areas

7. Residents can sometimes become frustrated with their hearing aids when they _____.

    a. experience the painful amplification of sounds from certain daily-use devices, like hair dryers and electric shavers

    b. have difficulty gripping the devices' small batteries

    c. forget how to adjust the volume

    d. all of the above

8. What can staff do to help residents care for their hearing aids?

    a. Clean them with thin, pliable objects, like toothpicks or paperclips

    b. Store them in the refrigerator to prevent their sensitive internal electronics from overheating

    c. Use hairs pray as an adhesive when they won't stay in a resident's ears

    d. Ensure they are regularly supplied with fresh batteries for optimum performance

9. Assistive devices used simply to make ADLs easier for residents are often called _____.

    a. mobility aids

    b. adaptive devices

    c. standalone devices

    d. reacher devices

10. Which of the following behaviors should staff NOT engage in?

    a. Facilitating residents' proper and safe usage of assistive devices

    b. Educating residents about why adjustments can't be made to their devices, even if they are experiencing discomfort

    c. Reporting improper or lack of device usage to supervisors

    d. Maintaining, cleaning, and caring for devices

CERTIFICATE OF COMPLETION

I hereby certify that

_____

has successfully completed the in-Service

Assistive Devices

_____

Signature _____

5

Understanding and Responding to Distress

Teaching Plan

To use this lesson for self-study, the learner should read the material, do the activity, and take the test. For group study, the leader may give each learner a copy of the learning guide and follow this teaching plan to conduct the lesson. Certificates may be copied for everyone who completes the lesson. The Medication of the Month feature may be used to teach workers that give or assist with medications.

Learning objectives

After this lesson, participants should be able to:

- List causes of behaviors

- State common triggers of agitation behavior

- Make changes in the environment to reduce agitation behavior

- Implement ways to overcome behavior problems

Lesson activities

Give each participant a card with a need, emotion or feeling written on it. For example: anger, sadness, hunger, need to urinate, thirst, pain, lost, wet, cold, hot, sad, confused, overwhelmed, anxious, or thoughtful. Play the game of Charades, with each participant taking a turn at acting out what they have on their card. Other participants try to guess what the person is trying to portray. You could divide participants into teams if you want to increase the competition.

Or ask participants to think of a time when they were feeling upset but weren't able to put words to their feelings. Ask them to talk about how they acted. Were other people able to see that they were upset, even though they didn't say anything to that person about it? If so, how? You will probably receive answers such as this: "I looked depressed or mad." Or "I was stomping my feet and slamming doors." Or "I refused to do my work." In other words, in some way their behavior changed because there was something going on inside them that they weren't able to talk about. It could be seen in their affect and their engagement.

Looking closely at a person's affect and their level of engagement can help give you clues and cues as to what they are feeling or experiences inside. Looking at the residents' affect and engagement can help the CNA be a bit of a detective to seek to understand, through empathy.

Mather LifeWays has studied observable quality of life for people with dementia, who have lost the ability to communicate their feelings with words. They have created tools to help us measure a person's affect and engagement. Their tools offer us a way to track the daily lived experiences of a person with dementia to see if we could bring more happiness to their day.

Affect: An expression of emotion or feelings seen through facial expressions, hand gestures, voice tone, and other emotional signs such as smiling or crying. A person's affect can be seen on their face and can also be referred to as body language. Affect can change depending on how the person is feeling emotionally. For example often just by looking at a person's affect you could see that they are experiencing pain.

Engagement: The person's participation in an activity, such as their level of participation in activities, ADLs, or conversations. Are they showing frustration, interest or enjoyment in the engagement? Is the experience one that helps the person feel positive or does it add to their distress.?

Following either activity, point out that people who have communication difficulties or, are disabled, suffering from dementia, or unable to communicate their needs (could be due to care partner speaking a different language than they do) well must find other ways to get what they want. Usually their needs, thoughts, and feelings are expressed through their behavior. It is our job as caregivers to try to determine the underlying cause of the behavior—what is our resident trying to tell us by this behavior?

The lesson

Review the material in the lesson with participants. Allow for discussion.

Conclusion

Have participants take the test. Review the answers together. Award certificates to those who answer 70% of the test questions correctly.

Test answers

1. communication	2. h	3. True	4. False	5. False
6. True	7. True	8. environment	9. True	10. True

Understanding and Responding to Distress

Learning Guide

Contents:

- What Is a Person Trying to Communicate Through Behavior?
  - Common triggers of agitation behavior in residents with dementia
- Dealing with Common Behaviors of Distress
  - Angry/agitated behavior
  - Repetitive phrases and actions
  - Paranoia
  - Wandering and pacing
  - Hoarding or gathering
  - Incontinence
  - Sleep disturbance or nighttime agitation
  - Communication
  - Simple interventions to ease agitation

What Is a Person Trying to Communicate Through Behavior?

Non-pharmacological considerations for specific behaviors	
Behavior	Consideration
Resisting care	Evaluate pain status Evaluate sleep patterns Provide positive distraction Provide consistent caregivers Personalize environment Allow time to process instructions Evaluate vision and hearing Provide simple cues
Disruptive in group activities	Determine whether toileting needs exist Provide rest periods Provide small group activities Provide activities that are broken into simple steps Provide snacks and refreshments Offer activities of preferences and interests or that are related to previous occupation Offer activities to promote calmness, such as slow tapping, drumming, clapping, rocking, or swinging
Verbally or physically abusive	Provide companionship Develop trust Avoid confrontation Provide massage or touch therapy Redirect to desirable activity or familiar activities (folding, sorting, matching) Decrease external stimuli Identify trigger and avoid trigger Provide favorite snack Review familiar photographs
Rummaging	Provide normalizing activities (sorting socks, folding towels) Provide rummaging areas such as dressers, purses, boxes Use "no entry" cues such as "do not disturb" signs
Sudden mood changes	Assess for impending acute condition Evaluate pain status Assess for hyperglycemia and hypoglycemia Accommodate customary schedule Provide consistent routines Provide consistent caregivers Decrease noise levels
Withdrawing from previous interests	Provide activities just before or after meals where meals are served Provide in-room visits Invite resident to special events Engage in activities that emphasize personal history and knowledge

Non-pharmacological considerations for specific behaviors	
Behavior	Consideration
Wandering/ elopement risk	Take resident for a walk
	Provide distraction of preferred activity
	Alleviate fears
	Provide space and environmental cues to reduce exit behavior (seating along walking path, objects to manipulate along the walking path, room with calm setting, rocking chairs, music)
	Aroma therapy
	Initiate conversations about what they are seeking
	One-on-one activities during active wandering times
	Provide pre-meal and post-meal activities
	Provide for toileting needs
	Provide room identifiers

Experts say that all types of behavior are forms of communication. Behavior problems surface for many reasons. If you can identify the reason for the behavior, you can know better how to handle it.

Common causes of behavior problems include:

- Fatigue

- Feeling overwhelmed or out of control

- Pain

- Medications

- Frustration

- Dementia/Alzheimer's disease (AD)/other brain disorders

- Established behavior patterns

- Anxiety

- Depression

Many times, dysfunctional behavior increases at the end of the day as stress builds and the person becomes tired. Pacing and wandering are clues that tension and anxiety are building. Certain stressors can trigger agitated behaviors. Many times you can recognize how a person is feeling by looking with empathy at his or her eyes, body language, and response to others around them.

Ignoring agitation behaviors is one of the worst things you can do. Try to discover the problem that is prompting the behavior, and intervene if you can. Always report these behaviors and symptoms to the nurse.

Common triggers of agitation behavior in residents with dementia

- Fatigue.

- Sudden or frequent changes in environment. Sameness and routine help to minimize stress.

- Pain. Unrecognized or undertreated pain can cause the person with dementia to respond with physical behaviors intended to stop you from touching him or her. Work with nursing to help create plans to address the person's pain.

- Feeling out of control. For example, if a person is awoken in the night for incontinence care, he or she might be frightened and feel in danger.

- Responses to overwhelming environmental stimuli.

- Excessive noise, commotion, or people. Large group activities can be disturbing.

- Excessive demands.

- Frustration. Caregivers and family must accept the fact that the person with dementia has lost and continues to lose mental functions. Doing too much for a person when he or she is trying to do it for him or herself can frustrate the person with AD who is trying to be independent.

When a person with AD is communicating that he or she is in distress, the first thing to ask yourself is "What would I be feeling if I was acting that way?" For instance, if you felt the need to physically grab another person, what would you be trying to tell that person? Perhaps you want the person to stop what he or she is doing because it hurts you. Perhaps you are afraid and need to feel safe. If someone is looking to go home, maybe that person is tired, misses loved ones, wants to be alone, or is feeling lonely. Understanding the communication behind the behavior is never easy, but it is worth it if you can help the resident with dementia feel safe, engaged, and comfortable. Use empathy and creativity, and keep an open mind. *If one strategy doesn't work, try another.*

Dealing With Common Behaviors of Distress

Angry/agitated behavior

- Determine whether medications are causing adverse side effects.

- Learn the person's history.

- Could the person be in pain?

- Reduce caffeine intake.

- In severe cases, and as a last resort, medication may be prescribed to keep a dementia resident calm.

- Reduce outside noise, clutter, or number of persons in the room. Keep objects and furniture in the same places.

- Help the confused person by making calendars and clocks available.

- Familiar objects and photographs may offer a sense of security and remind the person of pleasant memories.

- Gentle, soothing music, reading, or walks may help an agitated resident.

- Do not try to restrain a resident during an outburst.

- Keep dangerous objects out of reach.

- Acknowledge the resident's anger over the loss of control in his or her life. Say that you understand the person's frustration.

- Distract with a snack or an activity.

- Limit choices. Instead of asking "What would you like for lunch? Soup or a sandwich?" say "Here's a sandwich."

- Allow the person to forget the troubling incident that may have caused the behavior. Confronting a confused person may increase anxiety.

Repetitive phrases and actions

- Avoid reminding the resident that he or she just repeated the same phrase or asked the same question. Ignoring the repeated phrase or question may work in some cases.

- Use empathy to try to understand the meaning that the behavior is communicating.

- Agitated behavior or pulling at clothing may indicate a need to use the bathroom.

- Do not discuss plans until immediately prior to an event.

Paranoia

- Work with the care team to seek to understand the paranoia.

- Share paranoid behaviors with the resident's doctor.

- If the resident with dementia says money or an object is missing, assist him or her in locating it. Avoid arguing; instead validate the person's emotions and concerns with empathy. Try to learn his or her favorite hiding places.

Wandering and pacing

- A person who paces incessantly may burn off too many calories. Also, pacing may turn into wandering. Provide inviting places for the pacer to sit and relax.

- Ask nursing to assess for and treat pain; the person may be seeking comfort.

- Locking a resident in his or her room or restraining the resident in a chair is inappropriate. Implement activities and adjust the environment to promote meaningful engagement.

- Keep items such as coats, purses, or eyeglasses accessible to the person with dementia. Some people with dementia may be walking around looking for these "security" items. If you were unable to find your purse, you would be looking for it, too. Keeping the person feeling safe will help the person engage in other activities, which will bring more fulfillment and positive emotions.

- Provide for regular exercise and rest to minimize restlessness.

Hoarding or gathering

- Provide the patient with a safe place such as a canvas bag where he or she can store items.

- If there are items you know the person enjoys gathering, make it safe to do so. For example, if you know the person likes to take jewelry from her dresser and put it in a pocketbook, be sure to have lots of costume jewelry around for her to do this with. Then when she is engaged in other activities, place the jewelry from the pocketbook back into the dresser.

Incontinence

- Assist the resident to the bathroom every two hours (or ask family members to do so)

- Limit fluid intake in the evening before bedtime

- Place a commode at the bedside at night

- Use signs to indicate which door leads to the bathroom

Sleep disturbance or nighttime agitation

- Make sure the living quarters are safe—put away dangerous items and lock the kitchen door.

- Try soothing music.

- Keep the curtains closed to shut out darkness.

- If hallucinations are a problem, keep the room well lit to decrease shadow effects that can be confusing. Remove shadowy lighting, televisions, dolls, etc.

- Use medications as a last resort.

Communication

- Maintain eye contact to help keep attention.

- Use short, simple sentences and allow the person 20–90 seconds to respond.

- Avoid negative sentences such as "Don't go outside." Instead say, "Stay inside."

- Speak slowly and clearly.

- Encourage the resident to talk about familiar places, interests, and past experiences.

Simple interventions to ease agitation

A simplified approach to minimize or prevent distress is to make simple adjustments to the environment.

Adjusting the person's surroundings or activities can help. Some simple, basic interventions can be used to ease agitation behaviors.

- **Music as an intervention.** Some studies have shown that playing calming music can lead to a decrease in agitation. Music may be played during meals, baths, or relaxation. Creating silence is also beneficial at the right times.

- **Exercise and movement.** Light chair exercises can help to maintain function of limbs and decrease problem behaviors.

- **Activities.** Look for meaningful ways to engage the person. Learn the person's life story to find the things the person enjoyed in the past. From baking to classic cars, there are ways to include favorite hobbies into the day.

- **Socialization.** Connection with others is essential for people with AD. As the disease progresses, the person may no longer enjoy socializing in large groups. Try to find a volunteer who can converse, reminisce, or engage in meaningful activities with the person with AD. Sometimes videos are difficult for the person with AD because they have a hard time following the storyline.

Understanding and Responding to Distress

Test

Name _____ Date _____ Score _____

Directions: Fill in the blank with the correct answer, or circle the correct answer.
(Seven correct answers required.)

1. Behaviors are forms of _____.

2. A common cause of behavior problems is _____.

    a. fatigue

    b. pain

    c. medications

    d. established behavior patterns

    e. conflicts

    f. frustration

    g. dementia/AD

    h. all of the above

3. Many times, dysfunctional behavior increases at the end of the day.   True   or   False

4. It is best to ignore agitation behaviors.   True   or   False

5. It is wise to restrain a resident during an outburst.   True   or   False

6. Familiarity and routine help to minimize stress in people with dementia.   True   or   False

7.   A resident who paces incessantly may burn off too many calories, thereby requiring additional caloric intake to maintain good health.   True   or   False

8.   A simplified approach to managing agitation behaviors is to modify the _____ _____.

9.   If a resident is resisting care, you should stop and consider that the resident may be in pain. True   or   False

10.   All residents with AD benefit from a person-centered approach by their care givers. True   or   False

CERTIFICATE OF COMPLETION

I hereby certify that

has successfully completed the in-Service

Understanding and Responding to Distress

Signature

6

Bloodborne Pathogens and Standard Precautions

Teaching Plan

To use this lesson for self-study, the learner should read the material, do the activity, and take the test. For group study, the leader may give each learner a copy of the learning guide and follow this teaching plan to conduct the lesson. Certificates may be copied for everyone who completes the lesson.

Learning objectives

After this lesson, participants should be able to:

- Discuss harmful organisms that may be present in blood

- Demonstrate precautions to prevent the spread of bloodborne diseases

- Discuss procedures to follow after exposure to blood or body fluids

- Understand the importance of vaccination against hepatitis B

Lesson activities

Write this matching quiz on a board or poster. Have participants draw lines to match. The answer key is below.

1. Pathogens	a. There is no vaccine against it
2. Hepatitis B	b. These should be used with certain types of diseases
3. Hepatitis C	c. There is a vaccine against it
4. Standard precautions	d. This is the best way to prevent the spread of disease
5. Additional precautions	e. These are tiny organisms that can cause disease
6. Hand washing	f. These should be used at all times

Answer key

1. e	2. c	3. a	4. f	5. b	6. d

Ask a participant to draw one line matching an item in the left column with an item in the right column. Encourage the participant to ask others in the group for opinions if needed. Do the same thing with five other participants, until all the lines have been drawn connecting the phrases.

Hand out copies of the learning guide to participants. Lecture on the material in the guide, allowing for questions and discussion, or ask participants to read portions of the guide and tell the rest of the group what they learned.

Discuss the pyramid chart until everyone understands it. You may want to post it on a bulletin board as a reminder of infection-control precautions. If possible, demonstrate proper hand-washing technique and have participants practice.

Look at your matching quiz on the board again. Ask participants if they need to change anything. Correct anything that was not matched to the right phrase.

Administer the test and grade it.

The lesson

Review the material in the learning guide with participants. Allow for discussion.

Conclusion

Have participants take the test. Review the answers together. Award certificates to those who answer 70% of the test questions correctly.

Test answers

1. HIV, HBV, HCV	2. True	3. three	4. True	5. False
6. False	7. True	8. 10–15	9. d	10. a. Frequent, thorough hand washing; b. Wear gloves; c. mask, eye protection, gown; d. sharp items

Bloodborne Pathogens and Standard Precautions

Learning Guide

Contents:

Why Is It Important to Protect Yourself From Contact With Blood and Body Fluids?

Though they can't be seen, there are hundreds of tiny organisms living in blood and other body fluids that can cause disease in humans. These are called bloodborne pathogens.

Some of these organisms are harmless and can be handled easily by the body's immune system, but others can cause severe illness, such as hepatitis or AIDS.

Bloodborne Diseases: HIV/AIDS, Hepatitis B, Hepatitis C

Bloodborne pathogens include the hepatitis B virus (HBV), the hepatitis C virus (HCV), the human immunodeficiency virus (HIV) that causes autoimmune deficiency syndrome (AIDS), and others.

These pathogens are transmitted through contact with infected body fluids such as blood, semen, and vaginal secretions. Exposures occur (a) if the skin is punctured by a contaminated needle, razor, or other sharp item or (b) when broken skin or mucous membranes are splashed with blood or body fluid. Fortunately, most exposures do not result in infections.

Standard precautions are designed to prevent transmission of HIV, HBV, and HCV. Standard precautions must be observed in all situations where there is potential for contact with blood or other potentially infectious body fluids.

Standard precautions apply to:

- Blood

- Semen

- Vaginal secretions

- Saliva

- Cerebrospinal fluid

- Synovial fluid

- Pleural fluid

- Peritoneal fluid

- Pericardial fluid

- Amniotic fluid

- Feces

- Nasal secretions

- Sputum

- Sweat

- Tears

- Urine

- Vomitus

Treat all human blood and body fluids as if they are infectious. Remember who you are protecting—YOURSELF!

Standard precaution 1: Hand washing

Hand washing is the single most important thing you can do to prevent the spread of infection. Thorough hand washing removes pathogens from the skin.

Wash hands before and after all resident or body-fluid contact. Immediately wash hands and other skin surfaces that are contaminated with blood or body fluids. When wearing gloves, wash hands as soon as the gloves are removed.

Germicidal or alcohol-based handrubs are recommended *only* when you can't wash.

Proper hand-washing procedure

1. Remove watch or push it up your arm. You should not wear rings or bracelets at work.

2. Do not touch the sink with your hands while you are washing, and stand back from the sink to keep it from touching your clothes.

3. Use warm water. Hot water may dry skin.

4. Either bar soap or liquid soap is okay. If using a bar, rinse it first and hold it the whole time you are lathering. Soap does not have to be an antiseptic type, unless you are doing an invasive procedure such as catheterization.

5. Wet your wrists and hands.

6. Apply plenty of soap. Work up a thick lather all over your hands and wrists, between your fingers and thumbs, and on the back of your hands and wrists.

7. Vigorously rub all areas of your hands, fingers, and wrists for **a minimum of 10–15 seconds.** Sixty seconds is better. Friction helps remove dirt and microorganisms.

8. Clean under your nails by using the nails on your other hand, or rub your nails into the palm of your other hand. Clean around the top of your nails.

9. Rinse with warm water, letting water run down from wrists to fingertips and into the sink.

10. Dry with a clean paper towel and throw it away.

11. Turn off the faucet with a clean, dry paper towel and throw the towel away.

12. Use lotion on your hands to prevent irritation and chapping, which makes skin more prone to infection.

When hand-washing facilities aren't available, use an agency-approved antiseptic hand cleaner or an antiseptic towelette. As soon as possible, rewash your hands with soap and water following the correct hand-washing procedure.

Standard precaution 2: Gloves

- Use gloves in all situations where you may come in contact with blood or body fluids

- Use gloves for resident care involving contact with mucous membranes, such as brushing teeth

- Change gloves and wash hands between resident contacts

- Never wear gloves in the hallways

- Use gloves when you have scrapes, scratches, or chapped skin

- Do not wash or disinfect disposable gloves for reuse

Standard precaution 3: Protective barriers

Protective barriers, including gloves, reduce the risk of your skin or mucous membranes being exposed to potentially infective blood and body fluids. You should wear the appropriate barriers for the work you are doing. Always follow steps and special precautions to remove and discard all PPE to prevent contamination.

Employers must provide suitable personal protective equipment (PPE) in the right sizes. Protective equipment includes gloves, gowns, masks, eye protection, face shields, mouthpieces, resuscitation devices, and other things. Hypoallergenic gloves, glove liners, powderless gloves, or other alternatives must be available for those who are allergic to the regular gloves.

The equipment you need depends on your work. When splashing of blood or body fluids is likely, wear the following PPE in addition to gloves:

- Mask: if your face could be splashed with blood or body fluids

- Eye protection: if your eyes could be splashed with blood or body fluids

- Gown: if your clothing or skin could be splashed

Standard precaution 4: Proper disposal of sharp items

A sharp is any object that can penetrate the skin, such as a needle, a scalpel, broken glass, a broken capillary tube, and exposed ends of wires. A sharp is contaminated if it has been in contact with blood, body fluids, or body tissues.

Contaminated sharps must be disposed of properly. Follow your organization's policies. Although nursing assistants are not giving injections with syringes, it is important to know your organization's needlestick safety protocols.

Some protocols for syringe safety include, but are not limited to, the following:

- Be careful to prevent injuries from needlesticks and other sharp instruments after procedures and when disposing of used needles.

- It's best to use needleless injection systems or needles with injury protection. If you must use a regular needle, remember:

  - Do not recap or manipulate needles. If it is absolutely necessary to recap a needle, use one hand to slide the needle into a cap lying on a flat surface. Do not hold the cap in your other hand while recapping.

Tips

Use thick rubber household gloves to protect your hands during housekeeping chores or instrument cleaning involving potential blood contact
Treat all linen soiled with blood or body secretions as potentially infectious
Surfaces that have been contaminated with blood or body fluids should be cleaned with a disinfectant according to your organization's policies

**Figure 6.1: Centers for Disease Control
Two-Tiered System to Control Disease Transmission**

Everyone is a possible source of bloodborne infection.

Protect yourself!

**TIER 2:
Additional
Precautions**
Based on
Type of Disease and
How It Is
Transmitted:
1. Airborne
2. Contact
3. Droplet

TIER 1: Standard Precautions

Basic Precautions to Be Used at All Times,
with All Clients, to Prevent
Transmission of Bloodborne Diseases:
1. Frequent, thorough hand washing.
2. Wear gloves when you touch blood or body fluids.
3. When splashing of blood or body fluids is likely,
   wear the following, depending on the situation:
   a. Masks
   b. Eye protection
   c. Disposable Gowns
4. Safe use and disposal of sharp items.
   Do not recap needles at any time.

If an Exposure Occurs

Following your organization's exposure policy for blood or body fluids, immediately:

- Wash needlesticks and cuts with soap and water.

- Flush splashes to the nose, mouth, or skin with water.

- Irrigate eyes with clean water, saline, or sterile irrigants.

Next:

- Report the exposure at once. Treatment may be recommended, and it should be started as soon as possible. See a medical professional.

- Discuss the possible risks and the need for treatment with the person managing your exposure.

- Remember that mandatory testing of a resident for infection is not legal. Residents who might be the source of an infection must give consent to be tested.

Workers' rights

The Occupational Safety and Health Administration (OSHA) is a federal agency that guarantees rights to a safe workplace. Under OSHA's rules, workers who might be exposed to contaminated blood or body fluids have specific rights.

Employers must train workers that might be exposed to blood or body fluids about the hazards and how to protect themselves. This training must occur during working hours at no cost to employees, at orientation, and annually thereafter.

Standard precautions must be practiced at all times. Punctureproof and leakproof containers must be provided for disposal of sharp items. There must be a system for reporting exposures to blood or body fluids.

Employers must provide free hepatitis B vaccine, free protective equipment, and free immediate medical evaluation and follow-up for anyone exposed to blood or body fluids. Employees must receive confidential treatment, and their medical records must be protected.

Workers' responsibilities

- Always use standard precautions.

- Actively participate in evaluating safer equipment and encouraging your organization to purchase safer equipment. Be open to new products or practices that could prevent exposure and protect workers and residents.

- Be immunized against hepatitis B, getting the full series of three injections.

- Report all exposures immediately after cleaning and disinfecting the exposed skin or mucous membranes.

- Comply with postexposure recommendations of your organization.

- Support other workers who have been exposed. HIV-infected workers who continue working deserve support and confidentiality.

- Know your own HIV/HBV/HCV status. If you are positive for any of these viruses, you do not pose a risk for residents if you don't do invasive procedures.

Specific Exposure Risks and Treatments

Human immunodeficiency virus

HIV is the virus that causes AIDS.

Risk of infection after exposure:

- Needlestick is the most common cause of work-related infection.

- Risk factors include the amount of blood or fluid, the puncture depth, and the disease stage of the infected person.

- The average risk of HIV infection after a needlestick or cut exposure is 1 in 300. The risk after exposure of the eye, nose, skin, or mouth to positive blood is less than 1 in 1,000. If the skin is damaged, the risk may be higher.

Treatment after exposure:

- There is no vaccine against HIV.

- Postexposure treatment is not always recommended. A physician or exposure expert should advise you.

- Drugs used to prevent infection may have serious side effects.

- Perform HIV antibody testing for at least six months after exposure.

- 99.7% of needlestick/cut exposures do not result in HIV infection.

Hepatitis B virus

Risk of infection after exposure:

- Hepatitis B vaccine prevents this disease. Persons who have received the vaccine and developed immunity are at virtually no risk for infection. A series of three injections are required, given initially, then one to two months later, then four to six months after the first injection.

- Workers should be tested one to two months after the vaccination series to make sure the vaccination has provided immunity.

- For the unvaccinated person, the risk from a single needlestick or cut exposure ranges from 6–30%, depending on the level of virus in the infected person's blood. A higher concentration of virus makes it more likely that someone exposed to that blood will become infected.

Treatment after exposure:

- Everyone with a chance of exposure to blood or body fluids should receive hepatitis B vaccine, preferably during training, unless it is contraindicated because of allergies, pregnancy, or potential pregnancy.

- Hepatitis B immune globulin (HBIG) effectively prevents HBV infection after exposure. Recommendations for postexposure management of HBV may include HBIG and/or hepatitis B vaccine. The decision to begin treatment is based on several factors, such as whether the:

  - Source person is positive for hepatitis B

  - Worker has been vaccinated

  - Vaccine provided immunity

Hepatitis C virus

Infection with HCV carries a great potential for chronic liver disease and can lead to liver failure, liver transplants, and liver cancer.

Risk of infection after exposure:

- HCV is a growing problem

- The risk for infection after a needlestick or cut exposure to HCV-infected blood is approximately 1.8%

- The risk after a blood splash is unknown but is believed to be very small; however, HCV infection from such an exposure has been reported

Treatment after exposure:

- There is no vaccine against hepatitis C and no treatment after an exposure that will prevent infection.

- Immune globulin (HBIG) is not recommended.

- Following recommended infection-control practices is vital.

- There are several tests that should be performed in the weeks after an exposure and for four to six months afterward. Confer with a physician or an exposure specialist.

Additional Precautions for Infection Control

If you know or suspect that a resident has a disease that is spread in one of the following ways, use the following extra precautions, in addition to standard precautions.

Airborne germs can travel long distances through the air and are breathed in by people. Examples of diseases caused by airborne germs are tuberculosis (TB), chickenpox, and shingles. Precautions include the following:

- Wear a mask. If the resident has, or might have, TB, wear a special respiratory mask (ask your supervisor). A regular mask will not protect you.

- Remind the resident to cover nose and mouth when coughing or sneezing.

- Treat the resident's used tissues or handkerchiefs as infected material.

- If treating a person with TB in a hospital or skilled nursing facility, the person will be placed in a special room with negative air pressure.

Contact germs can cause the spread of disease by touch. Examples of diseases caused by contact germs are pink eye, scabies, wound infections, and methicillin-resistant *Staphylococcus aureus*. Precautions include the following:

- Wear gloves

- Treat bed linens, clothes, and wound dressings as infected material

- Wear a gown if the resident has drainage, has diarrhea, or is incontinent

- Use a disinfectant to clean stethoscopes, blood-pressure cuffs, or other equipment

- Dispose of equipment and PPE per policy and procedures

Droplet germs can travel short distances through the air, usually not more than three feet. Sneezing, coughing, and talking can spread these germs. Examples of diseases caused by droplet germs are flu and pneumonia. Precautions include the following:

- Wear a mask when working close to the resident (within three feet)

Bloodborne Pathogens and Standard Precautions

Test

Name _____ Date _____ Score _____

Directions: Fill in the blank with the correct answer, or circle the correct answer.

1. Name three bloodborne pathogens: _____, _____, and _____.
    (three points)

2. All workers with a chance of exposure to blood or body fluids should receive hepatitis B
    vaccine unless they shouldn't take it for medical or pregnancy reasons.   True   or   False

3. Hepatitis B immunization requires a series of _____ injections.

4. Persons who have received HBV vaccine and developed immunity are at virtually no risk for
    infection for hepatitis B.   True   or   False

5. There is a vaccine against HIV.   True   or   False

6. Most exposures lead to HIV infection.   True   or   False

7. There is no vaccine against hepatitis C and no treatment after an exposure that will prevent
    infection.   True   or   False

8. Proper hand washing requires lathering with soap for at least _____ seconds.

9. The first thing you should do if you are exposed to blood or body fluids is:

    a. Wash needlesticks and cuts with soap and water

    b. Flush splashes to the nose, mouth, or skin with water

    c. Irrigate eyes with clean water, saline, or sterile irrigants

    d. All of the above, depending on the area of the body exposed

10. Standard precautions involve four basic things. Fill in the blanks below (four points).

    a. _____, _____ _____.

    b. _____ _____ when might touch blood or body fluids.

    c. Wear _____, _____, or _____ when splashing of blood or body fluids is likely, depending on the situation.

    d. Safely use and dispose of _____.

CERTIFICATE OF COMPLETION

I hereby certify that

_____

has successfully completed the in-Service

Bloodborne Pathogens and Standard Precautions

_____
Signature

7

Communication

Teaching Plan

To use this lesson for self-study, the learner should read the material, do the activity, and take the test. For group study, the leader may give each learner a copy of the learning guide and follow this teaching plan to conduct the lesson. Certificates may be copied for everyone who completes the lesson.

Learning objectives

After this lesson, participants should be able to:

- State the meaning of communication
- Demonstrate how to be an active listener
- Demonstrate how to speak effectively
- List nonverbal ways of communicating
- List the five "don'ts" of communication
- Explain how to communicate in difficult situations

Lesson activities

1. Ask learners to work in pairs and take turns telling their partners about someone who is important to them, such as a child. After the first learners finish, their partners should tell them if their speech was effective, based on the five points in the section "Effective Talking." The learner who did the speaking should rate his or her partner as an active listener, based on the 10 points in the section "Active Listening." After everyone has had a turn, ask learners to share what they learned.

2. Ask your learners to look at you and say all the things they can think of that you are communicating to them. For example, are you happy today? How can they tell? Are you feeling stressed and tired? What makes them think that? See how many messages they can identify from your face, dress, posture, and body language.

3. Give the following lecture, in your own words:

"All of us are communicating all the time. As I speak these words to you, I am sending messages to you with my voice, my facial expressions, my posture, and my hand motions. Even the way I am dressed communicates something to you. You (the learners) are also communicating with me and with each other. By the looks on your faces and your body language, you tell me whether you are bored or interested. You communicate with me through words, but also by your dress and the way you do your job. "

"We communicate with our residents in all these ways, too, and we should be alert to what they are telling us through the various ways they try to communicate with us. For communication to occur, someone must send a message and someone must receive it. *If a message is not received and understood, then we are not communicating.* Communication requires you to deeply listen and understand what the other person is saying, not just waiting for your turn to talk. To be a good communicator, we must learn how to find out if our messages are received. We must learn how to ask questions and listen to *feedback* from our residents. For example, when you take the test at the end of this session, you will give me feedback about how well you understood the lesson. We must always be sure the receivers understand our message. Many things can hinder good communication. Eyesight and hearing problems, illness, stress, medications, emotions, fatigue, confusion, language or cultural differences, and even personality differences are some of the things that might affect how well a message is given and received. Learning how to communicate effectively can go a long way toward helping our residents feel happy and secure."

The lesson

Read the learning goals to the learners and proceed with the lesson.

Conclusion

Have participants take the test. Review the answers together. Award certificates to those who answer 70% of the test questions correctly.

Test answers

1. d	2. d	3. b	4. c		5. a
6. d	7. b	8. c	9. offer opinions, become defensive, make judgments, ask why, give empty assurances		10. a

Communication

Learning Guide

Contents:

- Active Listening

- Effective Talking

- Five "Don'ts" of Communication

- Seven Skills of Active Listening

- Expressions, Gestures, and Posture

- Barriers to Effective Communication

Active Listening

To communicate well, learn to listen well. Practice these listening skills:

- Make eye contact.

- Sit at eye level.

- Look relaxed and interested.

- Avoid making distracting movements.

- Lean toward the talker in a listening posture.

- Nod your head or make other understanding gestures.

- Make sounds of understanding and interest at appropriate intervals, such as "hmm" or "oh, my."

- Ask questions about what the speaker is saying, to clarify a point, focus the conversation, and show interest.

- Touch the speaker or hold his or her hand if appropriate.

- Use the seven skills of active listening.

- When talking to the person with dementia, allow 20–90 seconds for the person to respond.

- Avoid asking a lot of questions when the person is talking; it only distracts from the message they want to convey or the story they hope to share.

- Notice if you are listening with the goal of understanding, or simply waiting for your turn to speak.

Effective Talking

To get your message across, practice the following speaking skills:

- Speak clearly and distinctly

- Use simple words and sentences, and frame your message clearly

- Give all the information the person needs, such as who you are and what you are going to do

- Use descriptive gestures to reinforce your words

- Use humor when appropriate

- Use expressions, gestures, and body language that reinforce your message

Five "Don'ts" of Communication

To be an effective communicator, eliminate the following habits:

1. **Don't offer your opinions.** Help your residents make their own decisions; don't tell them what you think they should or shouldn't do.

2. **Don't become defensive.** When a resident criticizes you or someone else, reflect his concern back to him so you can learn more about the problem.

3. **Don't make judgments.** Instead of showing disapproval, ask the resident about his reasons for acting or feeling a certain way. Be open to differences of opinion.

4. **Don't ask "Why?"** "Why" questions make people feel defensive. Word questions in a non-threatening way, such as asking calmly, "What happened?" or "Can you tell me about it?"

5. **Don't give empty assurances.** "Everything's going to be fine" isn't necessarily true. Focus on helping the resident talk about his or her concerns.

Seven Skills of Active Listening

1. **Show interest.** Use encouraging sounds, and nod your head. Don't appear impatient or hurried.

2. **Be other-focused.** Ask questions so others will talk about themselves. Focus conversations on the person you are talking to, not on yourself.

> **Other-focused**
> Resident: "I have 15 grandchildren but Tommy lives closest to me."
> Staff member: "You have 15 grandchildren?! That's wonderful. Tell me about them."

3. **Reflect.** Keep conversations focused on the other person by reflecting back his or her thoughts and questions. Concentrate on the other person's feelings and concerns.

> **Reflect**
> Resident: "What should I do about my mother?"
> Staff member: "What do you think you should do?"

4. **Be quiet.** Sometimes people need some silence to gather their thoughts.

5. **Clarify.** Find out exactly what someone means when he or she says something. You can learn valuable information this way. Clarify anything that raises a question in your mind.

> **Clarify**
> Resident: "I'm too tired to take a bath today. Leave me alone."
> Staff member: "Can you tell me what you think is making you tired today?"

6. **Ask open questions.** Ask questions that require more than just a "yes" or "no" answer. You get more information that way. For example, rather than "Are you okay today?" ask "How are you feeling today?"

7. **Repeat.** To be sure you understand something, repeat what you hear in your own words and then ask if you repeated it correctly.

Expressions, Gestures, and Posture

The following are some tips on expression to communicate effectively:

- Make eye contact to show respect and interest

- Offer a gentle, respectful touch on the shoulder or the hand to give support and encouragement

- Sit at eye level if possible, and lean forward in an attitude of interest

- Demonstrate your words with hand motions that help show what you mean

In return, look for nonverbal messages in the face, hands, and body of those you talk with. Be aware of the nonverbal messages you are sending as well. If you are annoyed, you might be showing it more than you realize, with your hand on your hip and your eyes rolling. Pay attention to your body and correct any signals that might inhibit communication.

Barriers to Effective Communication

Sometimes, residents have trouble speaking, hearing, or understanding, or sometimes they get angry or emotional, making it difficult to communicate. The following are some tips to follow when you're in these situations:

- Allow plenty of time for the person to respond to something you say (20–90 seconds for the person with advancing AD).

- Turn off or remove distractions such as a television or radio. You might have to close the door to the room if there is noise in the hallway.

- Be sure to put your mobile phone away when you are talking with others. It is a symbol of distraction and disinterest in the person you are with.

- Stay on the resident's "good" side, where his or her hearing or speech is best. Let him or her see your mouth as you speak.

- Don't rush the person or finish his sentences for him, unless you can help by patiently supplying a word or two.

- When you are speaking, use the correct voice volume. You may have to be louder if the person is hard of hearing, but remember that individuals with dementia or people who have had a stroke aren't necessarily hard of hearing. A normal volume works best in these situations.

- Use short, simple words and phrases.

- Ask "yes" or "no" questions to make it easier for the resident to answer.

- When the person has difficulty finding the right words, ask him or her to point to words or pictures on a board or a piece of paper. Encourage the resident to use gestures such as head nodding and hand motions.

- When giving directions, state one instruction at a time. Break your directions down into simple steps.

- Keep your mood, facial expression, body language, and voice calm, quiet, and relaxed.

- Do not argue. This will only increase the individual's anger and cause the incident to get worse.

- Maintain eye contact even if someone is angry.

- Avoid touching an angry person.

- Keep a clear exit for yourself, being sure that the angry person doesn't block your way to the doorway.

- Use the skill of reflection. Reflecting is the process of paraphrasing and restating both the feelings and the words of the speaker.

- Don't pass judgment on someone's words or behavior. Stay open-minded and listen actively to hear the underlying feelings and concerns.

- After you have listened to the reasons for the person's anger, help him or her solve the problem or handle the situation.

Note: If these tactics don't work, or if you fear harm, you should leave the scene and notify your supervisor.

Communication

Test

Name _____ Date _____ Score _____

Directions: Circle the best answer.

1. Which of the following statements use the listening skill of reflection?

   a. "You seem worried about something."

   b. "What do you think is the best thing to do?"

   c. "So you think it might be hard to follow the doctor's orders?"

   d. All of the above

2. If a resident is having difficulty saying the right words, you should _____.

   a. be silent and allow time for the resident to think

   b. provide words or pictures on a board or paper for the resident to point to

   c. guess at what he or she is trying to say

   d. Both a and b

3. Open-ended questions are good for obtaining information, but it is better to ask questions that can be answered with a "yes" or "no" if _____.

   a. you are in a hurry

   b. the resident has difficulty speaking

   c. the resident has difficulty hearing

   d. you don't want too much information

4. Communication only occurs when _____.

   a. someone is talking

   b. someone is listening

   c. a message is both given and received

   d. the message is written down

5. Nonverbal communication occurs through _____.

   a. gestures, expressions, posture, and dress

   b. silence

   c. speech

   d. None of the above

6. If a resident says something that raises a question in your mind, you should _____.

   a. ignore it

   b. say he or she is thinking the wrong way

   c. offer your opinion

   d. clarify by asking the resident what he or she means

7. When a resident is angry, you should _____.

   a. give the resident a hug

   b. remain calm and ask what is wrong

   c. argue with the resident

   d. stay away

8. When speaking, it is important to _____.

   a. both c and d

   b. yell

   c. speak clearly and use simple words and phrases

   d. avoid looking directly at anyone

9. List the five "don'ts" of communication. Don't:

   _____   _____   _____   _____   _____

10. It is best if our conversations with residents focus on _____.

    a. the resident

    b. other people

    c. ourselves

    d. the organization

CERTIFICATE OF COMPLETION

I hereby certify that

_____

has successfully completed the in-Service

Communication

_____
Signature

8

Cultural Diversity

Teaching Plan

To use this lesson for self-study, the learner should read the material, do the activity, and take the test. For group study, the leader may give each learner a copy of the learning guide and follow this teaching plan to conduct the lesson. Certificates may be copied for everyone who completes the lesson.

Learning objectives

After this lesson, participants should be able to:

- Define cultural diversity

- Avoid stereotyping

- Communicate with residents of different cultures respectfully and effectively

Lesson activities

1. Engage your team in a discussion about their own cultural backgrounds. Invite clinicians and management to share in the discussion as well.

2. Encourage participants to discuss some past residents that they have worked with who had different cultural backgrounds and how this may have affected their roles in the home.

3. Obtain information about the makeup of your agency's resident population and provide tailored information on specific cultures to your agency.

The lesson

Review the material in the lesson with participants. Allow for discussion.

Conclusion

Have participants take the test. Review the answers together. Award certificates to those who answer 70% of the test questions correctly.

Test answers

1. d	2. a	3. c	4. a	5. b
6. d	7. False	8. True	9. b	10. False

Cultural Diversity

Learning Guide

Contents:

- Defining Cultural Diversity

  - Geographic culture

  - Religious culture

- Stereotypes

- Communication and Active Listening

  - Care partner's role

Defining Cultural Diversity

Culture is a social pattern of behaviors, beliefs, and characteristics of a group of people that are passed on from generation to generation. It is important to understand that cultural characteristics are different from physical characteristics. Many people who have similar physical characteristics do not always have similar cultural characteristics.

Cultural diversity is the variety of human societies or cultures in a specific region or in the world as a whole. There are also more obvious cultural differences that exist between people, such as language, dress, and traditions.

Geographic culture

Some culture originates from the area of the world that the person is from. This is called geographic culture. There are many geographic cultures, and they can greatly influence a resident's views on diet and medical care.

The following are some types of geographic cultures. They are listed here to give you a better idea of the variety within these cultures and not to provide specific information about an individual resident or family. Keep in mind that these are very general and will not apply to all residents.

Eastern Asian and Pacific Islanders

Eastern Asian and Pacific Islanders contain many different ethnic groups. These groups include, but are not limited to, Chinese, Korean, Japanese, Vietnamese, Hmong, Indonesian, Filipino, and Samoan people. Dietary habits are varied, based on the culture, and there are often special diets to be taken into consideration during illness. Fish, fruits, vegetables, and rice are the primary diet, along with small amounts of chicken, pork, or beef. In most of these cultures, a meal is almost like a ceremony and should not be interrupted. There are several religions practiced, including Confucianism, Buddhism, Taoism, Islam, Shintoism (Japan), and Roman Catholic. Medicinal herbs and folk remedies and rituals are commonly used to prevent or treat illness. Most believe that good health is a result of harmony and may use health healers and spiritual healers before seeking standard medical care. Drawing of blood is especially upsetting to many. There is a tendency to hide outward signs of pain, so it may be difficult to determine how much pain a resident is having. Many believe in some type of reincarnation.

Haitian, Puerto Rican, and Cuban

Generally, people of Haitian, Puerto Rican, or Cuban culture believe that diet is very important for maintaining good health. Many believe that foods have hot and cold properties, and these must be in harmony. Some believe that illness is supernatural and caused by evil spirits or enemies of deceased relatives. They may wear amulets to protect against evil spirits. Most consult folk healers or spiritualists before seeking standard medical care. Use of herbs and rituals for healing is common. Many are suspicious and fearful of hospitals. Cuban-Americans are most likely to use standard medical practices in combination with religious or home remedies.

Religious culture

In addition to cultures passed on from different geographic areas, there are many general religious cultural beliefs that you may find among your residents. Keep in mind that not all members of a particular religious group will hold the same beliefs. These are generally held beliefs and may not be those of each and every member.

Baptist

Almost all Baptist groups prohibit alcohol as a beverage. Many groups strongly believe in faith healing or "laying on of hands" by preachers or others empowered by God to heal. Many believe that when medical treatment cures them, it is because God is functioning through the doctors and nurses. They may refuse ventilators or resuscitation, believing it interferes with God's will. Mission work is very much part of most Baptist churches, because many of them believe that only Christians will go to Heaven.

Church of Jesus Christ of Latter Day Saints

People who practice at the Church of Jesus Christ of Latter Day Saints are commonly referred to as Mormons. While meat is not forbidden, members are encouraged to eat meat "infrequently," and they generally do not drink tea, coffee, or alcohol. Most will fast for 24 hours on the first Sunday of the month. They are strong believers in divine healing with anointing and "laying on of hands" by church elders but do not prohibit standard medical care. On their wedding day, they are given special undergarments that are always worn. Never remove these undergarments without discussing the process with the resident or family. The church headquarters is in Salt Lake City, Utah.

Islam

People who practice Islam are often referred to as Muslims or Nation of Islam. Muslims do not eat pork and pork products and generally do not use alcohol. During Ramadan (the last month of the Mohammedan year), they do not eat during daylight hours. They accept standard medical care and generally oppose faith healing. Muslims perform prayers five times daily. There is usually ritual washing after prayers. There are several different sects of Islam, and each is somewhat different.

Jewish

Dietary habits depend upon whether they are Orthodox, Reform, or Conservative. Jews do not eat pork; they eat only meat that comes from animals that eat vegetables, have cloven hooves, or chew their cud. Meat must be ritually slaughtered to make it "kosher." They do not eat seafood unless it has scales and fins. Orthodox and other Jews who strictly observe kosher laws never combine meat products and dairy products and do not store them together. They may have two sets of dishes—one for meat and one for dairy. During Passover, they do not eat any leavened bread (bread containing yeast or other ingredients to cause it to ferment and rise). Jews may refuse surgery during the Sabbath (sundown on Friday until sundown on Saturday). Because kosher foods are high in sodium, residents on low-salt diets do not have to use kosher meats. Jews generally oppose prolonging life with life support. Amputated limbs and other parts of the body removed by surgery are given to family for burial. There is no single Jewish authority over all Jewish synagogues. All congregations are independent and control their own activities. On the Sabbath, Orthodox Jews do not use cars, do not cook, and do not do work of any kind.

Roman Catholic

Catholics fast and do not eat meat on Ash Wednesday or Good Friday. Most still do not eat meat on Fridays during Lent, and some Catholics may still follow the old practice of not eating meat on any Friday during the entire year. The church does not approve of contraceptives, abortion, or fertility treatments. Most request anointing of the sick during major illness. Residents may refuse to eat or drink for an hour before someone is bringing them communion. The authority over all Roman Catholic churches is the Pope.

Stereotypes

All information in this lesson reflects general cultural beliefs of many geographic and religious cultures. That said, it is important to understand that not every person, even if they are of a particular culture, practices the same way. For example, someone may be Roman Catholic, but they may not go to church or take communion. Or maybe someone from Puerto Rico never eats the types of food from their region. Every person is different.

One thing that we must always be careful to never do is to stereotype residents based on their physical features or cultural backgrounds. Just because someone is from the Middle East, it does not mean that the person is Muslim; just because someone is Mormon, it does not mean that the person never drinks alcohol. There are many stereotypes in the world, and they are often reflected on TV, the Internet, and more. It is important to never assume and always make sure you listen and communicate with the resident so that you understand what cultural beliefs they hold.

Communication and Active Listening

Residents from different cultures will communicate in different ways. It is hard to know what is appropriate for residents of different cultural backgrounds. Observation between family members and nonverbal reactions to communication can be clues to aid you. Always address a person from a different culture by his or her formal name. In some cultures, direct eye contact may be considered disrespectful and communicating with eyes downcast is a sign of respect. Be aware of personal body space. Some cultures may see a close body space as threatening, whereas others may maintain a close body space. Cultures vary with regard to comfort with physical contact, especially when from someone of the opposite sex. When providing personal care for someone from a different culture, ask permission to touch or uncover areas of the body and expose only one area at a time.

It is so important for staff to listen to their residents. Many residents may not share their culture with you right away, but if they do, it is important to listen and retain that knowledge. An important part of effective communication is the art of active listening.

All of us are distracted by our personal lives and work responsibilities. This can interfere with our ability to be active listeners. Active listening does not always come easy. It is a technique that takes practice and a dedicated effort to maintain. But once you learn how to become an active listener, there is so much more information that can be gained from our residents or caregivers, and there is much more that we can do for them. Tools used in active listening are not complicated; they just take consistent use for them to become second nature.

The following are guidelines to use in active listening:

- Pay attention to what the resident or caregiver is saying

- Maintain eye contact

- Face the resident or caregiver directly

- Acknowledge that you are listening

- Do not interrupt the resident or caregiver when he or she is talking

- Do not talk when the resident or caregiver is talking

- Ask questions to clarify what the resident or caregiver said if you did not understand him or her

- Repeat back to the resident or caregiver what you thought you heard by paraphrasing

- Be aware of the resident or caregiver's nonverbal communication

- Be honest in your response

- Treat residents as you would want to be treated

Care partner's role

A person's culture is a part of them. As someone who cares for people in their homes, you may witness different cultures you have never encountered before.

Your role may include:

- **Respecting the resident's beliefs.** You may not always agree with a resident's values or lifestyle, but you must respect his or her beliefs, lifestyle choices, culture, attitudes, and other preferences. You must not be judgmental, and you must honor his or her choices.

- **Observing, reporting, and documenting.** Keen observation skills are important for anyone who works with residents in healthcare. Observation can be important to notice cultural practices. Residents may not always be open to communicate with you about their beliefs and rituals, but by observing the resident you may be able to understand them better. Sometimes residents will expect you to understand without communicating with you at all. Although this is unrealistic, you can get a head start to understanding by observing the resident. Report anything out of the ordinary to your supervisor, even if you don't think it's important. You should document anything that can improve care (types of food they don't eat, pray schedule, etc.). This is important information that should be documented. An example of when cultural diversity may need to be observed, documented, and reported is as follows:

A resident always prays at certain times during the day. Although he didn't mention his prayers to the staff member, he gets upset if he is busy during his prayer times. Once he even tried to get out of the bath in the middle of bathing to prepare to pray. The staff member tries to talk to the resident about it, but he does not want to talk about his religion, and there is a slight communication gap because of a language barrier.

Staff first need to respect the resident's choice to not discuss his religious practices. Since the resident doesn't communicate, you must observe the resident and help base his care on the observations. By observing the times that the resident prays, the staff can document and let the clinician know when the resident prefers to be visited and cared for. If there is a routine in the resident's prayer schedule, as there often is, make sure you document it. This information can make it easier for you and others caring for the person to schedule care and also make the resident happier.

Cultural Diversity

Test

Name _____ Date _____ Score _____

Directions: Circle the best answer.

1. Which of the following is a technique of active listening?

   b. Maintaining eye contact

   c. Acknowledging that you are listening

   d. Being aware of the resident or caregiver's nonverbal communication

   e. All of the above

2. Which of the following groups of people would make up a type of culture?

   a. Muslims

   b. Women

   c. Californians

   d. Nurses

3. How might the cultural beliefs of a resident affect a frontline staff member's job?

   a. If the resident's beliefs are wrong, then the staff member needs to correct them

   b. They won't

   c. The staff member may need to change meal preparation to respect the resident's cultural beliefs

   d. The staff member may need to pretend to follow the same beliefs

4. Which of the following cultures is generally opposed to taking medications?

    a. Christian Scientists

    b. Muslims

    c. Eastern Asians

    d. Mormons

5. Which of the following is *not* true about cultures?

    a. The beliefs are passed on from generation to generation

    b. Everyone within the culture is the same and will believe and practice exactly the same things

    c. Members of the same race often have great cultural differences

    d. Cultural characteristics are different from physical differences

6. Which of the following help define a culture?

    a. A social pattern of beliefs shared by a group of people

    b. A pattern of social characteristics shared by a group of people

    c. Beliefs that are passed on from one generation to another

    d. All of the above

7. As soon as you know a resident's cultural background, you will know all about his or her beliefs, since they will always be the same. True   or   False

8. One of your most important obligations as caregiver is to respect the rights of residents, including their cultural beliefs. True   or   False

9. What is a stereotype?

    a. An accurate description of a person's cultural beliefs

    b. A widely held but fixed and oversimplified image or idea of a particular type of person or thing

    c. A type of culture

    d. A type of stereo system

10. Observing a resident's cultural rituals is always a waste of time, and you shouldn't bother to pay attention, as it's important to always mind your own business. True or False

CERTIFICATE OF COMPLETION

I hereby certify that

_____

has successfully completed the in-Service

Cultural Diversity

_____

Signature _____

9 Caring for People With Dementia

Teaching Plan

To use this lesson for self-study, the learner should read the material, do the activity, and take the test. For group study, the leader may give each learner a copy of the learning guide and follow this teaching plan to conduct the lesson. Certificates may be copied for everyone who completes the lesson.

Learning objectives

After this lesson, participants should be able to:

- Know the definition and symptoms of dementia

- Know some good ways to approach people with dementia

- Know the importance of trying to understand what a resident with dementia is thinking and feeling

- Understand the difficulties faced by someone with dementia

Lesson activities

Give each learner a copy of the corresponding learning guide. Before beginning, assign one of the case studies to each of different learners. Ask them to be ready to present the case to the group.

Explain that the learners will be examining good ways to work with people that have dementia, and encourage the learners to ask specific questions about people they assist. Many times, other workers will have good ideas about how to help a specific patient, and they need opportunities to share this information with each other.

Section 1: Definition

1. Ask a learner to read the definition and causes of dementia from the learning guide. Determine whether the learners have any questions about this information.

2. Briefly review the "Important things to remember about dementia" section in the learning guide. Mention that it might seem time-consuming to try to figure out what a person with

dementia is thinking or feeling, but the person has the right to expect this from caregivers. In addition, spending the time to do this will often save time and difficulty later. Emphasize that there is not one right way to help, but that each individual person has special needs and special ways of relating that must be understood.

Section 2: Results and ways to manage

Discuss the section "The results of dementia" in the learning guide and lecture on the following ways to deal with symptoms:

1. Memory loss:

    a. Teach a skill by repeating the procedure in exactly the same way over and over again

    b. Provide opportunities for the patient to perform skills he or she remembers from before he or she developed his or her impairment (folding clothes, raking, sweeping, sanding wood, stuffing envelopes, playing piano)

2. Language loss:

    a. It is up to the caregiver to understand and be understood by the patient

    b. Ask direct, clear questions and leave 20–90 seconds for the person to respond

3. Attention loss:

    a. Remember that people hear what we say even if they don't seem to be listening

    b. Minimize distractions

4. Judgment loss:

    a. Respect the individual's right to make his or her own decisions as you gently guide him or her through each step of a decision

5. Loss of senses or perceptions:

    a. Provide strong visual cues. For example, silverware on a white tablecloth might be difficult to see, so use a colored tablecloth.

6. Loss of muscle organization:

a. Start an activity for the person at the beginning, and determine whether muscle memory will take over

b. Male residents may be unable to get in a car on the passenger side because of habit. Let them sit on the rear left side if leaving the facility.

Section 3: Communication—use the guide

Review communication tips and ways to help.

Section 4: Case studies—use the guide

Ask the different learners to present one of the case studies to the group. Allow for discussion.

Conclusion

Have participants take the test. Review the answers together. Award certificates to those who answer 70% of the test questions correctly.

Test answers

1. f	2. a	3. e	4. j	5. h
6. d	7. g	8. i	9. b	10. c

Caring for People With Dementia

Learning Guide

Contents:

- Introduction

- Symptoms

  - Important things to remember about dementia

  - The results of dementia

  - Communication tips

  - Ways to help a resident perform a task Case Studies: What Would You Do?

    - Case study 1: Mr. Blair

    - Case study 2: Miss Mead

Introduction

Dementia is an organic mental disorder involving a general loss of intellectual abilities and changes in the personality. (Organic means the disorder is caused by physical changes in the brain.) Dementia is a general term for a decline in mental ability severe enough to interfere with daily life.

Symptoms

Symptoms can vary greatly, but at least two of the core mental functions below must be significantly impaired to be considered dementia:

- Memory

- Communication and language

- Ability to focus and pay attention

- Reasoning and judgment

- Visual perception

Many different things cause dementia. The most common, in order of occurrence, are:

1. Alzheimer's disease

2. Strokes and other blood-vessel diseases

3. Parkinson's and other nervous-system diseases

4. Miscellaneous causes, such as alcoholism, malnutrition, head injuries, drug reactions, thyroid disease, brain tumors, and infections

Important things to remember about dementia

- Adults with dementia deserve the respect and status they have earned. They often do not know their abilities have changed and do not understand why people treat them differently. They must be given as many opportunities as possible to make decisions and retain control over their lives.

- With the right environment and support, a person with dementia's ability to function can be strengthened and improved. If those supports are removed, the patient's function will decline.

- The deficiencies caused by dementia affect all areas of a person's life. Although the disability is invisible, it affects the patient's ability to do even the smallest activities.

- The way a person with dementia behaves is not just the result of impaired brain functions. Behavior is often caused by efforts to meet needs while compensating for lost abilities.

- We can help people with dementia by trying to understand what they feel and think.

While people affected by Alzheimer's disease and other related dementias are losing abilities, many abilities remain. It is important for the care team to create the days' experiences in a way that draws out the things the person can do well, which will help keep the person feeling engaged and dignified. These abilities may change over the course of the person's disease, but they do include the ability to show love, enjoy humor, and feel helpful to others. The person will benefit from meaningful engagement and can feel the positive emotions that result from caregivers connecting his or her life story to the experiences in the skilled nursing facility.

The results of dementia

- Memory loss:

    - Affects recent memories the most

    - Makes it difficult to learn anything new or to follow instructions

- Language loss (the meaning of words):

    - Makes it difficult to recognize words and understand complex sentences

    - Makes if difficult to express ideas

- Attention loss:

    - Unable to start or stop a task

    - Easily distracted

- Judgment loss:

    - Cannot accurately assess circumstances

    - Unable to see consequences of actions

- Loss of perception or senses:

    - Unable to recognize things or people

    - Misinterpret what they see, hear, or feel

- Loss of muscle organization:

    - Unable to perform multiple-step tasks

    - Require prompts or cues for routine tasks

Communication tips

- Be open, friendly, and gentle at all times.

- Always address the person by name to get his or her attention at the beginning of an interaction.

- Give your full attention to the conversation or task. This helps the resident stay focused.

- Briefly introduce yourself and offer some cues when you approach, stating your name and relationship and the purpose of your visit.

- Speak slowly, and give 20–90 seconds for the person with dementia to respond.

- Use gentle touching or hand holding, but get permission first.

- Avoid arguing and attempts to reason with a person who is upset. Acknowledge the person's feelings and calmly distract him or her with something soothing, pleasant, and friendly.

Ways to help a patient perform a task

1. Explain each step in simple language, one thing at a time

2. Demonstrate each step, doing the task while he or she watches

3. Move the person through the steps of the task, placing arms and legs in the right positions

4. If the person is distracted, begin again at the beginning

5. Remember to be patient and unhurried

Case Studies: What Would You Do?

Case study 1: Mr. Blair

Mr. Blair is not normally incontinent. Recently, however, he has begun walking outside to relieve himself. Occasionally he wets himself. He has started to wander, and he often seems anxious and agitated.

What caregivers may assume: Mr. Blair has lost the ability to control his bladder and should be placed in adult incontinent briefs.

What is really happening: Mr. Blair cannot find the toilet. In his bathroom, the white toilet blends in with the cream-colored tiles and walls, and his visual loss is causing him to be unable to see them. He spends much of the day looking for a place to urinate, but when he can't find one he relieves himself outside, where there are more bright colors that are easy to see.

Try this: Place a brightly colored toilet seat or toilet cover on Mr. Blair's commode to help him locate it. When you see Mr. Blair wandering anxiously in the halls or acting agitated, ask whether you can help him find the bathroom and then guide him to it.

Case study 2: Miss Mead

Miss Mead was a nurse for 40 years. She refuses to eat in the dining room but insists on having a tray brought to her room. She doesn't eat the food you bring but places the dishes on her windowsills and cabinets "for the others." She is losing weight rapidly but refuses to eat.

What caregivers may assume: Miss Mead will have to be placed in a hospital and fed with a stomach tube because of her refusal to eat.

What is really happening: Miss Mead is concerned for the "others" that she sees in her room. She believes that her reflections in the mirrors and windows are actually people that need her to care for them. She will not eat until she feeds them first.

Try this: Ask questions to determine what Miss Mead is trying to do. Once you understand the situation, remove the mirrors from Miss Mead's room. Cover the windows with blinds or shades. You could provide two trays of food, one for Miss Mead and one for "the others."

Caring for People With Dementia

Test

Name _____ Date _____ Score _____

Matching test. Find the answer that best matches each situation.

1. In the case study about Mr. Blair, the caregivers helped him by providing what? _____

2. We can help people with dementia by doing what? _____

3. Many times, a person with dementia behaves in a difficult fashion because he or she is trying to do what? _____.

4. When a person with dementia can't remember how to get into a car or starts to brush his or her hair with a toothbrush, which of the six results of dementia is causing the problem? _____

5. You should do this when starting a conversation with a patient with dementia. _____

6. When a person can't think of a word, or the words come out wrong or in the wrong order, the person is experiencing which of the six results of dementia? _____

7. This is one way to help a person with dementia perform a task. _____

8. It is important that persons with dementia be allowed to do this as much as possible. _____

9. It is best to use these kinds of questions when dealing with people with dementia. _____

10. Dementia is a condition that is characterized by what? _____.

a. Putting ourselves in their shoes, and trying to understand what they feel and think

b. Direct, closed questions such as "Would you like to wear this red dress today?" instead of open-ended questions like "What would you like to wear today?"

c. Loss of intellectual abilities and personality changes

d. Language loss

e. Cope with or compensate for lost abilities

f. Strong visual cues (contrasting colors on things the patient uses)

g. Tell the person how to do each step in simple language, one thing at a time

h. Address the person by name, and briefly introduce yourself and state the purpose of your visit

i. Make decisions and retain control over their lives

j. Loss of muscle organization

CERTIFICATE OF COMPLETION

I hereby certify that

_____

has successfully completed the in-Service

Caring for People With Dementia

_____
Signature

10

Depression and Anxiety

Teaching Plan

To use this lesson for self-study, the learner should read the material, do the activity, and take the test. For group study, the leader may give each learner a copy of the learning guide and follow this teaching plan to conduct the lesson. Certificates may be copied for everyone who completes the lesson.

Lesson overview

- This lesson plan is about how to understand and provide care for people who suffer from depression or anxiety.

- You may use this in a group setting or for individual study. Every learner must read the material and pass the test before receiving the certificate. You may also use the test as both a pretest and posttest.

- Copy the learning guide, test, and certificate for each learner.

- Have a board or flipchart available.

- Prepare two workers in advance.

Learning objectives

After this lesson, participants should be able to:

- Define depression and anxiety and their causes

- Know the signs and symptoms of depression and anxiety

- Know some ways to prevent depression and anxiety

- Know how to care for people with depression or anxiety

- Know the warning signs of suicide and how to prevent it

Before the session

Ask two workers to prepare a brief presentation for the group meeting, using the "Definitions and Causes of Depression and Anxiety" section of the learning guide. Have one worker explain the definitions, causes, and symptoms of depression and another do the same for anxiety.

Introductory activity

Ask your learners if they know any depressed people. If they do, ask them to tell you some of the symptoms of depression. List these symptoms on a board or flipchart under the heading "Depression." Do the same thing for anxiety. Determine whether your learners can think of residents that may suffer from one of these conditions. Ask them what kinds of problems they have had taking care of people who are depressed or anxious.

Lesson activities

1. Ask the two workers who prepared in advance to share their information with the group. Allow for questions and discussion after each worker has finished.

2. Emphasize that depression and anxiety are treatable illnesses, not normal conditions. Give a brief lecture on prevention.

3. Discuss the ways to care for people with anxiety and depression, using the material under the section "What Should Be Done?" This is a good time for participants to share stories and examples from experience.

4. Review the information on suicide. Emphasize that workers are responsible for observing and reporting.

Conclusion

Have participants take the test. Review the answers together. Award certificates to those who answer at least 70% of the test questions correctly.

Test answers

1. d	2. Both	3. d	4. a	5. a	6. d	7. Both
8. a	9. depression	10. medication	11. anxiety	12. goodbye	13. guilty	14. weight

Depression

Learning Guide

Contents:

- Definitions and Causes of Depression and Anxiety
  - Depression
  - Anxiety
- Signs and Symptoms of Depression and Anxiety
  - Signs of depression
  - Signs of anxiety
- What Should Be Done?
  - Preventing depression and anxiety
  - Caring for people with depression or anxiety
- The Warning Signs of Suicide
  - Suicide prevention

Definitions and Causes of Depression and Anxiety

This lesson covers two separate problems that are very common among adults: depression and anxiety.

Depression

What it is: Depression is a mental disorder marked by a sad or irritable mood lasting more than two weeks.

What it is not: Everyone gets sad or irritable from time to time, but for most people these moods only last for a few hours or a few days. When these feelings last for several weeks without improving, a person's way of thinking can be altered and the person may become clinically depressed.

Who gets it: About 10% of U.S. adults suffer from depression, but this number can increase with age, disability, or illness. Some estimates of major depression in older people living in the community range from less than 1% to about 5% but rise to 13.5% in those who require healthcare.

What causes it: Depression has many different causes. The following are some:

- Medication side effects, particularly from drugs used to treat arthritis, heart problems, high blood pressure, or cancer

- Illnesses such as Alzheimer's disease, Parkinson's disease, stroke, hormonal disorders, and others

- Genetics—it may run in families

- A traumatic event, such as a death in the family

- Pain

- Changes or differences in brain chemistry

Anxiety

What it is: Anxiety is a feeling of concern or worry and includes increased alertness or awareness. It can be mild, moderate, or severe; when very severe, it can become a state of panic.

What it is not: Mild to moderate anxiety is a normal part of living and can even be helpful when we must focus on something urgent or important. As it is a normal reaction to a stressful situation, it helps us take action. When anxiety becomes a long-term condition, or becomes severe, the person becomes overly focused on specific details and can't think of anything else. In this case, most of the individual's behavior is directed toward relieving the anxiety.

Who gets it: Anxiety disorders are the most common mental illness in the U.S., affecting 19% of the adult population. It is a very common disorder in the elderly and is more common in women than men.

What causes it: Some of the many causes of anxiety are:

- Persistent stress

- Worrying about the future or fretting about the past

- Extreme change

- Illness, particularly cancer, heart disease, and chronic illnesses

- Chemical changes in the brain

- Abnormal brain functioning

- Medication side effects

- Pain

Signs andSymptoms of Depression and Anxiety

Signs of depression

If a person has four or more of the following symptoms lasting two weeks or more, he or she may be depressed:

- Sad, depressed, or apathetic mood. May cry a lot, or complain of feeling empty.

- Irritability, agitation, or grumpiness.

- Disturbed sleep—either difficulty sleeping or sleeping more than usual.

- Fatigue and loss of energy.

- Changes in appetite and weight—either increased or decreased.

- Loss of interest or pleasure in normal activities, such as self-care or social activities. Withdrawal from others.

- Feelings of worthlessness, guilt, helplessness, hopelessness, or self-reproach.

- Thoughts of death or suicide, or attempted suicide.

- Difficulty thinking, concentrating, focusing, or remembering.

- Slowed or agitated movements or speech.

- Complaining of aches and pains, dizziness, blurred vision, racing heart, anxiety, or vague discomforts.

- Constant complaining.

- Mood swings.

- Excessive alcohol use.

Signs of anxiety

There are five main types of severe anxiety, and each has different symptoms. The types are:

- **Generalized anxiety disorder:** This condition involves excessive and unreasonable anxiety and worry lasting at least six months. Signs include restlessness, fatigue, difficulty concentrating, irritability, muscle tension, shaking, crying, pacing, sweating, rapid breathing, rapid heartbeat, fearfulness, and sleep problems.

- **Panic disorder:** People with this condition have recurring attacks of panic. They may have dizziness, faint feelings, sweating, trembling, chills, flushes, nausea, numbness, heart palpitations, or chest pain. These attacks occur suddenly and last several minutes.

- **Obsessive-compulsive disorder:** This disorder causes recurrent and persistent thoughts, impulses, or images that are unwanted and inappropriate. The person performs repetitive behaviors in response to these thoughts.

- **Phobias:** These are irrational, intense fears of certain things or situations, which interfere with normal functioning.

- **Posttraumatic stress disorder:** This occurs after a person experiences or witnesses a traumatic event. Symptoms include recurring memories, nightmares, and flashbacks.

What Should Be Done?

Even though depression and anxiety are common, they are NOT normal, even among the disabled, ill, or elderly. Signs of these illnesses should always be reported to a physician.

Other diseases can cause some of these symptoms, so the doctor will have to decide on a diagnosis and a treatment. We must never assume that these signs are a normal part of disability, illness, or aging.

Preventing depression and anxiety

Although many types of depression and anxiety cannot be prevented, there are some general things that everyone can do to lower the risk of developing these conditions. They are as follows:

1. Keep and maintain friendships and social activities.

2. Develop enjoyable interests or hobbies.

3. Stay physically active. Exercise and stay physically fit.

4. Stay mentally active. Read, take classes, and learn new things.

5. Maintain contact with family members.

6. Eat a balanced and nutritious diet. Avoid sugar, caffeine, and alcohol.

7. If you take medicines that might have depression or anxiety as side effects, follow the doctor's directions on using the medicines to lower the risk of those side effects.

Caring for people with depression or anxiety

Depression: The goal of care is to lift the person's mood.

- Encourage depressed people to express their feelings. Listen to what they say. Accept them as they are without making judgments. Give them time to get their thoughts together and to tell you what they are thinking and feeling. Help them feel valued.

- Brighten the environment by hanging pictures, posters, or family pictures. Make family photo albums easily available. Keep the environment neat and clean.

- Encourage engagement in pleasant activities such as listening to music or having a hobby.

- Encourage socialization. Start with one-to-one conversations, and gradually help with participating in larger social events.

- Encourage daily exercise or activity. Even the disabled can usually move a few body parts.

- Encourage as much self-care as possible. Help the people you're caring for gain a sense of control by letting them make as many independent decisions as possible.

- Pay attention if someone talks of self-injury or suicide. Always report this to a supervisor.

- Be sure the person takes his or her medications in the correct way and at the correct time.

Anxiety: The goal of care is to lower the person's anxiety level.

- Listen to a person's fears and anxieties. Respond with reassurance and support.

- The environment should be quiet and less stimulating than normal.

- Many people will never become completely free from anxiety. Help them learn to accept and tolerate a certain level of worry and anxiety. If they believe that you will assist them with their problems and keep them safe, their anxiety may be relieved.

- Sometimes an anxious person can be distracted if you help them think about something pleasant or relaxing or have them picture a peaceful image. Help the person relax each muscle, guiding them to consciously and progressively relax every muscle from toes to head. Instruct them to breathe slowly and deeply.

- Help anxious people recognize that although their feelings are real, their fears are not based on reality. Gently point this out: "You're feeling anxious, but you are really okay."

- Ensure that medications are taken as prescribed.

The Warning Signs of Suicide

Sometimes anxiety and depression occur together, or one may lead to the other. People suffering from either one of these illnesses may decide that they want to end their life. It is important to be alert to things that might indicate a person is seriously considering suicide. The suicide rate is twice as high in people older than age 65 as it is in younger age groups. Untreated or mistreated depression can lead to suicide. Pay attention to the following warning signs and report them to a supervisor:

- Talking about suicide. Statements such as "I have no reason to go on living" are danger signs.

- Being preoccupied with death.

- Giving things away.

- Stockpiling pills or obtaining some sort of weapon.

- Refusing to follow doctor's orders about medications or diet.

- Making unusual visits or calls to family and friends, saying goodbye to loved ones.

- Getting affairs in order or making funeral arrangements.

- Losing interest in things or people that used to be important.

- Suddenly becoming happier and calmer after a period of depression or anxiety.

- Talking about how worthless or helpless they are, saying they have no hopes or plans.

Suicide prevention

The following are some things you can do to help prevent someone from taking his or her own life:

1. Recognize anxiety and depression in others and help them get appropriate treatment.

2. Remove any weapons and be sure the environment is safe and secure.

3. If you suspect someone is thinking about suicide, ask the person if he or she is thinking about suicide. Don't be afraid that you will be giving the person ideas. If the person tells you that he or she is having these thoughts, report it.

4. Be sure a depressed or anxious person is seeing the doctor as ordered and getting his or her medications.

5. Reassure a suicidal person of how much you care. Explain that depression is no one's fault, that it can be treated, and that suicidal thoughts are temporary and will go away.

6. Don't try to minimize the individual's problems. Don't tell the person how hurt his or her family will be or that he or she has everything to live for, because this just makes the person feel guilty and even more hopeless.

7. If you suspect someone is thinking about suicide, always report your suspicions to the appropriate person. Don't think that you are imagining things or getting worried for nothing. It is much better to be cautious in this situation than to ignore important warning signs.

If you are a direct caregiver in an agency, and one of your residents shows warning signs of suicide, contact your supervisor immediately—time could be very important. If you are the family member or friend of someone you think is suicidal, help the person get to a physician at once.

People commit suicide because they think it is the only way to stop the pain they are feeling. Our job is to help them find other ways to get rid of their pain, through appropriate care and treatment.

Depression and Anxiety

Test

Name _____ Date _____ Score _____

The following is a list of things that can be done to help people with depression or anxiety. Beside the things that are helpful for depression, write a "D." Beside the things that are helpful for anxiety, write an "A." If the item is helpful to both disorders, write "Both."

_____ 1. Keep the environment bright and clean.

_____ 2. Listen.

_____ 3. Encourage daily exercise.

_____ 4. Help the person breathe deeply and relax the muscles.

_____ 5. Reassure the person that you will help and keep him or her safe.

_____ 6. Encourage the individual to be with people and participate in social events.

_____ 7. Make sure medications are given as ordered.

_____ 8. Keep the environment quiet and nonstimulating.

Fill in the blanks in the statements below:

1. A person who feels unneeded or unwanted may be suffering from _____.

2. Illness, chemical changes in the brain, and _____ side effects can all cause depression or anxiety.

3. Someone who is constantly fearful or restless may be suffering from _____.

4. Saying _____ to loved ones could be a sign that a person is thinking about suicide.

5. Telling a suicidal person that he or she will hurt loved ones if he or she commits suicide only makes the person feel more hopeless and _____, thereby increasing his or her pain.

6. Losing or gaining _____ could be a sign of depression.

CERTIFICATE OF COMPLETION

I hereby certify that

_____

has successfully completed the in-Service

Depression and Anxiety

_____

Signature

11
▪ Diabetes

Teaching Plan

To use this lesson for self-study, the learner should read the materials, do the activity, and take the test. For group study, the leader should give every learner a copy of the learning guide and use the suggested group activities to teach the lesson. Certificates may be copied for everyone who completes the lesson.

Learning objectives

After this lesson, participants should be able to:

- Explain what diabetes is and does

- Describe the four key elements of treatment for diabetes

- List the symptoms of low blood sugar and high blood sugar

- Know how to respond to a diabetic emergency

Teaching Tip

When lecturing, move around the room a little to provide visual interest. Insert humor or interesting stories to keep the material engaging. Focus attention by writing main points on a board.

Lesson activities

Give the learners a copy of the case study activity. Ask them to read the case studies and think about their responses. Explain that they will learn answers to these problems today.

What diabetes is and does

Go over the material in the learner guide about what diabetes is, the two types of diabetes, and the long-term effects of diabetes. You can do this as a lecture. Point out that the pancreas is located behind the stomach, in front of the lower part of the backbone.

The four key elements of treatment

Review and discuss the material together, asking learners to read portions of the lesson aloud to the others. Emphasize the points that are of particular concern for your agency.

Diabetic emergencies

Ask the workers to study the symptoms of low blood sugar and high blood sugar for a minute. Quiz them by calling out a symptom and asking whether it means high blood sugar or low blood sugar. For fun, throw a small piece of candy to the first person to call out the correct answer. Observe that some similar symptoms occur in both conditions, but low blood sugar happens suddenly. High blood sugar symptoms usually appear gradually and become worse.

Ask the learners to tell you how to respond to each type of diabetic emergency. Be sure they know that low blood sugar can cause heart attacks and strokes if not treated promptly.

Conclusion

Have participants take the test. Review the answers together. Award certificates to those who answer 70% of the test questions correctly.

Test answers

1. 80–130; 100–150	2. a. Diet b. Exercise c. Medication d. Monitoring	3. b
4. False	5. c	6. True
7. 70	8. 180	9. False
10. True		

Diabetes

Learning Guide

Contents:

Introduction

Diabetes is a disease that changes the way our bodies use food. It causes the level of sugar in the blood to be too high. The extra sugar harms the blood vessels and other organs in the body over time. Diabetes can cause great damage before any symptoms appear.

When we eat, our bodies digest the food and turn it into sugar, or glucose. In a normal healthy person, an organ called the pancreas produces the hormone insulin. Insulin helps the body's cells use glucose to produce energy. The cells use this energy to keep our bodies healthy.

In someone with diabetes, either the pancreas is not producing enough insulin or the body does not use its insulin effectively. The cells cannot turn sugar into energy, and the sugar builds up in the blood. The cells are starved for energy, and the blood carries dangerously high levels of sugar that can't be used.

Main Types of Diabetes

Type I means that the pancreas is not producing insulin or is producing very little. This type requires shots of insulin injected into the body every day.

Type II means that the pancreas is producing insulin, but not enough, or that the body does not use its insulin effectively.

Nine out of 10 cases of diabetes are type II. It usually occurs in people over age 45 who are overweight. It can be treated by diet, exercise, and/or medications that are taken by mouth. Sometimes it also requires insulin injections.

Importance of Controlling Diabetes

The goal of treatment for diabetes is to keep the individual's blood sugar as close to normal as possible. Doing this will lower the person's chances of:

- Stroke

- Heart disease

- Kidney failure

- Stomach disease

- High blood pressure

- Eye disease, loss of vision, or blindness

- Nerve damage, with pain or loss of feeling in hands, feet, legs, or other parts of the body

- A high level of sugar in the blood over a long period of time can cause these problems

Diabetic Treatment

There are four parts to diabetic treatment:

1. Diet

2. Exercise

3. Medicine

4. Monitoring

Anyone who helps a person with diabetes should be familiar with the medicine, exercise regimen, monitoring program, and diet that the individual is supposed to follow.

Diet

There is no one diet designed for every person with diabetes. There are guidelines to help people with diabetes with food choices. These guidelines are very similar to the kind of eating that is healthy for anyone. The following are the main rules that should be followed:

1. Eat few sugary foods, and watch carbohydrate intake carefully

2. Eat less fat, especially saturated fat and cholesterol (butter, margarine, oils)

3. Eat a variety of fresh fruits, vegetables, lean meats, and fish

4. Eat just enough calories to stay at a healthy weight

The exact number of servings a person with diabetes should have from each food group depends on individual calorie and nutrition needs, weight goals, exercise level, and preferences.

Many people think that people with diabetes are not allowed to eat sugar of any kind. This is no longer required. Sugar is a carbohydrate, like bread or potatoes, and can be part of the food plan for people with diabetes. However, most sugary foods provide calories without many vitamins or minerals, and they are often high in fat. It is better to eat more foods rich in nutrients, like vegetables and fruits, and very few fatty, sweet foods like ice cream and candy.

Dietitians sometimes teach people with diabetes and those who care for them to use exchange lists. These lists are a way to plan meals by putting foods in a category, such as a starch exchange or fruit exchange. Foods on a list can be substituted for each other and sometimes for foods on other exchange lists. The person with diabetes eats only a certain number of each type of exchange every day, as ordered by a doctor or established by the dietitian.

Exercise

Exercise usually lowers blood sugar and may help insulin work better. It helps control weight, it improves blood flow, and it strengthens the heart. People with diabetes should exercise at least three times per week. Before a person starts a new exercise program, a doctor should approve the kind of exercise as well as the frequency and duration. Elderly and disabled people need to exercise also and should be helped to find an exercise they can do.

It is important that a person with diabetes not develop low blood sugar while exercising. Since the body burns sugar during exercise, the person should fuel up with a piece of fruit or half a sandwich within an hour before starting any exercise. It is also a good idea for the person to check his or her blood sugar level before starting exercise. If the blood sugar reading is less than 70, he or she should eat something and wait for the blood sugar level to come up over 70 before exercising.

If a person with diabetes feels faint, sweaty, dizzy, or confused while doing any activity, he or she should stop and immediately drink fruit juice or a sweet (not diet) soft drink. The person must respond quickly to this feeling, because it means his blood sugar level is too low.

Medication

People with diabetes might receive insulin shots or they may take pills by mouth. Only a doctor can decide what medication and how much of it the person should receive. It can be VERY dangerous to change the medication of a person with diabetes in any way unless it is ordered by a doctor. People with diabetes must receive the exact amount of medicine their doctor has ordered, at the times the doctor has ordered. Timing of medicine and meals is important to prevent low blood sugar.

Monitoring

Close monitoring of the person's blood sugar level is one of the best ways for him or her to prevent long-term complications from the disease. People with diabetes check their blood sugar by pricking a finger with a needle and testing a drop of blood with a special blood-glucose meter. The meter, also called a monitor, gives a number that tells the level of glucose in the blood. These monitors must be kept clean and should be checked for accuracy periodically.

Most people with diabetes need their blood-sugar level tested at least once per day, usually in the morning before breakfast. Depending on the type of diabetes, the age of the person, and other factors, the individual may need his or her blood glucose tested as much as five times per day. Sometimes insulin dosages are adjusted depending on the blood-sugar level. This chart from the National Diabetes Education Program shows the recommended blood-sugar levels at different times of the day:

Before meals	80–130
At bedtime	100–150

A doctor must set the acceptable ranges *for each person,* and *they might differ from the normal ranges* given in the chart. When a blood-glucose level falls outside the range set by the doctor, the doctor must be notified as soon as possible. If you are assisting a person with diabetes with monitoring his or her blood sugar, be sure you know the correct range for the person.

Another important part of monitoring is watching the person's feet and skin. Diabetes can turn a small sore or wound into a very large problem. Sores, blisters, and wounds on a resident's feet and skin must always be reported to your supervisor or a nurse.

Diabetic Emergencies and How to Respond

Diabetes can cause both long-term and short-term problems. Blood sugar that is too low or extremely high can lead rapidly to unconsciousness and even death. You must know the symptoms of both conditions and know how to respond.

Hypoglycemia means that the level of sugar in the blood is too low (less than 70). Too much insulin or oral medication, too much exercise, not eating enough food, or drinking alcohol can cause it. Hypoglycemia can cause strokes and heart attacks in the elderly. This problem is also called **insulin reaction** or **insulin shock**.

Low blood sugar

Symptoms

The following symptoms occur suddenly and without warning:

- Shaky, nervous

- Sweaty and cold

- Pale, clammy skin

- Weak and tired, drowsy

- Sudden hunger

- Blurred or double vision

- Tingling of hands, lips, or tongue

- Confusion

- Personality change

- Slurred speech

- Loss of consciousness

- Dizziness or a staggering walk

- Nausea

- Headache

- Fast heartbeat

- Itching

Note: Elderly people and people with other diseases and disabilities can be especially sensitive to low blood sugar, and it can be very dangerous for them. Some people may have a reaction even when their blood sugar is not below 70. Any person with diabetes suddenly showing any of the signs listed must receive *immediate* attention.

Treatment

- Follow the care plan for interventions ordered by the resident's doctor.

- Such interventions may include medication or assisting the person to drink a sweet drink, such as sugar-sweetened coffee or tea, orange juice, or nondiet soda. Or, the diabetic could eat sugar, corn syrup, or candy or take glucose tablets.

High blood sugar

Hyperglycemia means that the level of sugar in the blood is too high (above 180). It can be caused by infections, illness, stress, injury, not enough insulin, not enough exercise, or eating too much food. Very high levels of sugar can cause coma and death.

Symptoms

The following symptoms occur gradually and get worse over time:

- Extreme thirst and/or hunger

- Rapid weight loss

- Frequent urination

- Vision changes

- Dry skin and mouth

- Fatigue, drowsiness

- Nausea

- Fruity-smelling breath

- Very deep, gasping breathing

- Unconsciousness

Treatment

The first seven symptoms in this list should be reported to your supervisor or a nurse as soon as possible. Fruity-smelling breath, deep, gasping breathing, and unconsciousness are emergency symptoms that can lead quickly to death. Call 9-1-1 or access emergency medical care at once.

Case Study Activity

The following case studies are examples of things that sometimes happen to those receiving care in their homes. Read each case study and discuss possible ways of handling the situation. If you are doing this lesson by yourself, think about what you should do and how you would respond to these situations. You can write your ideas below.

Case study 1: Mrs. Jarvis

Mrs. Jarvis is diabetic. One day, as you are assisting her with her shower, you notice that she seems confused. She doesn't seem to understand what you say to her, and she acts nervous. Her skin feels cool and damp and looks paler than usual.

What do you think might be happening to Mrs. Jarvis? What, if anything, should you do?

Case study 2: Mr. Young

One morning, Mr. Young's blood sugar reading is 250. He seems fine and says he feels great. Mr. Young's doctor said his blood sugar should not go above 220.

What should you do in this situation?

Case study 3: Mrs. Bond

Mrs. Bond checks her blood sugar and gives herself insulin every morning. You are supposed to remind her to do this. When you remind her, she always tells you that she has done it or is about to do it. Lately you've noticed that Mrs. Bond seems to be losing weight. You watch to be sure she is eating, and you see that she is eating a large amount of food. She has started urinating on herself sometimes, and when you help her get cleaned up, she says that she is urinating a lot and sometimes she just can't make it to the bathroom. When you suggest that she should cut back on the water she is drinking, she tells you that she is thirsty all the time.

What is going on with Mrs. Bond? What action, if any, should you take?

Case Study Activity Answers

The following are the suggested answers for the case study activity. You might need to add additional information because of specific protocols and procedures at your agency.

Case study 1 answer: Mrs. Jarvis

Mrs. Jarvis is probably suffering from low blood sugar. She should be given a drink of fruit juice or other sweetened drink (tea or coffee with sugar, nondiet soda) or assisted to take some sugar cubes or glucose tablets. If possible, her blood sugar should be checked.

If Mrs. Jarvis does not get better, if she gets worse, or if her blood sugar is outside her approved range and does not improve when rechecked, medical assistance should be summoned.

Case study 2 answer: Mr. Young

Mr. Young's blood sugar is too high and must be reported to his physician. Even though he has no symptoms, this condition could worsen without treatment. In addition, a blood sugar this high is causing hidden long-term problems in his body. Follow your agency's protocol for notifying your supervisor, a nurse, or the doctor.

Case study 3 answer: Mrs. Bond

Mrs. Bond might have an inaccurate glucose monitor machine, she might not be taking her insulin correctly, or she might be forgetting to take it in spite of your reminders. Her symptoms indicate that her blood sugar is too high. Her blood sugar should be checked. Even if her blood sugar is normal, these symptoms must be reported to her doctor.

Diabetes

Test

Name _____ Date _____ Score _____

Directions: Fill in or circle the best answer. (12 points required).

1. Fill in the chart of normal recommended blood-sugar levels with the missing numbers: (two points)

Before meals	
At bedtime	

2. Write the four parts of diabetic treatment: (four points)

   a. _____ b. _____ c. _____ d. _____

3. If a person with diabetes becomes weak, tired, and dizzy, you should first _____.

   a. alert the nurse

   b. have the person lie down until it wears off

   c. give the person something sweet to drink

4. People with diabetes should never eat candy, ice cream, or cake. True   or   False

5. You should alert the nurse if a person with diabetes has the following symptoms:

   a. Confusion and personality change

   b. Weakness and dizziness

   c. Fruity-smelling breath or deep, gasping breathing

   d. Itchy skin

6. Having high levels of sugar in the blood over a long period of time can cause heart disease, blindness, and loss of feeling in the feet. True   or   False

7. For most people, blood sugar is too <u>low</u> if it reads less than _____ on a glucose meter.

8. For most people, blood sugar is too <u>high</u> if it reads more than _____ on a glucose meter.

9. All people with diabetes must take insulin shots. True or False

10. All people with diabetes should monitor their blood sugar, control their diet, exercise, and take their medicines. True or False

CERTIFICATE OF COMPLETION

I hereby certify that

_____

has successfully completed the in-Service

_____

Diabetes

_____
Signature

Dysphagia

Teaching Plan

To use this lesson for self-study, the learner should read the material, do the activity, and take the test. For group study, the leader may give each learner a copy of the learning guide and follow this teaching plan to conduct the lesson. Certificates may be copied for everyone who completes the lesson.

Learning objectives

After this lesson, participants should be able to:

- Define dysphagia

- Recognize causes and symptoms of dysphagia

- Understand effective management of dysphagia

Lesson activities

Have everyone as a group match situations and solutions using Figure 12.1. Discuss any questions or concerns that come up during the activity, using the learning guide as a reference.

The lesson

Review the material in the lesson with participants. Allow for discussion.

Conclusion

Have participants take the test. Review the answers together. Award certificates to those who answer 70% of the test questions correctly.

Test answers

1. True	2. d	3. b	4. True	5. True
6. d	7. True	8. d	9. False	10. True

Dysphagia

Learning Guide

Contents:

- Introduction

- What Causes Dysphagia?

- How Is Dysphagia Diagnosed?
  - Symptoms of dysphagia

- Treatment of Dysphagia
  - Speech pathology exercises
  - Care partners' roles in effective dysphagia management

Introduction

People with dysphagia have difficulty swallowing and may experience pain while swallowing (odynophagia). It is most frequently found in older adults and is common in residents who have experienced strokes. Due to the high prevalence of dysphagia, frontline staff must be able to recognize its symptoms and work with residents for treatment.

What Causes Dysphagia?

Dysphagia occurs when there is a problem with the neural control or structures involved in any part of the swallowing process. The muscles and nerves that help move food through the throat and esophagus don't work right. Any condition that weakens or damages the muscles and nerves used for swallowing may cause dysphagia. For example, people with diseases of the nervous system, such as cerebral palsy or Parkinson's disease, often have problems swallowing. Weak tongue or cheek muscles may make it hard to move food around in the mouth for chewing. Additionally, stroke, head injury, or other nervous-system disorders, such as muscular dystrophy, may weaken or affect the coordination of the swallowing muscles or limit sensation in the mouth and throat. Another difficulty is when weak throat muscles cannot move all of the food toward the stomach—a problem that sometimes occurs after cancer surgery.

Some of the signs of dysphagia include taking a long time to begin a swallow; food leaking from the nose or mouth; coughing or choking on food, fluids, or saliva; or a feeling of fullness, tightness, or pain in the throat or chest when swallowing.

How Is Dysphagia Diagnosed?

A thorough assessment and testing may be done by:

- An otolaryngologist (a physician who treats the ear, nose, and throat)

- A speech-language pathologist (a specialist who evaluates and treats swallowing problems)

- A neurologist (a physician who treats problems of the brain, nervous system, and spinal chord)

Symptoms of dysphagia

Food or liquids may be aspirated when swallowing or when food is coming up, such as during vomiting or reflux (heartburn). When a resident aspirates, the lungs recognize the substance as foreign material. This should cause the resident to reflexively cough or gag. If he or she successfully coughs the substance out, no airway damage occurs. If the food or liquid remains in the lungs, however, the stage is set for a chemical reaction that may lead to pneumonia or even death.

Frontline staff can help residents by recognizing the many signs and symptoms of dysphagia. These symptoms include:

- Difficulty controlling liquids and secretions in the mouth, drooling, or food falling out of the mouth

- A wet or gurgly-sounding voice

- A weak voice in combination with other signs or symptoms

- Taking a long time to begin a swallow

- Swallowing several times for a single bite of food

- Food leaking from the mouth or nose

- Frequent throat clearing

- Lack of a gag reflex

- Weak cough before, during, or after a swallow

- Coughing or choking on food, fluids, or saliva

- Pocketing food

- A feeling of fullness, tightness, or pain in the throat or chest when swallowing

- A sensation of food or saliva sticking in the esophagus or sternal area

- Feeling as if a foreign body or lump is sticking in the throat

- Drooping appearance of lower face in combination with other signs or symptoms

- Asymmetrical appearance of face in combination with other signs or symptoms

- Spitting food out or refusing to eat

- Recurrent upper respiratory infections or persistent low-grade fever

- Unintentional weight loss

- Signs and symptoms of malnutrition or abnormal or inadequate nutrition

If a resident experiences any of these signs or symptoms, you should notify the care team and physician. An isolated symptom such as coughing or refusing to eat is likely not a problem. Having a pattern of problems, or many signs and symptoms, suggests dysphagia. Consultation with a speech-language pathologist is needed.

Treatment of Dysphagia

There are different treatments for various types of dysphagia. Medical doctors and speech-language pathologists who evaluate and treat swallowing disorders use a variety of tests that allow them to look at the stages of the swallowing process. One test, the flexible endoscopic evaluation of swallowing with sensory testing (FEESST), uses a lighted fiber-optic tube, or endoscope, to view the mouth and throat while examining how the swallowing mechanism responds to stimuli, such as a puff of air, food, or liquid. A videofluoroscopic swallow study (VFSS) is a test in which a clinician takes a videotaped x-ray of the entire swallowing process by having a resident consume several foods or liquids along with the mineral barium to improve visibility of the digestive tract. The x-ray helps identify where in the swallowing process the resident is experiencing problems. Speech-language pathologists use this method to explore strategies that will allow a resident to swallow food safely.

There are several steps, under the direction of the speech therapist, that can be taken to assist residents with dysphagia. The resident's food may be changed, either through altering its texture or cutting the food into smaller pieces. The resident may adjust his or her head and neck posture or use maneuvers such as chin tucking (which helps ensure food and other substances do not enter the trachea when swallowing). A resident can also perform muscle exercises to strengthen weak facial muscles or improve coordination. If a resident is unable to swallow safely despite rehabilitation strategies, short-term medical or surgical intervention may be necessary as the resident recovers.

In progressive conditions such as amyotrophic lateral sclerosis (ALS, or Lou Gehrig's disease), a feeding tube in the stomach may be necessary for the long term.

Speech pathology exercises

Speech-language pathologists usually work with residents in treating dysphagia. The therapist will develop a plan that may include changing food texture to an easily swallowable consistency. The speech-language pathologist will recommend resident-specific techniques for improving swallowing and preventing aspiration. Common approaches are:

- Tucking the chin

- Turning the head

- Avoiding eating when fatigued

- Swallowing twice with each bolus of food

- Performing strengthening exercises for the muscles used with swallowing

Your restorative program may involve working with the resident on these exercises, because most residents with dysphagia require one-to-one supervision during meals. The resident's care plan may include the following:

- Making sure the resident is fully awake and alert before beginning a meal.

- Adopting a "So what?" attitude for spills and food messes.

- Positioning the resident upright, providing support if necessary.

- Positioning the head facing forward, with the neck flexed forward slightly, avoiding extending the neck. This technique changes the position of the airway, which is effective for some, but not all, types of dysphagia. In some residents, it may actually increase the risk of aspiration.

- Minimizing conversation.

- Limiting environmental distractions as much as possible. Focus the resident on eating.

- Cutting the food into small (dime-size) pieces.

- Directing the food to the unaffected side of the mouth if the resident has had a stroke.

- Encouraging the resident to eat slowly, taking small bites.

- Reminding the resident to chew thoroughly.

- Instructing the resident to cough or clear the throat after each bite of food.

- Checking to be sure the mouth is empty before adding more food.

- Using straws with caution; they may cause the resident to drink at an unsafe speed and volume.

- Following the therapist's instructions for tucking the chin during swallowing. For some resident, the head should be slightly down during swallowing. With others, it should be slightly back or turned to one side.

- Instructing the resident to avoid swallowing when the head is tipped back.

- Checking the mouth for food particles after meals, and assisting with oral hygiene.

- Monitoring the resident, because swallowing problems often worsen when the resident is tired.

The speech-language pathologist may order other special positions, exercises, and techniques, depending on the resident's needs. For example, the muscle activity involved in swallowing food is slightly different than that involved in swallowing liquid (the latter is more difficult), and the resident may have difficulty adjusting the swallowing muscles if trying to switch between the two. The speech-language pathologist may recommend consuming food and fluid separately. For items such as soup, taking in one consistency at a time may work best. If this does not work, serve food with mixed consistency (e.g., soup, cereal with milk) separately. The resident may need to avoid very dry foods entirely; they are difficult to swallow, and crumbs may end up in the airway. Moistening dry foods with gravy or cream-based soup may also help.

Care partners' roles in effective dysphagia management

The speech-language pathologist may order a particular consistency of food, or a dysphagia diet, to effectively treat a resident with dysphagia. One of the following four diet levels is usually ordered:

- **Level 1: Dysphagia pureed.** Foods in this level are pureed or of similar consistency, cohesive, and pudding-like.

- **Level 2: Dysphagia mechanically altered.** Foods in this level are cohesive, moist, and semisolid, requiring some chewing ability. They include ground or minced meats as well as fork-mashable fruits and vegetables. Some examples of excluded foods are most bread products, crackers, and other dry foods.

- **Level 3: Dysphagia advanced.** Foods in this level are soft-solid and require more chewing ability. They include easy-to-cut meats, fruits, and vegetables. Disallowed foods include hard, crunchy fruits and vegetables, as well as foods that are sticky or very dry.

- **Level 4: Regular.** Any solid textures.

Nursing and dietary personnel must work closely with the speech-language pathologist and dietitian to ensure altered food remains acceptable to the resident. Attractive food appearance, taste, and proper temperature are important. Some residents refuse pureed food, for example, because it resembles baby food. Generally speaking, pureed diets should not be watery or runny. Creative ideas for pureed-meal recipe planning can be found on the Internet. When properly prepared, regular pureed items should be about the consistency of pudding and support a plastic spoon in the upright position.

It is important for staff to understand that the goal of food preparation is to ensure that the food:

- Is the proper consistency to meet the resident's needs and reduce the risk of aspiration

- Looks appetizing and tastes delicious

- Is altered in consistency as little as possible; sometimes extra gravies or sauces are all that is needed

The speech-language pathologist will work with the resident and nursing staff to teach individualized approaches for eating and drinking. He or she may recommend using food thickeners to slow the movement of food and fluid through the esophagus. Thickeners can alter the consistency of food and liquid to resemble nectar, honey, or pudding. Applesauce, soft fruits, and instant potatoes may be used to thicken some foods, as can corn starch and gelatin (which will continue their thickening action as the food sits). However, commercial thickeners such as powders work best.

When thickening liquids with powder, keep in mind that the consistency of the liquid depends on the amount of powder added. Additionally, the viscosity (thickness) of a liquid changes as its temperature changes. As the item cools, less thickener is needed, so more thickener is needed for hot liquids than for cold liquids. There is a great margin of error in mixing powdered thickeners, so it is important for the staff member to follow the therapist's instructions exactly.

Dysphagia can be serious. Someone who cannot swallow safely may not be able to eat enough of the right foods to stay healthy or maintain an ideal weight. Dysphagia can also lead to additional major medical problems. You are an important partner in managing each individual's dysphagia symptoms and treatment plan.

Figure 12.1: Solve the Problem

Directions: Match the situation on the left with the best solution on the right.
Put the letter of the solution in the blank next to the problem.

1. Your resident has dysphagia and is embarrassed by spitting food out accidentally.	a. Remind your resident that extending his head back might make him choke or aspirate, and remind him to follow the therapist orders (which are usually to tuck the chin, turn the head slightly back or turn the head).
2. Your resident is supposed to have pureed food but doesn't find the "baby food" appealing.	b. Position your resident upright, providing support if necessary.
3. Your resident keeps choking on his favorite crackers.	c. It may be helpful to have the resident consume food or drink separately.
4. Your resident is having trouble eating his watery and runny pureed food.	d. Encourage quiet during eating.
5. Your resident is in bed eating but having difficulty staying upright and is choking on his food at every bite.	e. Try to thicken the food per a therapist's instructions. Food shouldn't be watery.
6. Your resident keeps choking when you give him his juice with a cup and straw.	f. While keeping in line with orders, try to allow the food to taste as close to normal as possible, and if permitted, add gravies or sauces.
7. Your resident has started to show signs of dysphagia and continues to see meals as socializing time.	g. Talk to your supervisor and alert him or his that your resident might be suffering from dysphagia.
8. Your resident has started to drool a bit while eating and is taking a long time to swallow and clears his throat often.	h. Adopt a "So what?" attitude toward spills and messes.
9. Your resident tries to help himself to swallow by extending his head way back when he eats.	i. Remove the straw to slow down drinking or monitor very closely and remind them to slow down.
10. Your resident is eating his lunch and juice but seems to have a problem switching between different consistencies.	j. Ask your resident if he'd like something else, or pour gravy (if orders allow) on his favorite snack to help it go down.

Solve the Problem Answer Key

1. h	2. f	3. j	4. e	5. b
6. i	7. d	8. g	9. a	10. d

Dysphagia

Test

Name _____ Date _____ Score _____

Directions: Circle the best answer.

1. Dysphagia occurs when there is a problem with the neural control or structures involved in any part of the swallowing process. True or False

2. When caring for a resident with dysphagia, a staff member should _____.

    a. position the resident lying down

    b. become offended during the meal

    c. try to engage in a full conversation

    d. make sure the resident is fully awake and alert before beginning a meal

3. All of the following are signs associated with dysphagia, *except* _____.

    a. coughing or choking on food

    b. a feeling of emptiness

    c. food leaking from the nose or mouth

    d. pain in the throat or chest when swallowing

4. One of the main concerns with dysphagia is the potential for aspiration.
   True or False

5. Speech-language pathologists typically work with residents in treating dysphagia.
   True or False

6. Dysphagia can be a result of _____.

    a. stroke

    b. cancer surgery

    c. Parkinson's disease

    d. all of the above

7. For a resident with dysphagia, liquids can often be the most difficult to swallow. True or False

8. The goal of food preparation for a resident with dysphagia is to _____.

   a. change the food consistency as much as possible

   b. make the food look and taste completely different

   c. use solids to help boost consistency

   d. make the food the proper consistency to meet the resident's needs

9. There are two levels of diet for dysphagia residents. True or False

10. Speech-language pathologists often use two different tests, FEESST or VFSS, to examine how the swallowing mechanism responds to various stimuli. True or False

CERTIFICATE OF COMPLETION

I hereby certify that

_____

has successfully completed the in-Service

Dysphagia

_____

Signature

13

Elder Abuse and Neglect: Preventing, Recognizing, and Reporting

Teaching Plan

To use this lesson for self-study, the learner should read the material, do the activity, and take the test. For group study, the leader may give each learner a copy of the learning guide and follow this teaching plan to conduct the lesson. Certificates may be copied for everyone who completes the lesson.

The topic of this lesson is required by many state regulatory agencies on an annual basis for staff that care for the elderly. It covers the prevention, recognition, and reporting of elder abuse and neglect.

Learning objectives

After this lesson, participants should be able to:

- Define different kinds of abuse and neglect

- Identify symptoms of caregiver stress that could lead to abuse or neglect

- List ways to prevent abuse and neglect

- Recognize signs of abuse and neglect

- Know how to report elder abuse and neglect

Lesson activities

Introduce the lesson to your learners by asking them to do the matching activity in the "Ways Elders Are Abused" section in the learning guide, either individually or as a group. The answers to the activity are:

1. d	2. c	3. b	4. e	5. a	6. f

Ask if anyone can add anything to the "Other Ways Elders Are Abused" section.

Who are the victims?

State that the typical abuse victim lives with and depends on a family member for daily care, but abuse is also a problem in institutional settings. Most victims are female, age 75 or over, with a mental or physical illness. Most are completely dependent on the abuser.

Who are the abusers?

State that most abusers are relatives who take care of the elderly person. The abusers may have problems such as alcohol or drug dependence, emotional or mental illness, or stress. Many times, the abusers need as much help as the victims.

Caregiver stress

Explain that caregiver stress can be a problem for anyone caring for the elderly, and that this can lead to abuse in an institutional setting. Instruct the learners to fill out the questionnaire "Are You an Overly Stressed Caregiver?" Ask for discussion. Point out that this questionnaire could be used for family caregivers as well.

Preventing abuse and neglect

Point out the ideas for preventing abuse at the bottom of the learning guide's first page. Explain the following:

1. Professional caregivers have valuable skills to care for the elderly. Work is less stressful when we know how to do it well. We can also teach these skills to family members.

2. We can help each other by listening while we vent frustrations and by working together to solve problems. We can help family members by listening to their frustrations.

3. We must observe the elderly person's rights at all times and teach them to others.

Recognizing abuse and neglect

Review the signs of abuse and neglect, and point out that some of these could happen even to an agency that cares for the elderly. Everyone should be alert to the signs.

Reporting abuse and neglect

Explain your agency's and your state's reporting procedures, giving the appropriate regulatory agency's name and number to the learners.

Give learners a copy of the statement of resident or elder rights for your state.

The lesson

Review the material in the lesson with participants. Allow for discussion.

Conclusion

Have participants take the test. Review the answers together. Award certificates to those who answer 70% of the test questions correctly.

Test answers

1. c	2. a, b, c	3. b	4. c	5. a, b
6. b, c	7. a, c	8. True	9. b	10. respect

Elder Abuse and Neglect: Preventing, Recognizing, and Reporting

Learning Guide

Contents:

- Introduction

- Ways Elders Are Abused

  - Other ways elders are abused

- Are You an Overly Stressed Caregiver?

- Signs of Elder Abuse and Neglect

- Reporting Abuse and Neglect

- Prevention

Introduction

> **Elder abuse:** Any mistreatment or neglect of an elderly person. Everyone has the right to be treated with respect.

There is no acceptable excuse for abuse and neglect of the elderly, but recognizing and preventing the problem of caregiver stress may help prevent some elder abuse.

Ways Elders Are Abused

Match the definition to the term:

1. _____ Psychological abuse

2. _____ Neglect

3. _____ Physical abuse

4. _____ Rights violations

5. _____ Financial abuse

6. _____ Sexual abuse

    a. Stealing or mismanaging the money, property, or belongings of a person. Also called exploitation.

    b. Using physical force to cause physical pain or injury.

    c. Failing to provide something necessary for health and safety, such as personal care, food, shelter, or medicine.

    d. Causing emotional or psychological pain. Includes isolation, verbal abuse, threats, and humiliation.

    e. Confining someone against his will, or strictly controlling the elder's behavior. Includes improper use of restraints and medications to control difficult behaviors.

    f. Forcing sexual contact without the person's consent, including touching or sexual talk.

Other ways elders are abused

- Overmedicating

- Denying aids such as walkers, eyeglasses, or dentures

- Dirty living conditions

- Inadequate heating and air conditioning

Are You an Overly Stressed Caregiver?

Answer these questions with "yes" or "no."

1. I am frequently unable to sleep because I have so much on my mind. _____

2. Most of the time I don't feel very good. _____

3. I have difficulty concentrating and often forget to do routine tasks. _____

4. I feel depressed or sad much of the time. _____

5. I feel worried and anxious almost all the time. _____

6. I lose my temper easily and become angry at other people. _____

7. I don't think there's anything wrong with me; I just wish everyone else would stop doing things that upset me. _____

8. Most days I feel irritable and moody, often snapping at others. _____

9. I feel tired almost all the time, and just drag myself through my days. _____

10. I'm too busy to do anything fun or to go out with my friends. _____

Any "yes" answers could be a sign of excessive stress. More than three "yes" answers should prompt you to talk to your supervisor or physician about the way you are feeling.

Signs of Elder Abuse and Neglect

As people age, they may become frail and experience hearing and vision loss. They may become unable to think as clearly as they once could. This leaves them open for people to take advantage of them.

Types of elder abuse include:

- Physical abuse

- Emotional abuse (including fear of retaliation)

- Sexual abuse

- Neglect and abandonment by a caregiver

- Financial exploitation

- Healthcare fraud and abuse

Be concerned if you see an elderly person showing the following new behaviors or signs:

- General abuse signs:

    - Becoming withdrawn, unusually quiet, depressed, or shy

    - Becoming anxious, worried, or easily upset

    - Refusing care from caregivers

    - Not wanting to be around people and not wanting to see visitors

- Physical abuse signs:

    - Bruises or burns

- In a woman, vaginal bleeding or bruising of the genitals or thighs

- Fractures

- Unreasonable or inconsistent explanations for injuries

- Frequent emergency room visits

- Caregiver refusal to allow the nurse to see the resident alone

- Emotional abuse signs:

    - Belittling, threatening, or controlling behavior by the caregiver in your presence

    - Behavior from the resident that mimics dementia (e.g., rocking or mumbling)

    - Afraid of retaliation by caregiver if abuse is reported

- Financial abuse signs

    - Items or cash are reported missing from the home

    - Unnecessary goods or services or numerous subscriptions

- Healthcare fraud signs:

    - The resident complains about duplicate billing for the same service provided

    - Evidence of the resident being overmedicated or under medicated

- Signs of possible neglect:

    - Weight loss, malnutrition, or dehydration

    - Insufficient clothing, shoes, or basic hygiene items

    - Medications not filled or taken

    - Doctor visits not scheduled or kept

    - Unclean appearance or smell

    - Skin ulcers or sores

    - Declining health

    - Unsafe living conditions

While most of these are controlled in an institution, it is possible for any of them to occur anywhere. Abusive or neglectful caregivers can be professionals as well as family members. It is important for everyone to be alert to the signs of abuse and neglect.

Reporting Abuse and Neglect

Anyone who knows of an elderly person being abused or neglected is obligated to notify the proper authorities. Reporting procedures vary by state. Staff who suspect abuse of a resident by either a family member or another professional caregiver should first report it to supervisors. You should become familiar with any statements of rights that your state has issued to protect residents—ask your supervisor for a copy. It is the responsibility of every staff member to report any suspected abuse or neglect, of any type. It is not the staff member's responsibility to investigate or confirm the abuse or neglect; the supervisor, leadership, and/or human resources will follow up with an investigation. If you believe that an employee in a supervisor/management/leadership role is committing abuse or neglect, find another person to report your suspicion to. Follow organizational policies for reporting structures.

Every state has an office or department that deals with abuse and neglect of the elderly. There are different names for these offices: Human Services, Adult Protective Services, Health and Welfare, Department of Aging, etc. Write the name and number of your state agency here:

_____

This is the place to call when you know of, or suspect, elder abuse or neglect.

Prevention

You can help prevent abuse and neglect by:

- Listening to the residents and caregivers

- Intervening when abuse or neglect is suspected

- Educating the residents and caregivers on how to recognize abuse and neglect

Elder Abuse and Neglect: Preventing, Recognizing, and Reporting

Test

Name _____ Date _____ Score _____

Directions: Circle the correct answer(s); some questions have more than one correct answer.

1. If you know of or suspect abuse or neglect of a resident, you should first _____.

   b. confront the staff member or family member that you suspect of committing the abuse

   c. call the state agency that accepts abuse reports

   d. report it to your supervisor

2. Some causes of abuse and neglect are _____.

   a. caregiver stress

   b. emotional or mental illness

   c. alcohol or drug use

3. Threatening a resident with punishment for not doing what you tell them to is _____.

   a. acceptable if done with a soft tone of voice

   b. verbal abuse, and it is never acceptable

   c. useful in disciplining an older person

4. Exploitation is a form of abuse that involves _____.

   a. physical harm

   b. emotional harm

   c. misuse or theft of money, property, or other financial assets

5. Some good ways to help prevent abuse are _____.

   a. education, counseling, and support groups

   b. listening, teaching caregiving skills, and communicating

   c. none of the above

6. Symptoms of possible abuse include _____.

   a. dementia

   b. becoming unusually quiet or withdrawn

   c. bruises or burns

7. Symptoms of possible neglect include _____.

   a. necessary medical visits not scheduled or kept

   b. too many outside activities

   c. lack of basic hygiene items and adequate clothing

8. It is the responsibility of everyone working in a skilled nursing facility to report suspected abuse or neglect to a supervisor.   True or False

9. Improper use of bedrails or other restraints is considered _____.

   a. physical abuse

   b. rights violation

   c. emotional abuse

10. Abuse and neglect will not occur if we remember that everyone has the right to be treated with _____.

CERTIFICATE OF COMPLETION

I hereby certify that

has successfully completed the in-Service

Elder Abuse and Neglect

Signature

14

End-of-Life Care

Teaching Plan

To use this lesson for self-study, the learner should read the material, do the activity, and take the test. For group study, the leader may give each learner a copy of the learning guide and follow this teaching plan to conduct the lesson. Certificates may be copied for everyone who completes the lesson.

Learning objectives

After this lesson, participants should be able to:

- Discuss the difference between curing and caring

- Know the goals of end-of-life care

- Understand the rights, issues, and decisions of end-of-life care

- Know the meaning and purpose of advance directives

- Be able to describe his or her role in end-of-life care

Lesson activities

Introductory activity: Beliefs about dying

Ask your learners to fill out the end-of-life issues quiz (Figure 14.1), answering the questions with their own personal thoughts and ideas. There are no right or wrong answers to this quiz. Ask if anyone is willing to explain some of his or her answers to the group. Encourage the learners to discuss the questions.

Lesson activities

1. Remind your learners that everyone's life will end someday. When we work with people who are disabled, ill, or elderly, it is likely that from time to time, someone we care for will die. Death is an inevitable part of life. We need to consider how we can help people through this period at the end of life.

2. Help your workers go over the information in the section "Two Ways to View the End of Life."

3. Provide your learners with posterboard and markers, and ask them to make a poster about one of the rights of a dying person. If appropriate for your agency, post these in your training room as reminders.

4. Review the section "Goals of End-of-Life Care," and then discuss the section "Important Issues and Decisions" in the learning guide.

5. Emphasize ways caregivers can help a terminally ill person, using the concepts on the last page of the learning guide. After the discussion, ask your learners whether any of them have changed their ideas or beliefs about the end of life.

Conclusion

Have participants take the test. Review the answers together. Award certificates to those who answer 70% of the test questions correctly.

Test answers

1. life-sustaining	2. caring	3. pain	4. emotional	5. oral hygiene
6. accept	7. depression	8. instructions	9. decrease	10. food

Figure 14.1: End-of-Life Issues Quiz

End-of-Life Issues Quiz

1. Why is the end of life an important period of an individual's life?

2. What are some of the rights of the dying patient?

3. Should someone's pain or suffering be considered in deciding when the patient and/or family are ready for the hospice level of care?

4. How does the teaching of your faith or religion, if you have one, influence your feelings about death?

5. What are some of the comfort measures you, as home health staff, can provide—and teach a caregiver to provide—to the patient to assist with pain relief and discomfort during a terminal illness?

End-of-Life Care

Learning Guide

Contents:

- Two Ways to View the End of Life

  - Curing

  - Caring

- Hospice Care

- The Rights of a Dying Person

- The Goals of End-of-Life Care

- Important Issues and Decisions

  - Life-sustaining therapies

  - Withholding and withdrawing treatment

  - Do not resuscitate

  - Advance directives

- Your Role in Caring for Someone at the End of Life

  - Acceptance

  - Relief of suffering through effective care

Two Ways to View the End of Life

Curing

The medical model of dying says there comes a time when all possible treatments have been tried and there is nothing left to do that will prevent death. In this view, we must give up fighting against death when we have no other choice.

When doctors, nurses, and direct caregivers think this way, they might quit giving good care to a dying person because they feel there is nothing more that can be done. They feel they have lost control because they can't fix the problem and may feel helpless and guilty. These feelings can lead them to avoid the dying person. People at the end of life can sense this in their caregivers, and they may fear being abandoned. This fear increases their loneliness and discomfort.

Caring

The caring model of dying says the end of life is an important period of an individual's life. During this final phase, curing the problem is no longer possible, and the focus shifts to caring for the person. When caregivers think this way, they concentrate on the many things they can do to make a dying person comfortable, to improve the quality of the dying person's life, and to provide opportunities for the person to meet his or her final life goals.

When caregivers focus on caring, they shift their energies from *whether* the person will die to *how* the person will die. Helping to relieve pain and other symptoms, giving emotional and spiritual support, and providing family time are all things that caregivers can do to care for a dying person.

Hospice Care

According to the National Hospice and Palliative Care Organization's web site (*www.nhpco.org*), hospice is considered to be the model for quality, compassionate care for people facing a life-limiting illness or injury, hospice care involves a team-oriented approach to expert medical care, pain management, and emotional and spiritual support expressly tailored to the patient's needs and wishes. Support is provided to the patient's loved ones as well. At the center of hospice and palliative care is the belief that each of us has the right to die pain-free and with dignity, and that our families will receive the necessary support to allow us to do so.

How does hospice care work? Hospice focuses on caring, not curing, and in most cases, care is provided in the patient's home. Hospice care also is provided in freestanding hospice centers, hospitals, and nursing homes and other long-term care facilities. Hospice services are available to patients of any age, religion, race, or illness. Hospice care is covered under Medicare, Medicaid, most private insurance plans, HMOs, and other managed-care organizations.

The Rights of a Dying Person

A dying person has the right to:

- Decide how to spend the final phase of his or her life

- Refuse treatment (including food and water) and to decide how much treatment to have

- Be relieved from pain and suffering, as much as is medically and legally possible

The Goals of End-of-Life Care

Each individual should decide what his or her goals are for the final phase of life. Caregivers can help people identify and achieve these goals. The goals may include things like:

- The individual's personal goals and desires, such as personal choices about living, continued personal growth, and things he or she wants to accomplish

- Relief from pain and other uncomfortable symptoms

- Relief from emotional and spiritual distress

- Enrichment of personal and family relationships

- Transition of individual and family toward death

Important Issues and Decisions

Sometimes people with terminal illnesses have to make decisions about how much treatment they want to have and how long they want to prolong life. Family members may have to make these decisions when the individual is too ill to decide. We must respect and support these decisions even if we do not agree with them—adults have the right to make these decisions.

Life-sustaining therapies

A life-sustaining treatment is anything used to maintain one or more physical functions in a terminally ill person. This includes machines that breathe for the person, usually called respirators or ventilators. It also includes feeding someone by artificial means, such as through the veins or through a tube into the stomach. Therapies like this keep a person alive when they can no longer eat or drink or breathe without this kind of assistance.

Withholding and withdrawing treatment

Sometimes a terminally ill person (or the family) may decide to let a doctor start a treatment that will keep the person alive. Then, after a time, it might become obvious that the therapy is not meeting the goals of care or is doing more harm than it is good. For example, feeding someone through the veins or through a stomach tube can cause swelling, choking, difficulty breathing, discomfort, restlessness, nausea, constipation, and increased pain. If the life-sustaining treatment is causing this kind of discomfort for a terminally ill person, the person and/or his family may decide that they want to stop the therapy and let the illness take its natural course toward death.

Stopping a life-sustaining therapy is legally and ethically acceptable. It is also acceptable not to start the therapy at all, if the terminally ill person and/or his family decide that the treatment is not in the person's best interests. The benefits of treatment should be compared to the burdens of treatment when making these decisions.

Do not resuscitate

A do-not-resuscitate (DNR) order means the person does not want cardiopulmonary resuscitation (CPR) performed if his or her heart stops and he or she stops breathing. It does not affect anything else about the person's care. An individual with a DNR order may still want every other kind of life-sustaining treatment, such as tube feeding.

Advance directives

Advance directives are any oral or written instructions that a person has given about future medical care. These instructions are to be used if the person becomes unable to speak for himself or herself.

There are two kinds of advance directives: a living will and a medical power of attorney. A living will states the person's medical treatment wishes in writing. A medical power of attorney (or durable power of attorney for healthcare) appoints someone to make decisions about medical care when the person cannot make them. If there is no living will or medical power of attorney, the spouse, children, or parents of an individual will make medical decisions when the person cannot make them. This person is called a surrogate. The surrogate is supposed to make healthcare decisions that the terminally ill person would have made if possible and to act in the person's best interests.

Every state has different rules about advance directives. Federal law requires healthcare facilities and agencies that receive Medicaid or Medicare funds to inform residents of their right to issue advance directives.

Your Role in Caring for Someone at the End of Life

You should remember two important concepts when caring for someone who is terminally ill: acceptance and relief of suffering.

Acceptance

The first thing you must do when caring for someone who is at the end of life is to get to know the person's life story and accept the person and the choices they make about how to live and how to die. You must accept the person's religious beliefs, cultural and ethnic background and values, and wishes about what he or she wants to do and whom he or she wants to see. You must accept the person without judging his or her decisions. Your job is to listen, encourage, and support the decisions he or she makes.

If you find that it is impossible for you to support a dying person because you feel strongly that his or her decisions or beliefs are wrong, you must tell your supervisor about it. Sometimes it is necessary for the supervisor to transfer your responsibilities for the dying person to another caregiver. A terminally ill person will probably know when a caregiver disagrees with his or her choices, and this can cause the person to feel afraid, abandoned, or defensive. In this case, it is best for someone else to care for the person if possible.

Relief of suffering through effective care

Good care can relieve much of the pain and discomfort that a person may experience during a terminal illness. You should always be checking to determine whether the person is uncomfortable and finding ways to improve the comfort level. Some things you can do include:

- Position pillows comfortably

- Moisten lips and mouth

- Rub lotions on the skin

- Position body comfortably

- Provide good oral care

- Watch for skin breakdown; give skin care

Pain is not the only symptom that should be relieved. Nausea, constipation, anxiety, depression, difficulty breathing, and other symptoms should be reported to your supervisor so they can be treated with medications and other therapies.

When a person is dying, the need and the desire for food and water decrease. You should not force food or water on someone who doesn't want it. Remember that competent adults have the right to refuse any treatment, including food and water. Often, a terminally ill person will have a craving for a particular food, but when it is brought to him or her, he or she will take only one or two bites and say he or she is finished. The best thing to do is get the resident the food he or she wants if at all possible, but don't force him or her to eat it. One bite may satisfy the craving.

A dying person may not want to drink anything, but the lips, mouth, and throat might get dry. You can relieve this discomfort with small sips of liquid, ice chips, hard candy, and oral hygiene. You should not force someone to drink more than he or she wants.

Don't be worried about starving someone to death if the person is dying from a terminal illness. The illness is causing death; death is not caused by the decrease in food and water. If the person is allowing the natural processes of death to occur, they will want only enough food and water to be comfortable. Giving food and water only when it is wanted can allow chemical processes to occur in the body that actually decrease pain and discomfort. Forcing food and water on a dying person can greatly increase pain and suffering and cause a more difficult death.

End-of-Life Care

Test

Name _____ Date _____ Score _____

Directions: Fill in the blanks in the statements below.

1. A _____-_____ treatment is anything that maintains one or more bodily functions in a terminally ill person.

2. The _____ model of dying says that the end of life is a time when we concentrate on making a dying person comfortable, improving the quality of life, and providing opportunities for the person to meet goals.

3. A dying person has the right to relief from _____ and suffering.

4. One of the goals of end-of-life care is relief from _____ and spiritual distress.

5. You can relieve the discomfort of a dry mouth with small sips of liquid, ice chips, hard candy, and _____ _____.

6. You must _____ a terminally ill person without judging his or her decisions.

7. Nausea, constipation, anxiety, _____, difficulty breathing, and other symptoms should be reported to your supervisor so they can be addressed with medications or treatment.

8. Advance directives are any oral or written _____ that a person has given about future medical care.

9. Giving food and water only when it is wanted can allow chemical processes to occur in the body that actually _____ pain and discomfort.

10. Competent adults have the right to refuse any treatment, including _____ and water.

CERTIFICATE OF COMPLETION

I hereby certify that

has successfully completed the in-Service

End-of-Life Care

Signature

15
■ Ethics

Teaching Plan

To use this lesson for self-study, the learner should read the material, do the activity, and take the test. For group study, the leader may give each learner a copy of the learning guide and follow this teaching plan to conduct the lesson. Certificates may be copied for everyone who completes the lesson.

Learning objectives

After this lesson, participants should be able to:

- Define the term ethical

- State three ethical standards

- Explain the process for making ethical decisions

- Describe three signs of ethical problems in the workplace

Lesson activities

1. Discuss personal experiences with ethical issues in healthcare

2. If the agency has an ethics committee, invite a member of the committee to discuss the process for addressing ethical dilemmas

The lesson

Review the material in the lesson with participants. Allow for discussion.

Conclusion

Have participants take the test. Review the answers together. Award certificates to those who answer 70% of the test questions correctly.

Test answers

1. d	2. c	3. True	4. d	5. a
6. True	7. c	8. a	9. False	10. True

Ethics

Learning Guide

Contents:

- Introduction

- Basic Ethical Standards

- Ethical Requirements in Healthcare

  - Ethical dilemmas in healthcare

  - Professional and organizational ethics

  - Personal ethics and responsibilities

- Staff Role in Ethics

  - Maintain knowledge of employee requirements

  - Uphold professional behavior

  - Provide personal care

  - Offer support

  - Observe and report

  - Participate in team meetings

  - Reinforce education

Introduction

Healthcare workers face ethical issues in every setting. This is especially true in skilled nursing where the facility is a home that fosters person-centered care and independence of residents and empowerment of the care providers. This makes identifying and dealing with ethical issues a challenge.

For skilled nursing staff, ethical issues may be due to resident-care concerns, resident choice, family involvement, and the staff member's personal involvement and compliance with agency policies and laws. To understand the risk involved and act responsibly, the staff member must have an understanding of ethics and be able to recognize and report potential ethical issues.

Ethics can be defined as the study of the difference between right and wrong. Ethics is closely related to human behavior, values, and morality. Over time, many people have accepted basic beliefs about right and wrong. Those common beliefs are known as **ethical standards** or **principles**.

The common standards, as well as a person's own standards, guide the way that person acts. Actions can show a person's understanding of right and wrong and his or her beliefs about ethics. Staff must also be aware of the ethical standards, or requirements, of their roles and their workplace. Those standards are used to guide ethical actions while providing care. Staff must also think about how well those standards match their own understanding of ethical actions.

Key Terms to Aid Your Understanding

Bioethics: healthcare ethics; the ways the standards of right and wrong are used in healthcare

Code: a set of written rules

Compliance: following the rules, doing what is expected

Morality: acting in ways that agree with customs and traditions, often in relationship to personal or religious beliefs

Standards: requirements for the way something should be done; in ethics, standards are also called principles

Values: beliefs that are important to a person or group of people

Basic Ethical Standards

There are several ethical standards that revolve around the simple concept of doing good, which can be described by the following guidelines:

- Be kind to others

- Do no harm

- Treat people fairly

- Respect the rights of others to make their own choices

- Keep promises

- Tell the truth

- Respect privacy and personal property

Most people agree to follow those guidelines and try to live by them each day. In many cases, "doing good" can be quite simple, such as donating food or helping a neighbor.

Doing good and doing no harm are two concepts that go hand in hand. Sometimes it becomes harder to tell the difference between doing good and avoiding harm.

It's usually good to tell the truth. Occasionally, though, telling the truth might hurt someone's feelings, especially if it concerns something such as the person's weight or new hairstyle. When healthcare issues are involved, telling the truth can become even more difficult.

Ethical Requirements in Healthcare

Healthcare professionals encounter situations daily that require ethical behavior and decision-making. These may involve resident care, families, or a healthcare staff member's personal behavior. Additionally, sometimes there are ethical and legal requirements affecting the same situation, making it difficult to tell the difference between the two. For example:

- **Resident care.** When caring for residents, it is normal for healthcare workers to want to do the right thing and avoid harming those residents. Following policies and procedures helps ensure that care is provided properly. However, resident care questions may occur, such as how to care for a resident who refuses to eat. Healthcare workers often find themselves wondering whether to support the resident's right to make choices when it seems that the resident is making a poor choice.

- **Advance directives.** Residents may sign these documents to indicate their choices about care at the end of their life. These statements are signed in advance, because the resident may not be able to make choices when they reach the final stages of illness. Healthcare workers are required by laws and ethical standards to follow advance directives.

- **Resident mental status.** There are a number of ethical questions healthcare workers must answer when a resident's mental status changes and the resident begins having problems making decisions and choices. To meet basic ethical standards, the team of care providers must often work together. Sometimes obtaining legal advice is necessary.

- **Families.** Working with families also requires understanding ethical, and sometimes legal, standards. The Health Insurance Portability and Accountability Act (HIPAA) is a law that protects resident information. Doing the right thing means allowing the resident to decide how much information is shared with family members.

- **Personal behavior.** In addition to ethical concerns about resident care, care providers must be aware of their own behavior as employees. This includes telling the truth when documenting care and reporting the number of hours worked. It also includes behavior toward residents and their families, as well as protecting property that belongs to the resident or the employer.

- **Billing and finance.** A healthcare organization's billing practices receive a great deal of attention. Organizations must follow ethical standards when billing residents and insurance companies, including the Medicare and Medicaid programs. This means accurate reporting of time and services, along with accurate charges. Every employee who is involved with billing or reporting the amount of care given to a resident must act ethically. When unethical practices occur, individual employees and entire organizations can be charged with legal offenses.

- **Compliance with laws.** In addition to the regulations for accurate billing, hospitals, homecare agencies, and skilled nursing facilities must meet many other federal and state regulations and requirements for providing care. Hospitals, homecare agencies, and skilled nursing facilities usually have a compliance plan, which explains how employees will meet these requirements.

Ethical dilemmas in healthcare

Ethical conflicts, or disagreements, occur when people have different beliefs about what is right and wrong. This happens in both personal lives and in the professional world. When different beliefs and backgrounds are combined with the many choices and new technologies, it's easy to understand how there can be disagreement.

Sometimes the disagreement occurs because a healthcare choice can have both positive and negative results. People may follow ethical standards but still find that there is no correct answer. This is known as an ethical dilemma.

Think about ethical dilemmas in healthcare by comparing actions that seem to agree with standards but also have both good and harmful effects or may conflict with the resident's rights. The following situations describe potential ethical dilemmas (Figure 15.1).

Figure 15.1: Examples of Ethical Dilemmas

Ethical standard	Example of following ethical standard	Possible dilemma
Do good.	Give someone a heart transplant.	The family of another patient who is brain dead must decide whether to end life support and allow the patient to die and provide a heart to the transplant patient.
Do no harm.	Do not give fatty food to a patient with a heart conditions.	This may conflict with the patient's right to choose and request the type of food he desires.
Tell the truth.	A physician informs a wife that her husband will not recover from his heart condition.	The wife feels very sad and it seems that telling the truth caused harm to the wife.
Respect the right of others to make their own choices.	A patient has an advance directive, so as a nurse, you do not resuscitate him when he stops breathing.	A family member may not agree with the patient's choice and may feel that the patient was "left to die."
Respect privacy and personal property.	Following HIPAA guidelines, do not release patient informations except as allowed.	A daughter says she wants to help her father but needs information in order to do so. The patient has refused to release information. The patient may be harmed by not accepting the daughter's help.

In each of these situations, following the ethical standard can seem to conflict with doing the right thing. Good communication is most important. A review of the different possibilities and viewpoints of those involved is necessary. Healthcare organizations, such as hospitals, homecare agencies, and skilled nursing facilities, usually have an ethics committee that will help staff discuss these types of difficult situations and make the best decision possible.

Educating those involved in ethical dilemmas about different options is helpful, although these situations also involve human emotions. It's important to be concerned about both the type of information communicated and the way communication occurs.

Professional and organizational ethics

Most healthcare professions have a written code of ethics, such as the American Nurses Association (ANA) Code of Ethics for Nurses. A code contains guidelines that members of a profession have created over time. The guidelines, or standards, help staff members understand the expectations for their daily work, as well as how to make decisions when facing ethical dilemmas.

Job descriptions often include statements that are similar to ethical standards. Organizations, such as homecare agencies, may choose to use basic ethical standards and professional codes when creating job descriptions. An example of a job description statement that includes a requirement for ethical behavior is:

> *The certified nursing assistant (CNA) will function according to the organization's code of conduct. The CNA will demonstrate this by maintaining confidentiality, acting with ethics and integrity, protecting the property of the organization, reporting noncompliance, and adhering to applicable federal and state laws and regulations and accreditation and licensure requirements.*

Staff will be evaluated according to whether they meet the requirements of the job description. However, even the job description cannot include guidelines for all the situations that might occur while working.

Personal ethics and responsibilities

Healthcare workers must recognize that there are times when their own actions or the actions of co-workers, residents, and families may be questioned. As you've seen, there are times when even doing something good may cause other people harm or may conflict with someone's rights. Cultural differences, personal background, religion, and other beliefs may also affect actions and the way actions are judged by others.

Organizations have policies that require ethical actions. Some situations may be addressed by policies that require discipline or termination of employment if an employee does not meet standards, such as the following:

- It is unethical to become involved socially with residents or family members, such as dating a resident's son while responsible for the resident's care. This situation may make it difficult to make good decisions about the resident's needs.

- Staff members are required to protect resident property, which includes not stealing or even borrowing from residents. Staff members should also avoid any involvement with a resident's finances.

- It's normal for residents and families to want to reward good care, but most agencies have specific guidelines for accepted tips, etc. (For example, a box of cookies may be accepted, but a check for $50 could not be accepted.)

- Even though residents may have personalities that make it difficult to care for them, it's always right to "do good" for each resident as well as "do no harm." This means never physically or emotionally abusing a resident. In addition, there are ethical and legal requirements to report suspected abuse of residents.

- Ethical behavior requires respect for each resident. As long as care can be provided in a safe manner and the resident is safe, staff members must respect the resident's lifestyle and never try to force one's own beliefs and needs on the resident.

Ethical decision-making[1]

When faced with a potential ethical problem, there are steps you can take to help make the best decision possible.

Before acting, ask yourself the following questions:

- Is it right?

- Is it fair?

- Will someone get hurt?

- If my actions were reported in the newspaper, would I be embarrassed?

- Would I tell someone else, especially a child, to do the same thing?

- Does this "smell" right? (Your common sense may tell you that there's something wrong.)

Staff Role in Ethics

Ethical standards are part of everything you do as a staff member. Understanding the basic ethical standards helps you care for residents appropriately while also meeting the agency's employee standards.

Maintain knowledge of employee requirements

Even though you understand basic ethical standards, it's important to know how your organization includes those standards in its policies. Read your job description and ask questions about any requirements you don't understand.

Stay up to date with changes in agency policies, especially those that affect ethical and legal requirements. Read each new message or policy change that is posted. Attend meetings and complete annual education requirements. This might include annual training about HIPAA, the agency's compliance plan, or identifying and reporting abuse.

When you understand your organization's polices and standards, you will be better prepared to make good decisions about the care you provide, as well as respond properly to unexpected situations that you may face.

Uphold professional behavior

Recognize that your own personal problems may affect your reactions to work requirements. It may be tempting to talk about your own personal problems with residents and their families, but doing so places a burden on those who are already branded with illness and their own problems. Ethical standards for doing good, treating residents fairly, and showing respect require that you focus your attention on them while caring for them.

Provide personal care

The primary role of nursing assistants is personal care. Since personal care is a very intimate activity and may even be embarrassing to the resident, it's important to follow the care plan and organization's procedures carefully. Be sure that you understand the requirements of the care plan, and ask questions if any part of the assignment does not seem to fit the needs of the resident. By acting in this way, you'll make sure that all your actions are good for the resident.

Offer support

Many residents have a need for emotional support. They may be lonely, dealing with a difficult diagnosis, or in pain. As a result, they may be weepy, overly dependent on you, or demanding. Keeping in mind that you want to do good, you will also need to balance requirements to allow the resident to make choices and to be fair to all residents.

You can show your support by listening carefully when residents talk with you and by showing kindness through gentle touch and paying attention to details while providing care. If a resident likes to be covered with two blankets after a bath, or to be left with the television on when you leave, he or she will feel supported when you remember to do those things.

Remember to remain professional; while you may feel as though you're a family member, you are not. Performing your duties in an ethical manner is easier when you maintain your separate role as a caregiver.

Observe and report

Since you may be involved in ethical dilemmas at any time or you may see situations that appear to be questionable, it's important to observe for changes in a resident's physical status, changes in a resident's behavior, or changes in plans that residents may tell you about. Report these changes to your supervisor. In particular, if a resident tells you about a new advance directive or a change in how he or she wishes to be cared for, report this to your supervisor immediately.

Participate in team meetings

Team meetings are a time to discuss new information and different points of view. If ethical dilemmas already exist, attending the meeting can bring new ideas to light and team members can provide support to one another. Sharing information about resident care problems that you're having can also help you understand how to handle a situation and avoid future ethical issues.

Reinforce education

Supporting a resident's right to make his or her own choices depends on ensuring that the resident has the right information. If a resident has questions or does not seem to understand information, follow up with the nurse or therapist about possible problems you've observed.

1. Bowditch & Buono, 1997, as cited in Sellers, 2008, in P. Kelly (ed.), Nursing leadership and management (2nd ed., p. 523). Clifton Park, NY: Delmar Learning: Thomson.

Ethics

Test

Name _____ Date _____ Score _____

Directions: Circle the best answer.

1. Ethics involves which of the following?

   a. Human behavior

   b. Values

   c. Morality

   d. All of the above

2. Which of the following is *not* a basic ethical standard?

   a. Do no harm

   b. Be fair

   c. Save time

   d. Do good

3. Ethics is about telling the difference between right and wrong. True or False

4. Which of the following situations requires ethical decision-making?

   a. Honoring a resident's advance directive

   b. Not accepting gifts from residents beyond what's allowed by the organization

   c. Protecting a resident's privacy

   d. All of the above

5. Which of the following would cause an ethical dilemma?

   a. A family's decision to ask the physician for a DNR order

   b. Talking with a resident about the care plan

   c. Both a and b

   d. None of the above

6. An organization's policies and job descriptions often contain expectations for ethical behavior. True or False

7. What ethical action should staff members avoid?

   a. Caring for the resident according to the care plan

   b. Talking about resident issues during team meetings

   c. Becoming too socially involved with a resident or family

   d. Making a resident happy by paying attention to details

8. Which group is most likely to be involved in decision-making when an ethical dilemma affects resident care?

   a. Regulatory compliance committee

   b. Agency ethics committee

   c. American Nurses Association

   d. Education committee

9. It's acceptable to perform extra duties that are not on the care plan, as long as it makes the resident happy. True or False

10. When you understand your organizations' polices and standards, you will be better prepared to make good decisions about the care you provide, as well as respond properly to unexpected situations that you may face. True or False

CERTIFICATE OF COMPLETION

I hereby certify that

_____

has successfully completed the in-Service

Ethics

_____

Signature

16

Heart Disease and Health

Teaching Plan

To use this lesson for self-study, the learner should read the material, do the activity, and take the test. For group study, the leader may give each learner a copy of the learning guide and follow this teaching plan to conduct the lesson. Certificates may be copied for everyone who completes the lesson.

Learning objectives

After this lesson, participants should be able to:

- Understand how the heart functions

- Identify potential problems with heart function

- Identify treatment and care for the heart to prevent heart problems

Lesson activities

For an introductory activity, review the "How the Heart Works" section in the learning guide. Have your learners fill in the blanks with these words: "When the heart muscle contracts, pumping blood out, it is called systole. When the heart muscle relaxes, it fills up with blood again. This is called diastole." Ask your learners if they recognize these terms. Point out the information about blood-pressure measurement numbers and what they mean.

Heart failure and heart attack

1. Assign half the learners to read the "Heart failure" section in the learning guide and half to read the "Heart attack" section.

2. Ask learners from each group to tell the rest of the class what they learned in their reading.

3. Emphasize the fact that a heart attack is an emergency situation requiring immediate medical care. Be sure your learners know the signs of a heart attack and how to respond.

4. Discuss the symptoms of heart failure. Ask your learners to think about the residents who have heart failure. Is there anything that your learners should change in their care of these residents?

Prevention

1. Review the guidelines for a healthy heart. Point out that following these guidelines also lowers the risk of certain other diseases, such as diabetes and some cancers.

2. Deliver a lecture on the information in the learning guide about diet and exercise.

3. Ask your learners how they can use this information to assist your residents in achieving or maintaining optimum health.

Conclusion

Have participants take the test. Review the answers together. Award certificates to those who answer 70% of the test questions correctly.

Test answers

1. muscle; pump	2. True	3. c	4. False	5. a, b, c, e
6. Eat a variety of foods Engage in regular physical activity Achieve and maintain a healthy weight Limit total salt (sodium) consumption to less than one teaspoon a day Eat foods low in fat and cholesterol Limit sugar intake Eat plenty of vegetables, fruits, and whole-grain products If you drink alcohol, consume no more than one drink per day Do not smoke Monitor blood pressure and keep it within healthy limits				
7. False	8. Blood supply (or blood flow)	9. b	10. hour	

Heart Disease and Heart Health

Learning Guide

Contents:

- How the Heart Works

- What Can Go Wrong With the Heart?

  - Heart failure

  - Heart attack

  - Causes and risk factors of heart failure and heart attacks

  - Preventing heart disease

- Guidelines for a Healthy Heart

  - Fat and cholesterol

  - Exercise guidelines

How the Heart Works

The heart is a bag made out of muscle, with blood vessels leading in and out. It works like a large pump, pushing blood from the bag and through the blood vessels that run throughout the body. The blood carries oxygen, nutrients, and waste products.

Blood is pumped from the heart to the lungs, where it picks up oxygen. The blood then returns to the heart, where it is pumped out to the rest of the body. The blood delivers its oxygen to the tissues and picks up and distributes nutrients and waste products and then returns to the heart and gets pumped back to the lungs.

Figure 16.1: Understanding the Heart

When the heart muscle contracts,
pumping blood out, it is called _____.

The top number of a blood pressure reading measures the heart when it beats.
This is the systolic pressure.

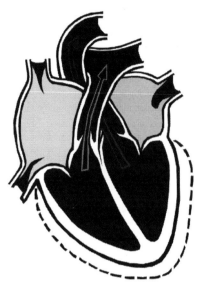

When the heart muscle relaxes, it fills up with blood again. This is called _____.

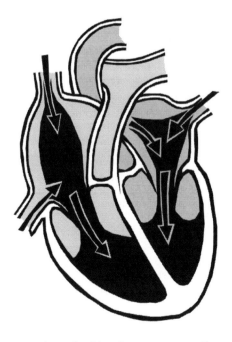

The bottom number of a blood pressure reading measures
the heart at rest. This is the diastolic pressure.

What Can Go Wrong With the Heart?

We will look at two different unhealthy heart conditions: heart failure and heart attacks.

Heart failure

Heart failure is a condition in which the heart doesn't pump as well as it should. The heart has not actually "failed," but it is not pumping enough blood to meet the requirements of the body's tissues and organs. The blood flow slows down, causing a backup of fluid and waste products and depriving the tissues of oxygen and nutrients.

Heart failure is not a disease in itself but is caused by underlying problems like high blood pressure or clogged arteries. It is often called congestive heart failure (CHF) because of the excess fluid or congestion that tends to build up in the lungs and in tissues throughout the body. This excess fluid creates symptoms like swollen ankles and shortness of breath.

Heart failure is usually a long-term condition that gradually becomes worse. The heart tries to make up for its loss of power by enlarging its chambers, developing more muscle mass, and pumping faster. The body tries to compensate in other ways. Blood vessels narrow, and blood is diverted away from less important tissues and organs to maintain flow to the heart and brain.

The most common signs and symptoms of heart failure are:

- Fatigue, weakness, feeling tired

- Shortness of breath during activity

- Unable to breathe well when lying flat

- Edema: swelling in feet, ankles, legs, or abdomen

- Rapid weight gain

- Lack of appetite, full feeling in stomach, nausea

- Memory loss, disorientation, confusion

- Heart palpitations, heart racing

- Irregular heart beat

- Anxiety, restlessness

- Decreased urine output

- Cold, sweaty skin that might look gray or bluish in color

- Persistent coughing or wheezing, possibly with white or pink blood-tinged foamy phlegm

Heart attack

A heart attack is an injury to the heart muscle caused by a loss of blood supply. It occurs when an artery that feeds blood to the heart becomes blocked. The blockage is usually due to a blood clot that forms where one of these arteries has been narrowed by a build up of cholesterol and fat.

A heart attack is also called a myocardial infarction, or MI. *Myo* means muscle, *cardio* means heart, and *infarct* means that some heart tissue has died from lack of oxygen.

A heart attack usually occurs over a time period of four to six hours. With each minute, more heart tissue is deprived of oxygen and is damaged or dies. The only way to help the individual suffering a heart attack is to restore blood flow before too much damage is done.

Heart attack symptoms in women, the elderly, and people with diabetes tend to be less pronounced. Some people have no symptoms at all. While heart attacks usually occur suddenly, about half of all victims have warning symptoms in advance.

All heart attacks are emergencies. Early treatment, including cardiopulmonary resuscitation (CPR) if the heart stops, is essential to survival. Everyone should learn CPR and be able to use it. Recognizing symptoms of a heart attack and helping the person get emergency care can save a life.

Warning signs of a heart attack include:

- Pressure, fullness, uncomfortable squeezing or pain in the middle of the chest that lasts beyond a few minutes

- Pain spreading beyond the chest to the shoulders, neck, arms, or back, and sometimes to the teeth and jaw

- Pain in the upper abdomen that lasts for more than a few minutes (sometimes people think they are having indigestion or heartburn)

- Shortness of breath, difficulty breathing

- Intense sweating

- Fainting, unsteadiness, lightheadedness

- Nausea and vomiting

- Confusion

- Sense of anxiety or impending doom

- Angina: a type of chest pain caused by the heart temporarily not getting enough blood flow; angina of increasing frequency may be a warning sign of a heart attack

People that die from heart attacks usually die within the first hour after symptoms start. If you suspect that someone might be having a heart attack, call emergency medical personnel immediately.

Causes and risk factors of heart failure and heart attacks

The main causes of heart failure are the same things that can cause heart attacks, such as smoking, eating fatty foods, not exercising, and being overweight. Other causes include birth defects and viruses that damage the heart valves or muscles. Someone who experiences a heart attack will often develop heart failure because part of the heart muscle has been damaged, making the heart work harder.

The following are the main risk factors for heart disease:

- High blood pressure

- High blood-cholesterol levels

- Smoking

- Lack of exercise

- Obesity

- Diabetes

- Stress

- Alcohol

- Family history

- Abnormal heart valves

- Coronary artery disease

- Heart muscle disease

- Congenital heart disease

- Severe lung disease

Preventing heart disease

Some of the things that cause heart disease can't be easily changed, such as diseases caused by viruses or birth defects. Many of the causes and risk factors, however, can be improved with diet and activity changes. Everyone can benefit from following the "guidelines for a healthy heart."

Guidelines for a Healthy Heart

- Eat a variety of foods

- Engage in regular physical activity

- Achieve and maintain a healthy weight by controlling calorie intake

- Limit total salt (sodium) consumption to less than one teaspoon per day

- Eat foods low in fat and cholesterol

- Limit sugar intake

- Eat plenty of vegetables, fruits, and whole-grain products

- If you drink alcohol, consume no more than one drink per day

- Do not smoke

- Monitor blood pressure and keep it within healthy limits (less than 140 systolic and 90 diastolic for most people, or 140/90)

Fat and cholesterol

Cholesterol is a waxy substance made in the body (mostly in the liver). Our bodies use it to make some of our hormones and tissues. Foods that come from animals also contain cholesterol, so we add cholesterol to our body's supply when we eat things like eggs and meat. A high level of cholesterol in the blood is a major risk factor for heart disease.

A high intake of fatty foods is another risk factor for heart disease. There are three kinds of fat: saturated, polyunsaturated, and monounsaturated. Saturated fat is the chief culprit in raising blood cholesterol and increasing the risk of heart disease. The main source of saturated fat is animal foods such as meat, eggs, cream, cheese, and butter. Some plant oils, such as coconut oils and cocoa butter, are also high in saturated fats. Foods that are high in saturated fat are usually high in cholesterol as well. The two unsaturated fats (poly and mono) may help lower blood cholesterol when used in place of saturated fats. Unsaturated fats are found in certain plant oils, such as corn, safflower, olive, and peanut oils. Total intake of all three kinds of fat should be less than 30% of your total calories.

Two other substances connected with cholesterol are of concern in heart health. Low-density lipo-proteins (LDL) and high-density lipoproteins (HDL) carry cholesterol through the blood. LDL is the main cholesterol carrier, and if too much of it circulates in the blood, it can slowly build up in the arteries that feed the heart and brain, causing the arteries to clog. HDL is the other cholesterol car-rier, and it takes cholesterol away from the arteries and back to the liver, where it is taken out of the body. To maintain a healthy heart, you want to have a low level of LDL and a high level of HDL.

To keep your dietary intake of fats and cholesterol at the right levels, follow these guidelines:

- Get two to four servings of fat-free or low-fat milk and dairy products (yogurt, cheese) daily.

- Eat no more than six ounces (cooked) of lean meat, poultry, and seafood a day. Include fish in your diet several times per week.

- Get five or more servings of vegetables and fruits every day.

- Eat six servings of grains (breads, cereals) and starchy vegetables (beans, potatoes) daily.

- Limit your intake of saturated fats like shortening, fried foods, whole milk, ice cream, and butter.

Exercise guidelines

Physical activity does not have to be strenuous to bring health benefits. The important thing is to do a moderate amount of physical activity every day. Regular exercise helps control weight, raises HDL levels in some people, strengthens the heart muscle, and promotes good circulation. Keep the following in mind:

- Older adults and people with disabilities should talk to their doctors before beginning a new physical activity

- Choose an activity that is rhythmic and repetitive and improves the circulation, like walking

- Find an activity that is enjoyable and can be done year-round

- Wear comfortable clothes and shoes

- Exercise with a friend or a group

- When walking, choose a smooth, soft surface that is well lit

- Take time to warm up before exercising and cool down afterward

- When stretching, stretch muscles slowly and gently

- Start exercising slowly and progress gradually

- Drink water at least every 15 minutes while you are exercising

Heart Disease and Health

Test

Name _____ Date _____ Score _____

Directions: Circle the correct answer or fill in the blank with the correct word.

1. The heart is a bag made out of _____ that works like a large

   _____ .

2. Someone with heart failure might have swollen ankles or difficulty breathing because the heart is not pumping well, so blood flow slows and fluid backs up in the lungs and body tissues. True or False

3. Warning signs of a heart attack include:

   a. Fatigue, coughing, and swollen ankles

   b. Headache and back pain

   c. Chest pain and shortness of breath

   d. Excessive urination

4. It is impossible to do anything to prevent heart disease. True or False

5. Circle the four risk factors for heart disease in this list:

   a. Smoking

   b. Obesity

   c. Inactivity

   d. Old age

   e. High blood pressure

   f. Being male

6. List at least four things people can do to prevent heart disease:

    1. _____

    2. _____

    3. _____

    4. _____

7. Exercise is good for younger people, but older people won't benefit from it. True   or   False

8. A heart attack is caused by a lack of _____ to the heart.

9. Which type of fat is the main cause of blockages in the arteries that feed blood to the heart?

    a. Polyunsaturated fat, which is mostly from plant oils

    b. Saturated fat, which is mostly from animals

    c. Monounsaturated fat, which is mostly from plant oils

10. People that die from heart attacks usually die within the first _____ after symptoms start.

CERTIFICATE OF COMPLETION

I hereby certify that

_____

has successfully completed the in-Service

Heart Disease and Health

_____

Signature

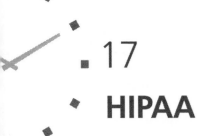

17

HIPAA

Teaching Plan

To use this lesson for self-study, the learner should read the material, do the activity, and take the test. For group study, the leader may give each learner a copy of the learning guide and follow this teaching plan to conduct the lesson. Certificates may be copied for everyone who completes the lesson.

Learning objectives

After this lesson, participants should be able to:

- Uphold the privacy, confidentiality, and security of residents' protected information

- Summarize the critical components of the Health Insurance Portability and Accountability Act (HIPAA)

- Define consent and authorization

Lesson activity

Do this activity first to get participants thinking about issues of privacy and confidentiality.

Use the situations in the section "Activity: What Should You Do If…?" Cut each situation out, fold it, and put it in a container (without the answers). Ask each participant to draw one of the situations, read it to the group, and explain the best thing to do in that situation. If the participant does not know what to do, he or she can ask others for opinions. You may give the correct answers at this time or tell the participants to keep the situations and determine whether they can find the correct answers as the lesson proceeds. The answers are provided to assist you in guiding the discussion.

Activity answers

1. Refer the resident to your supervisor. Your organization must allow a person to view and photocopy his record if requested, except in certain special circumstances.

2. If the resident has signed a consent form releasing the information, you may fax the information, using a cover sheet marked "Confidential."

3. Politely explain that you cannot discuss a resident's health condition with others.

4. The resident must sign a special authorization for anyone to see his record other than for purposes of providing healthcare (for which he must sign a consent).

5. Go to a private area where you cannot be overheard by others.

6. Remind your coworker that you should not discuss residents where others can hear you, and you should only discuss residents when it is important for providing care.

7. Put the record away immediately, out of sight of unauthorized persons.

8. Turn the computer screen so unauthorized persons cannot see it and/or clear the information from the screen if you are able to do so safely.

9. If the individual on the phone is authorized to access the resident's information, you may give the information as long as no one else can overhear you. If the resident has not signed a consent form or a specific authorization, you may not give the information.

The lesson

Bring copies of your organization's privacy and confidentiality policies and procedures to the training session for the employees to keep and review. Discuss the information in the learning guide and in your policies and procedures with the participants. Be prepared to answer specific questions about your policies.

For more information about HIPAA, go to *www.hhs.gov/ocr/hipaa*.

Conclusion

Have participants take the test. Review the answers together. Award certificates to those who answer at least seven (70%) of the test questions correctly.

Test answers

1. d	2. b	3. False	4. True	5. c
6. True	7. b	8. True	9. d	10. c

Activity: What Should You Do If . . .

Directions: Discuss each scenario.

1. A resident asks to see or copy his resident record.

2. A doctor's office asks you to fax them something from a resident's record.

3. A resident or a friend of a resident asks you about another resident's condition.

4. A resident's family member asks to see the resident's record.

5. A coworker wants to talk to you about a resident.

6. A coworker wants to talk to you about a resident while you are at a restaurant.

7. You notice a resident's record sitting open and out where others can see it.

8. A computer screen that can be seen by others is on, displaying resident information.

9. You answer the phone and someone asks for information about a resident.

HIPAA

Learning Guide

Contents:

- HIPAA History and Overview

    - The American Recovery and Reinvestment Act of 2009 and the HITECH Act

    - Why do we need HIPAA?

    - Who is required to follow the HIPAA rules?

    - What else are covered entities required to do?

- Information Protected Under HIPAA

- Protecting Resident Records

    - What is the difference between consent and authorization?

    - May a person see his or her personal PHI and make changes?

- Exceptions to the HIPAA Privacy Rule

- Protection of Resident Privacy and Confidentiality

    - Mobile and online considerations

- Consequences

HIPAA History and Overview

Congress passed HIPAA to require the security, confidentiality, and privacy of every person's health information.

- **Privacy** relates to who should and should not have access to health information. Residents have the right to privacy, meaning that information about them should only be available to people who need it to provide care.

- **Confidentiality** relates to preventing someone from hearing or seeing a person's private health records and information without the proper authorization. All health information is confidential. Anyone who possesses personal health information (PHI) is responsible for protecting it.

- **Security** is the means used to provide privacy and confidentiality. The purpose of security is to ensure that only those persons having authorization may access PHI.

Frontline staff should remember the general HIPAA rule of thumb: **the right information, to the right person, for the right reasons.**

The American Recovery and Reinvestment Act of 2009 and the HITECH Act

On February 17, 2009, the American Recovery and Reinvestment Act of 2009 became a federal law. A subset of that law, called the HITECH Act, enhances and expands the HIPAA Privacy and Security Rules and adds requirements for breach notification. The HITECH Act not only makes privacy regulations more strict, but it gives more power to federal and state authorities to enforce privacy and security protections for patient data, and it raises the fines for noncompliance.

The 2013 Omnibus Privacy, Security, Enforcement, and Breach Notification Rule (Omnibus Rule) implements many of the HITECH Act provisions for PHI protection.

Why do we need HIPAA?

More and more health information is in the form of electronic data, either instead of or in addition to paper files. We must protect data in any form. Federal laws make sure every state and every provider follow the same rules for privacy, confidentiality, and security.

Who is required to follow the HIPAA rules?

The following public and private organizations must follow the HIPAA rules:

- **Health plans and health insurance companies**, such as health maintenance organizations (HMO) and preferred provider organizations (PPO)

- **Healthcare clearinghouses**, such as billing services

- **Healthcare providers**, such as doctors, dentists, chiropractors, therapists, hospitals, nursing facilities, clinics, pharmacies, home health agencies, hospices, and long-term care or personal care facilities of any type or size

The HIPAA rules call these organizations **covered entities**.

What else are covered entities required to do?

Covered entities are required to communicate how HIPAA is implemented to both residents and frontline staff. They must:

- Notify residents about their privacy rights and give a clear, written explanation of how the provider may use and disclose residents' health information. This notifies residents of their right to view their own records, obtain copies, have copies sent to another person or organization, request restrictions on how their PHI is used and disclosed, receive confidential communications, receive a report of certain disclosures of their PHI, and request amendments to their information. The privacy notice must also let residents know how to file a complaint with the entity or with the Office for Civil Rights.

- Adopt written privacy procedures that define who has access to protected information, how the entity will use the information, and when the entity might disclose the information to others.

- Train employees in the privacy procedures.

- Implement safeguards to prevent intentional or accidental misuse of PHI.

- Appoint an individual to make sure that employees follow the privacy procedures.

- Give an accounting of instances where the entity has disclosed PHI for purposes other than treatment, payment, or healthcare operations.

Information Protected Under HIPAA

The privacy protections of HIPAA apply to PHI, which is information:

- Created or received by a covered entity or an employer that relates to a person's past, present, or future health condition, health treatment, or payment for healthcare services

- That could identify an individual, such as name, address, telephone number, date of birth, diagnosis, medical record number, Social Security number, employer, position, or other identifying data

PHI can be in any format: paper, electronic, or oral. The most common example of PHI is the resident record.

Protecting Resident Records

Although the HIPAA Privacy Rule specifies that obtaining a patient's consent is optional when a covered entity discloses PHI to another party for treatment, payment, and healthcare operations (e.g., a resident's doctor shares PHI with a second doctor who can provide valuable input on care strategies), some facilities may choose to implement policies that require this additional safeguard. These expectations may direct the resident to sign a consent form prior to disclosure, though the HIPAA Privacy Rule states that the specifics of this process are at the discretion of the covered entity.

However, there is much less flexibility if a facility wants to disclose a resident's PHI for a purpose other than providing care. In such cases, it needs that person's specific authorization.

Only authorized personnel should enter confidential medical information into a computer-based resident record. Computer systems should be password protected to help guard against unauthorized access and use.

What is the difference between consent and authorization?

- To give **consent,** a resident must sign a consent form. The resident needs to sign the consent only one time for each provider. The consent will apply whenever that provider discloses the person's PHI for purposes of providing healthcare.

- Specific **authorization** is required when a covered entity wants to use or disclose a person's PHI for purposes not related to providing healthcare. The person must sign an authorization form for each specific instance.

May a person see his or her personal PHI and make changes?

A covered entity must allow a person to view and photocopy his or her PHI if that person submits a request. The organization may charge the person for copies of these records.

- In a few special circumstances, such as when a covered entity has compiled information for use in a civil, criminal, or administrative proceeding, that entity does not have to give a person access to his or her PHI.

- A covered entity may deny a person access to his or her PHI if the entity has reason to believe that access would create a risk of danger to that person's health.

- If a person believes that his or her PHI contains information that is incorrect, the person may ask the covered entity to make changes. The covered entity may deny the request if they believe the current information is accurate and complete, or if they did not create the information.

Exceptions to the HIPAA Privacy Rule

The HIPAA Privacy Rule permits covered entities to disclose a person's healthcare information without that person's specific authorization in certain situations, depending upon state or local law, such as:

- Emergencies

- Public health needs (such as infectious-disease registries)

- Mandatory reporting of child or elder abuse and neglect

- Judicial and administrative proceedings

- When there are substantial communication barriers

If there is no state or local law specifically requiring disclosure of information in the instances listed above, covered entities are required to use "professional judgment" in deciding whether to disclose information and how much to disclose.

Protection of Resident Privacy and Confidentiality

Quality resident care requires communication between care workers. Computers, the Internet, emails, and faxes make it easier to share resident records. However, this information is then often readily available to anyone who walks by the fax machine or logs on to the computer. Some people fear that the exposure of their PHI could result in job discrimination, personal embarrassment, or the loss or denial of health insurance.

Important HIPAA considerations

Remember that confidentiality of information, whether in written, electronic, or verbal form, is a priority. Confidentiality should extend to all health information.

Handle all resident records as confidential at all times. Do not leave them open where unauthorized persons can see them.

Learn the safeguards your organization requires for the use, disclosure, and storage of PHI. Know your organization's privacy policies and procedures.

Remember that individuals have the right to decide and to know who may have access to their health information and under what circumstances they may have it.

Discuss resident information in a private place so others cannot overhear the conversation.

Accompany all faxed information with a cover sheet marked "Confidential."

Remove any detailed identifying information when emailing information about a resident. For example, refer to the resident by initials or by the internal resident number, instead of by full name.

Remember that only authorized personnel should enter confidential medical information into a computer-based resident record. Computer systems should be password protected to help guard against unauthorized access and use.

Use only objective, precise language when documenting in the resident record. Avoid casual remarks and abbreviations that might be misunderstood.

Always take the utmost care to protect the privacy and confidentiality of all health information. Be aware of who is around you while you are working and do not allow unauthorized people to hear or see PHI.

Think about how you would want your PHI treated, and give your residents that much protection and more.

Always obtain permission from residents before sharing PHI with their family or friends.

Do not share information you learned about a resident while performing your job with the resident's family or friends.

Mobile and online considerations

Properly managing your electronic passwords, preventing the spread of computer viruses, logging off your computer, protecting your tablet and smartphone (if used for resident care), and being aware of and responsible for any resident information taken or accessed off-site are important ways you can contribute to information security. You should know and understand your facility's policies on which devices can be used for work and in what manner.

Remember that HIPAA applies to *all* communication. This includes any and all types of social media: Facebook, Twitter, LinkedIn, Instagram, text, etc., are no places to share any kind of resident information. This includes text and pictures.

Before quickly sharing information you might think is innocent on your smartphone at lunch, realize that if you are in any way identifying a resident's health information, you could find yourself in serious trouble.

Consequences

Covered entities are required to have a sanctions policy covering employees and other workforce members who violate HIPAA privacy and security regulations. Violating HIPAA's Privacy, Security, or Breach Notification Rules can result in civil or criminal penalties for an individual or group of individuals, and the facility will also encounter severe consequences.

HIPAA

Test

Name _____ Date _____ Score _____

1. HIPAA stands for:

   a. Health Inclusion Portability and Assurance Act

   b. Health Information Protection and Assurances Act

   c. Health Identification Protection and Accountability Act

   d. Health Insurance Portability and Accountability Act

2. _____ refers to preventing someone from hearing or seeing a person's private health records and information unless he or she has the proper authorization.

   a. Privacy

   b. Confidentiality

   c. Security

   d. None of the above

3. HMOs are not considered "covered entities" under HIPAA. True or False

4. The resident record is included in the protected health information (PHI). True or False

5. If a frontline staff member wants to disclose a person's PHI for purposes of providing healthcare, the provider needs to obtain the person's _____.

   a. electronic health record

   b. authorization

   c. consent

   d. None of the above

6. A covered entity must allow a person to view and photocopy his or her PHI if that person submits a request. True or False

7. Skilled nursing facilities and other covered entities are required to do all of the following *except*_____.

a. notify residents of their privacy rights

b. maintain all residents' printed records under lock and key

c. train employees so that they are fully aware of the privacy procedures

d. implement safeguards to prevent intentional or accidental misuse of PHI

8. A cover sheet marked "Confidential" should accompany all faxed information. True or False

9. Even if frontline staff are certain that the person they are speaking with is permitted to hear certain information, they should not discuss a resident's PHI _____.

a. on Facebook

b. at parties

c. in restrooms of public buildings

d. All of the above

10. If uncertain as to whether a family member needs to know information about a resident, staff members should _____.

a. consult with other frontline staff

b. notify the resident

c. check with their supervisor

d. ask the family member whether they are permitted to know the information

CERTIFICATE OF COMPLETION

I hereby certify that

_____

has successfully completed the in-Service

_____

HIPAA

_____
Signature

18

Incontinence and Constipation

Teaching Plan

To use this lesson for self-study, the learner should read the material, do the activity, and take the test. For group study, the leader may give each learner a copy of the learning guide and follow this teaching plan to conduct the lesson. Certificates may be copied for everyone who completes the lesson.

This lesson discusses urinary incontinence, bowel incontinence, and constipation. The Agency for Healthcare Policy and Research (AHCPR) and the American Society of Colon and Rectal Surgeons provided much of the information presented here. The AHCPR's urinary incontinence guidelines are part of the recommended or required standards for care facilities in many states. You and your staff can make a big difference in your residents' lives by helping them overcome incontinence and constipation through the use of these guidelines.

Learning objectives

After this lesson, participants should be able to:

- Know the causes of common urinary and bowel elimination problems

- State the best ways to help residents with these problems

- Understand various behavioral, nutritional, and care interventions for urinary and bowel incontinence and constipation

Lesson activities

1. Ask your learners, "How many of you think that being unable to control your bladder or your bowels is a normal part of aging?" This is a common misconception, and it is likely that many of your learners will agree that your statement is true. Then ask, "Do you think anything can be done to improve the problem in older people?" Many times we just accept there is nothing that can be done for these conditions except to wear protective clothing. However, there are things that can be done by caregivers that can help control these problems, thereby improving the resident's quality of life.

2. Ask your learners to study the learning guide. Review the uses of scheduled toileting, prompted voiding, and habit training. Discuss how you could use these techniques with your residents.

3. Go over the material in the learning guide. Discuss dietary management and how your workers can assist residents with diet, habit training, exercises, toileting, and skin care.

4. If you will use it, go over the sample bladder record, or review the one already in use in your facility.

Conclusion

Have participants take the test. Review the answers together. Award certificates to those who answer 70% of the test questions correctly.

Test answers

1. a	2. b	3. a	4. c	5. True
6. False	7. True	8. True	9. True	10. True

Incontinence and Constipation

Learning Guide

Contents:

- What Causes Urinary Incontinence (UI)?

- What Are the Symptoms of UI?

- What Can You Do to Help a Resident With UI?

- Retraining Your Bladder: Information for Caregivers/Residents

    - Scheduled toileting

    - Prompted voiding

    - Habit training

    - Things to remember

    - Other ways to help residents with UI

- What Causes Bowel Incontinence?

    - What can you do to help a resident with bowel incontinence?

    - What causes constipation?

    - What can you do to help a resident with constipation?

- Dietary Management for Urinary Incontinence

- Dietary Management for Bowel Incontinence and Constipation

- Bowel Retraining for Bowel Incontinence and Constipation

    - Food sensitivities

    - Habit training

    - Exercises

What Causes Urinary Incontinence (UI)?

People who cannot control when or where they urinate suffer from UI. There are things that can be done to improve this condition, but it is important to know what the cause is so the right care and treatment can be given. This condition is not the person's fault, and it is not a necessary or normal part of growing older. It is not caused by laziness or meanness. UI is a health problem with a number of possible causes. Some of the most common causes include:

- Urinary tract infections (UTI)

- Confusion and forgetfulness

- Muscle weakness

- Vaginal problems (in women)

- Prostate problems (in men)

- Medication reactions

- Problems with clothing

- Trouble getting to the bathroom

- Constipation

What Are the Symptoms of UI?

Any residents who ever wet the bed or themselves, leak urine on the way to the bathroom, or have to use protective pads or padded briefs are suffering from UI. If you notice a resident, a bed, or a room that has urine stains or a urine odor, then you know the resident needs help with this condition. However, you probably don't know what kind of UI the resident might have. You can often determine this by watching the resident closely and keeping track of his or her urinating habits on a bladder record. There is an example included with this learning guide. It shows regular daily habits as well as accidents. Keeping a bladder record is an excellent way to get information about a resident's UI so ways can be found to treat it.

There are three different types of UI:

1. **Urge incontinence** may cause people to leak urine on their way to the bathroom, after they drink just a little bit of liquid, or as soon as they feel the urge to go.

2. **Stress incontinence** may cause urine to leak when people sneeze, cough, or laugh or when they exercise or move a certain way (getting out of bed, up from a chair, walking, lifting). This type of UI is common in women.

3. **Overflow incontinence** causes people to feel they need to urinate again right after going, to feel as though they never totally empty the bladder, or to pass small amounts of urine without feeling any need to go. It may be a sign of prostate problems in men.

What Can You Do to Help a Resident With UI?

Your first responsibility is to report UI to your supervisor, the nurse, or the resident's doctor, who will begin the assessment and care plan process. A doctor or nurse should check a resident with UI, and your observations about the resident, such as a those kept on bladder record, will help them determine the cause and type of UI (Figure 18.1).

Figure 18.1 Sample Bladder Record

NAME: _____

DATE: _____

INSTRUCTIONS: Place a check in the appropriate column next to the time you urinated in the toilet or when an **incontinence** episode occurred. Note the reason for the **incontinence** and describe your liquid intake (for example, coffee, water) and estimate the amount (for example, one cup).

Time interval	No incontinence	Small incontinence episode	Large incontinence episode	Reason for incontinence episode	Type/amount of liquid intake
6–8 a.m.					
8–10 a.m.					
10 a.m.–noon					
Noon–2 p.m.					
2–4 p.m.					
4–6 p.m.					
6–8 p.m.					
8–10 p.m.					
10 p.m.–midnight					
Overnight					
No. of pads used today:			No. of episodes:		

Comments: _____

The three treatments for UI are:

1. Medicine.

2. Surgery.

3. Behavioral treatments. These treatments help people control their urine and use the toilet at the right time. They work well for residents who have problems getting to the bathroom or are not able to tell you when they need to urinate. We will discuss three behavioral treatments for UI that you can assist with:

   • Scheduled toileting

   • Prompted voiding

   • Habit training

Retraining Your Bladder: Information for Caregivers/Residents

It is possible to retrain your bladder if you have trouble controlling your urine flow.

First, keep a record of your normal drinking and urinating patterns. Next, schedule your urination at regular intervals and begin to gradually increase the amount of time between urinating. Eventually, you want to train yourself to urinate no more than once every three to four hours.

Follow these steps:

1. Keep a record—write everything down on the bladder record.

2. Schedule urination.

   a. Begin by going to the bathroom every hour or two, whether or not you feel the need.

   b. If you feel the need to urinate more often than that, practice tightening your pelvic muscles to hold the urine. Relax, concentrate, and breathe slowly and deeply until the urge decreases or goes away.

   c. After the urge goes away, wait a few minutes, then go to the bathroom and urinate, even if the urge has passed. Don't wait for the next urge, because it may be difficult to control.

   d. After a week of this kind of training, if you are able to wait for two or three minutes easily, increase the waiting time (between feeling the urge and using the bathroom) to five minutes and then to 10 minutes.

e. Work toward intervals of three or four hours between urination. If you have an accident, don't let it discourage you. Just keep trying.

3. Helpful hints:

a. Be sure you can reach your bathroom or commode easily.

b. Walk to the bathroom slowly.

c. Urinate just before going to bed.

d. Set an alarm clock to remind you when to use the toilet. Do this in the daytime and also once or twice at night.

e. Drink eight to 10 glasses of fluid every day to prevent urinary tract infections and constipation.

f. Avoid caffeine drinks and alcoholic beverages.

g. Do your Kegel exercises to increase bladder tone (ask the nurse to teach you how).

Scheduled toileting

Use scheduled toileting for residents who can't get out of bed or can't get to the bathroom alone. To do this treatment, assist the resident to the bathroom every two to four hours on a regular schedule. If the resident has dementia, he or she may need your assistance with cues to find the location of toilets.

Prompted voiding

Use prompted voiding for residents who know when they have a full bladder but do not ask to go to the bathroom. To do this treatment:

1. Check the resident often for wetness.

2. Ask "Do you want to use the toilet?"

3. Help the resident to the toilet.

4. Praise the resident for being dry.

5. Tell the resident when you will come back to take him or her to the bathroom again.

Habit training

Use habit training for residents that tend to urinate at about the same time every day. To do this:

- Watch the resident to learn what times he or she urinates. A bladder record can help you do this.

- Take the resident to the bathroom at those times every day.

- Praise the resident for being dry and using the toilet.

Things to remember

For all behavioral treatments, remember the following things:

- Be patient. These treatments take time.

- Treat the resident as an adult.

- Do not rush the resident.

- Give the resident plenty of time to completely empty his or her bladder.

- Give privacy by closing the door, even if you must stay in the bathroom.

- NEVER yell or be angry with the resident if he or she is wet. Say, "You can try again next time."

- Respect dignity and confidentiality.

Other ways to help residents with UI

- Pelvic exercises can make muscles around the bladder stronger and help with UI. These are called Kegel exercises, and to do them the person tightens the pelvic muscles that stop and start the flow of urine. The muscles should be squeezed tightly for a few seconds and then released, up to 10 times at one sitting, four times every day. Then, whenever the person feels that urine might leak, he or she tightens those same muscles and prevents urine from leaking.

- People that can't get out of bed or can't get to the bathroom for some reason may need to use a bedpan, urinal, or bedside commode. These articles, if needed, should be kept by the bed.

- If a resident uses a wheelchair, walker, or cane to get to the bathroom, you can help by keeping the item near the bed, keeping the path to the bathroom clear and well lit, and answering calls for assistance as soon as possible.

- Encourage the resident to wear clothes that are easy to remove and have simple fasteners.

- If a resident needs to wear special pads or clothing to help keep the skin dry, they should be changed often. Use soft pads and clothing, keep them wrinkle-free, keep the skin clean and dry, and use protective skin creams if allowed. Remember that wet skin can develop sores and rashes.

- If the resident wets the bed at night, it might be helpful to restrict evening liquids, but you should only do this if a doctor or nurse orders it. This is usually done in the three hours before bedtime. The resident should use the bathroom just before going to bed.

- Some residents need to use a urinary catheter, which is a tube inserted into the bladder by a doctor or nurse. It drains urine into a bag. Sometimes men use a condom catheter that fits over the penis. Catheters can cause infections, and condom catheters that are too tight can be harmful. Catheters should be checked often. They are not recommended for most incontinence problems.

What Causes Bowel Incontinence?

People who cannot control when or where they pass gas or stool suffer from bowel incontinence. There are things that can be done to improve this condition, but it is important to know what the cause is so the right care and treatment can be given. This condition is not the person's fault, and it is not a necessary part of growing older. It is a health problem that is not caused by laziness or bad behavior.

Some of the most common causes include:

- Incorrect diet or fluid intake

- Confusion and forgetfulness

- Muscle injury or weakness (affecting the anal muscles)

- Nerve injury

- Medication reactions or laxative abuse

- Trouble getting to the bathroom

- Constipation or impaction

- Diarrhea

What can you do to help a resident with bowel incontinence?

Your first responsibility is to report episodes of bowel incontinence to your supervisor, the nurse, or the resident's doctor. A doctor or nurse should check the resident, and your observations may help them determine the cause of the problem. Treatments for bowel incontinence include:

- Medicine

- Surgery

- Dietary management

- Bowel management and retraining, with establishment of a habit regimen

- Biofeedback

Two of these treatments involve the care you provide: diet management and bowel retraining. These treatments are the same as those used to help people with constipation, so we will discuss the treatments together after examining the issue of constipation.

What causes constipation?

People usually say they are constipated when they are having infrequent bowel movements, but constipation is also used to refer to a sense of bloating or intestinal fullness, a decrease in the amount of stool, the need to strain to have a bowel movement, or the need to use laxatives, suppositories, or enemas to maintain regular bowel movements. It is normal for most people to have bowel movements anywhere from three times per day to three times per week, but some people may go a week or longer without discomfort or harmful effects. Many things can cause constipation, but the most common causes include:

- Inadequate fiber and fluid intake

- Inactivity or a sedentary lifestyle

- Change in routine

- Abnormal growths or diseases

- Damaged or injured muscles (sometimes from repeatedly ignoring the urge to go)

- Medication side effects and laxative abuse (it is NOT necessary to have a bowel movement every day)

Constipation may be diagnosed if movements occur fewer than three times weekly on an ongoing basis.

What can you do to help a resident with constipation?

Your first responsibility is to report a resident's constipation problems to your supervisor, the nurse, or the resident's doctor. A doctor or nurse should check the resident, and your observations may help them determine the cause of the problem. Treatments for constipation include:

1. Medicine

2. Surgery

3. Dietary management

4. Bowel management and retraining, with establishment of a habit regimen

Two of these treatments involve the care you provide: diet management and bowel retraining.

Dietary Management for Urinary Incontinence

While there is no dietary treatment for urinary incontinence, some foods and drinks can irritate the bladder, such as sugar, chocolate, citrus fruits (oranges, grapefruits, lemons, limes), alcohol, grape juice, and caffeinated drinks like coffee, tea, and cola. Residents with UI could try eliminating these foods and beverages from their diet and determine whether the condition improves.

Dietary Management for Bowel Incontinence and Constipation

The average American diet contains 10 to 15 grams of fiber per day. The amount of fiber recommended for good bowel function is 25 to 30 grams per day, plus 60 to 80 ounces of fluid. Look at the table below to get an idea of the amount of fiber in different foods. Most people can successfully treat their bowel irregularities, both incontinence and constipation, by adding high-fiber foods to their diets, along with increasing fluid intake to desired levels. Increase dietary fiber slowly to give the bowel time to adjust.

People with diverticulosis or diverticulitis should not consume a high-fiber diet. Figure 18.2 shows alternatives to a high fiber diet.

Figure 18.2 High-Fiber Diet Alternatives

Type of Food	Lower-Fiber Foods	Fiber grams	Higher-Fiber Alternatives	Fiber grams
Breads	White bread, 1 slice	0.50	Whole wheat bread, 1 slice	2.11
Cereals	Corn flakes, 1 oz.	0.45	Oat bran cereal, 1 oz.	4.06
Rice	White rice, ½ cup	1.42	Brown rice, ½ cup	5.27
Vegetables	Lettuce, ½ cup raw	0.24	Green peas, ½ cup	3.36
Beans	Green beans, ½ cup	1.89	Pinto beans, ½ cup	5.93
Fresh Fruits	Banana, 1 medium	2.19	Blackberries, 1 cup	7.20

Bowel Retraining for Bowel Incontinence and Constipation

Food sensitivities

Some people are sensitive to, or even allergic to, certain foods, which can cause them constipation or diarrhea. Dairy products such as milk and cheese, wheat products such as bread, and foods containing chocolate are some of the more common problem foods. A physician should evaluate a resident who seems to have particular food sensitivities.

Habit training

Habit training means designating a specific time each day to have a bowel movement. Keep a record of the resident's bowel habits, just as you do with a bladder record. If a pattern develops, that pattern can be used to set up a habit regimen that will reinforce a scheduled time each day to have a bowel movement. If no pattern can be seen in the resident's bowel activities, then a regimen can be established by selecting a convenient time each day, or even three times per day in the case of someone with bowel incontinence, for the resident to try to have a bowel movement. Be sure to help the resident stick with this schedule, even when he or she does not feel the need to go. Over time, the body will develop a habit that conforms to the scheduled routine.

Exercises

The Kegel exercises that are used to prevent urinary incontinence can be slightly modified to strengthen the anal muscles that control the outflow of stool. To do them, the person tightens the muscles around the rectum. The muscles should be squeezed tightly for a few seconds and then released, up to 10 times at one sitting, four times every day.

Incontinence and Constipation

Test

Name _____ Date _____ Score _____

Directions: Circle the best answer.

1. What are some causes of both bowel and urinary incontinence?

    a. Muscle weakness, confusion, or medication reactions

    b. Laziness, poor manners, or meanness

    c. Stupidity, uncooperativeness, and sloppiness

2. Scheduled toileting, prompted voiding, and habit training are _____.

    a. not encouraged by physicians, nurses, or state regulations

    b. planned interventions that the nursing assistant will participate in

    c. recommended behavioral treatments for urinary incontinence

    d. too time-consuming to be practical

3. For the best bowel function, we should consume how much dietary fiber every day?

    a. 10 to 15 grams

    b. 25 to 30 grams

    c. 45 to 50 grams

4. Kegel exercises are done by _____.

    a. circling the ankles around and around and then up and down

    b. lowering the chin to the chest, then turning the head side to side

    c. tightening the pelvic muscles that control the flow of urine

5. Urinary catheters are often recommended to treat urinary incontinence. True or False

6. Bowel retraining and behavioral treatments for urinary incontinence usually work quickly, fixing the problem within a week or less. True or False

7. Most fruits and beans contain higher dietary fiber than white breads and rice. True or False

8. It is important to keep residents with urinary or bowel incontinence clean and dry so their skin is protected from developing sores. True or False

9. Scheduled training, prompted voiding, and habit training can be used to help both urinary and bowel incontinence. True or False

10. Stress incontinence might cause urine to leak when someone sneezes or laughs. True or False

CERTIFICATE OF COMPLETION

I hereby certify that

_____

has successfully completed the in-Service

Incontinence and Constipation

_____
Signature

19

Infection Control: Guidelines for Standard and Additional Precautions

Teaching Plan

To use this lesson for self-study, the learner should read the material, do the activity, and take the test. For group study, the leader may give each learner a copy of the learning guide and follow this teaching plan to conduct the lesson. Certificates may be copied for everyone who completes the lesson.

Learning objectives

After this lesson, participants should be able to:

- Understand the four disease transmission categories

- Understand standard precautions and how and when they should be used

- Understand additional precautions and how and when they should be used

- Apply this understanding at work

Lesson activities

Begin by asking the learners to tell you what they already know about universal precautions or standard precautions. Ask if any learner can give an example of an incident that taught him or her the importance of following infection control guidelines. Have your own example ready as an illustration if no one volunteers.

Explain the content in the lesson overview and list the learning goals, using a blackboard, grease board, or flip chart if available.

Section 1: Disease transmission

1. Explain that diseases are transmitted from one person to another by four basic methods. Ask your learners to refer to the learning guide and tell you what those methods are.

2. Briefly discuss each of the four methods of disease transmission, allowing for input and questions.

3. Ask your learners to fill out the matching quiz in the learning guide. Discuss the answers: 1. C; 2. A; 3. D; 4. B.

Matching quiz

What kinds of germs are being spread in the following cases? Match the activity with the type of transmission by writing "A," "B," "C," or "D." (for Airborne, Bloodborne, Contact, or Droplet)

1. Changing the bed linens of a resident with a rash, without wearing gloves. _____

2. Keeping a fan blowing and the door open when a resident has shingles. _____

3. A resident who has a cold sneezes on others sitting at her table. _____

4. Wipe urine off the floor without gloves. _____

Section 2: Standard precautions

1. Explain that standard precautions are basic infection control guidelines. They should be used at all times as you perform your work. They protect us and others from diseases that are spread by bloodborne transmission.

2. Indicate the list of standard precautions on the handout. Ask learners to read parts of the list to the group.

3. Demonstrate proper hand washing with these three rules:

   - Use friction (rub hands together)

   - Wash for 10 seconds (sing "Happy Birthday" while washing; it takes 10 seconds to sing)

   - Use soap and water (disinfectant gels are not adequate)

4. Show your learners how to use standard precautions when using and cleaning resident care equipment—refer to the learning guide and your facility's procedures for specifics.

5. Allow for comments and discussion.

Section 3: Additional precautions

1. Review the additional precautions for the three types of transmission included in the learning guide

2. Ask the learners for examples of when these precautions should be used

Conclusion

Have participants take the test. Review the answers together. Award certificates to those who answer 70% of the test questions correctly.

Test answers

1. c	2. b	3. a	4. d	5. d
6. False	7. airborne, bloodborne, contact, droplet	8. wash hands; wear gloves; wear gown, mask, goggles (if risk of getting splashed); keep everything clean	9. False	10. True

Infection Control: Guidelines for Standard and Additional Precautions

Learning Guide

Contents:

- Disease Transmission

    - **A**—Airborne transmission

    - **B**—Bloodborne transmission

    - **C**—Contact transmission

    - **D**—Droplet transmission

- Standard Precautions

    - Standard precautions for handling objects

- Additional Precautions

Disease Transmission

There are four ways diseases are transmitted, or passed around.

A—Airborne transmission

Airborne germs can travel long distances through the air and are breathed in by people.

Examples of diseases caused by airborne germs are tuberculosis, chickenpox, influenza, and certain types of pneumonia.

B—Bloodborne transmission

If the blood of an infected person somehow comes in contact with the bloodstream of another person, germs can travel from the infected person into the other person's bloodstream. Blood and bloodborne germs are sometimes present in other body fluids, such as urine, feces, saliva, and vomit. Examples of diseases caused by bloodborne germs are HIV/AIDS and viral hepatitis.

C—Contact transmission

Touching certain germs can cause the spread of disease. Sometimes you touch an infected person, having direct contact with the germ. Sometimes you touch an object that has been handled by an infected person, having indirect contact with the germ. Examples of diseases caused by contact germs are pink eye, scabies, wound infections, and methicillin-resistant *Staphylococcus aureus*.

D—Droplet transmission

Some germs can only travel short distances through the air, usually not more than three feet. Sneezing, coughing, and talking can spread these germs. Examples of diseases caused by droplet germs are flu and pneumonia.

Standard Precautions

You should wash you hands:

- After touching blood, body fluids, or objects contaminated by blood or body fluids. Do this even if you were wearing gloves.

- After removing gloves.

- Between each resident's care.

- Before and after personal bathroom use or eating.

Wear gloves:

- Whenever you touch blood, body fluids, or contaminated objects.

- Before touching a resident's broken skin or mucous membranes (mouth, nose); put on clean gloves.

- Change gloves between tasks and between each resident's care. Dirty gloves spread germs, just like dirty hands!

- Do not wear gloves in the hallway unless there is an emergency in the hall. Wearing gloves you donned to use in the bedroom into the hall may cause contamination.

Wear a gown, mask, and goggles:

- If you know you might get splashed with blood or body fluids. Use a waterproof gown if you might get heavily splashed.

- Remove dirty protective clothing as soon as you can, and wash your hands afterward.

As a last precaution, keep everything clean and clean up spills as soon as possible.

Use standard precautions for all resident care. This is basic infection control for bloodborne diseases—to protect you and your residents.

Standard precautions for handling objects

- Clean any equipment that has been used by one resident before giving it to another resident. Follow your facility's cleaning procedures.

- Use disposable equipment only once.

- Dirty linens should be rolled, not shaken, and should be held away from your body. Linens soiled with body fluids can be washed with other laundry, using your facility's procedures.

- No special precautions are needed for dishes or silverware. Normal dish soap and hot water (water temperature must be hot enough to meet state requirements) will kill germs.

- Change cleaning rags and sponges frequently.

- Stethoscopes, blood pressure cuffs, and thermometers should be cleaned between each use, using your facility's procedures.

- Dispose of dangerous waste, such as razors or needles, VERY CAREFULLY. Needles and other sharp devices should go into clearly marked, punctureproof containers, NOT the regular trash container! Nurses are taught that they DO NOT RECAP used needles. Instead, they put them in the punctureproof container without the cap on.

- Trash that is contaminated with germs, such as wound dressings, should be disposed of according to your facility's procedures.

- Any container marked "Biohazard" is only for discarding contaminated waste—don't remove anything from it! If you must handle anything in the container, always use gloves. Don't put your hand in anything that contains needles or other sharp objects.

- Check your gloves and other protective clothing frequently. If you see tears or holes in your gloves, remove them, wash your hands, and apply clean gloves.

TIP: Don't touch your face (nose, mouth, eyes) when giving resident care, unless you remove your gloves and wash your hands first. Protect yourself from infection.

Additional Precautions

Use additional precautions in addition to standard precautions when a resident has an illness requiring extra infection control measures. If you know that a resident has a disease that is spread in one of the following ways, use these extra precautions:

- Airborne:

    - The resident should have a private room, possibly one with a special air filter.

    - Keep the resident's room door closed.

    - Wear a mask. If the resident has, or might have, tuberculosis, wear a special respiratory mask (ask your supervisor). A regular mask will not protect you.

    - Remind the resident to cover the nose and mouth when coughing or sneezing.

    - Ask the resident to wear a mask if he or she wants or needs to be around others.

- Contact:

    - The resident should be in a private room, but the door may stay open.

    - Put gloves on before entering the room.

    - Change gloves after touching a contaminated object (bed linens, clothes, wound dressings).

    - Remove gloves right before leaving the room. Don't touch anything else until you wash your hands. Wash your hands ASAP!

    - Wear a gown in the room if the resident has drainage, has diarrhea, or is incontinent. Remove the gown right before leaving the room.

    - Use a disinfectant to clean stethoscopes, blood pressure cuffs, or any other equipment used on the infected resident.

- Droplet:

    - The resident should be in a private room, but the door may stay open.

    - Wear a mask when working close to the resident (within three feet).

    - Ask the resident to wear a mask if he or she wants or needs to be around others.

Hand washing rule: Rub hands together with soap and running water for at least 10 seconds. Germicidal gels are not enough!

Infection Control: Guidelines for Standard and Additional Precautions

Test

Name _____ Date _____ Score _____

Directions: Circle the correct answer.

1. If a resident has the flu, you should use the following additional precautions:

    a. No additional precautions are necessary

    b. Wear a mask, gown, gloves, and goggles whenever you are in the resident's room

    c. Wear a mask when working close to the resident

    d. Isolate the resident from all contact with others

2. You should use standard precautions when _____.

    a. a resident appears to be sick

    b. doing all resident care

    c. you are sick

    d. you know the resident has AIDS or hepatitis

3. When disposing of a needle or other sharp object, always _____.

    a. place it carefully in a biohazard punctureproof container without touching the sharp end

    b. recap it very carefully

    c. leave it alone and tell your supervisor

4. When changing a bed or handling linens, the correct standard-precautions procedure is to
   _____.

   a. shake out the linens to remove any objects or dirt

   b. place the used linens on the floor or a table

   c. wash linens soiled with body fluids separately from other laundry

   d. roll the dirty linens up and hold them away from you until they can be placed in a
   laundry bag

5. If a resident has an infected wound, use the following additional precautions:

   a. Standard precautions are good enough

   b. Wear a gown, gloves, mask, and goggles while in the resident's room

   c. The resident should not go to the dining room until the wound is healed

   d. Put gloves on before entering the resident's room and remove them right before leaving

6. Residents may share walkers, wheelchairs, and other equipment without worrying about
   cleaning it between residents. True or False

7. List the four types of disease transmission:

   _____

   _____

   _____

   _____

8. List the four basic rules of standard precautions:

    _____

    _____

    _____

    _____

9. Standard precautions protect only against airborne diseases. For bloodborne, contact, and droplet transmission, additional precautions must be used. True   or   False

10. Airborne germs, like tuberculosis, can travel long distances through the air. True   or   False

CERTIFICATE OF COMPLETION

I hereby certify that

_____

has successfully completed the in-Service

Infection Control

_____

Signature

20

Kidney Disease

Teaching Plan

To use this lesson for self-study, the learner should read the material, do the activity, and take the test. For group study, the leader may give each learner a copy of the learning guide and follow this teaching plan to conduct the lesson. Certificates may be copied for everyone who completes the lesson.

Learning objectives

After this lesson, participants should be able to:

- State the function of the kidney

- Define kidney disease

- Identity tests and abnormal test results for kidney function

- Recognize prevention and treatment strategies

- Understand conditions related to kidney disease

Lesson activities

1. What are some strategies you can use to help educate your residents on the risk factors related to kidney disease? As a group, create a list of tips and resources you can use and/or give to residents to help inform them about the condition.

2. Play Kidney Disease BINGO by using Figure 20.1. Directions are included in the figure.

The lesson

Review the material in the lesson with participants. Allow for discussion.

Conclusion

Have participants take the test. Review the answers together. Award certificates to those who answer 70% of the test questions correctly.

Test answers

1. d	2. a	3. c	4. d	5. True
6. b	7. c	8. a and c	9. False	10. d

Kidney Disease

Learning Guide

Contents:

- Introduction

- Understanding Kidney Disease

- Help Keep Residents Healthy

  - Symptoms and diagnosis

  - Tests for kidney disease

  - Kidney failure

  - Early treatment

  - Medications

  - Treatment for later stages

  - Age and kidney function

  - Additional conditions

Introduction

The kidney is a bean-shaped organ that is about the size of a fist. Everyone has two kidneys, which are located in the middle of the back, on the left and right of the spine, just below your rib cage.

The main function of the kidneys is to filter the blood, removing wastes, minerals, and excess water to create urine. These organs also help control blood pressure and produce hormones that the body needs to stay healthy. When the kidneys are damaged, however, wastes can build up within the body, and this deterioration in function is known as kidney disease.

Without significant early symptoms, kidney disease is impossible to diagnose without completing blood and/or urine testing. Unfortunately, many sufferers do not complete these tests until the disease has already caused significant damage to their kidneys, affecting their overall health. Understanding the risk factors for kidney disease is a vital step in preventing the disease and getting early diagnosis and treatment.

Without intervention, kidney disease can progress into kidney failure, which may ultimately lead to death. In this lesson, you will learn about the risk factors and signs of kidney disease. You will read about the different urine and blood testing used for diagnosis of the condition. You will also explore the different treatment options available for residents who are in the various stages of kidney disease, including dialysis and kidney transplant.

Understanding Kidney Disease

Kidney disease is the result of damaged kidneys that can no longer remove wastes and excess water from the blood as they should. According to the Centers for Disease Control and Prevention, more than 20 million Americans (about 10% of adults in the United States) may have kidney disease.

The main risk factors for developing kidney disease are:

- Diabetes

- High blood pressure

- Cardiovascular disease

- A family history of kidney failure

Every kidney contains around 1 million filtering units composed of blood vessels, known as glomeruli. Conditions such as diabetes and high blood pressure can damage these blood vessels, but this damage often occurs slowly, over many years. This gradual deterioration is called chronic kidney disease. As glomeruli are damaged, kidneys become less effective at maintaining proper health.

Help Keep Residents Healthy

Help residents at risk for kidney disease keep their kidneys healthy with the following steps:

- Ensure that residents are informed and educated about blood and urine testing for kidney disease

- Monitor and manage conditions such as diabetes, high blood pressure, high cholesterol, and heart disease

- Encourage a healthy diet with fresh fruits, vegetables, whole grains, low-fat dairy foods, and limited salt

- Encourage physical activity and weight loss, as appropriate

- Assist and educate residents in taking medications as prescribed by their physician

Following these steps and limiting risk factors can delay or even prevent kidney failure.

Symptoms and diagnosis

Kidney disease is often called a "silent" disease, because most people have no symptoms with early kidney disease. Unfortunately, it is possible for those with kidney disease to "feel fine" until the kidneys have almost completely stopped working.

Blood and urine tests are the only way to check for kidney damage or measure kidney function. If a resident has any of the risk factors outlined above, testing for kidney disease may be recommended.

Tests for kidney disease

The sooner kidney disease is diagnosed, the sooner proper treatment can be implemented to delay or prevent kidney failure. Helping residents understand the tests that are available is vital for prevention and treatment.

Blood testing for kidney disease checks estimated glomerular filtration rate (eGFR)—a measure of how much blood the kidneys filter each minute. This test will indicate how well the kidneys are working. The results are as follows:

- An eGFR of 60 or higher is in the normal range

- An eGFR below 60 may indicate kidney disease, but because GFR decreases as people age, other information may be needed to formally diagnose kidney disease

- An eGFR of 15 or lower may indicate kidney failure

Although eGFR cannot be increased, proper intervention may keep it from dropping further.

The urine test will uncover albumin, a type of protein, in your urine. While a healthy kidney will not let albumin pass into the urine, a damaged kidney may.

Help limit confusion during kidney testing by informing residents of the different names and terms associated with urine testing for kidney disease. Residents may be told that they are being screened for "proteinuria," "albuminuria," or "microalbuminuria." Or they could be told that their "urine albumin-to-creatinine ratio" is being measured. This all refers to the same type of testing.

- A urine albumin result below 30 is normal

- A urine albumin result above 30 is abnormal and may indicate kidney disease

Note that a *low* number for urine albumin is better, while a *higher* number for eGFR is better.

Kidney failure

Kidney disease can get worse over time, ultimately leading to kidney failure. Kidney failure is advanced kidney damage where kidneys perform at less than 15% of the normal function. End-stage renal disease (ESRD) is kidney failure treated by dialysis or kidney transplant. If the kidneys fail, treatment options such as dialysis or a kidney transplant can help replace kidney function.

Early treatment

There are several types of treatments related to kidney disease. During the early stages of kidney disease, medications and lifestyle changes help maintain kidney function and delay kidney failure.

Lifestyle changes recommended during the early stages of kidney disease include:

- Making heart-healthy food choices and exercising regularly to maintain a healthy weight.

- Effectively monitoring and managing diabetes or high blood pressure can keep them from causing further damage to your kidneys.

- Consuming less than 1,500 milligrams of sodium each day.

- Eating the right amount of protein. Excess protein makes your kidneys work harder. Eating less protein may help delay progression to kidney failure.

- Quit smoking. Cigarette smoking can make kidney damage worse.

Medications

Certain medications can also help keep kidneys healthier longer. Two types of blood pressure medications have been shown to slow down kidney disease and delay kidney failure. These medications are:

- Angiotensin-converting enzyme (ACE) inhibitors

- Angiotensin receptor blockers (ARB)

The most important step a resident can take to treat kidney disease is to control his or her blood pressure. Many people need two or more types of medications to keep their blood pressure below recommended levels to keep the kidneys healthy.

It is common for older adults to be taking medications for other conditions. As kidney disease progresses, it is vital for physicians to monitor and adjust the dosages of all medications that affect the kidney or are removed by the kidney, as needed.

Treatment for later stages

If kidney disease progresses to kidney failure, the goal of treatment changes. There are two main options for kidney disease in this stage: dialysis and transplantation. Residents suffering from kidney failure should be educated on their treatment options.

Dialysis

Dialysis is a treatment that takes waste products and extra fluid out of the body. There are two main forms of dialysis—hemodialysis and peritoneal dialysis.

- In **hemodialysis,** the blood passes through a filter located outside of the body, where the blood is cleaned and returned to the body.

- **Peritoneal dialysis** uses the lining of a resident's abdominal cavity (the space that holds organs such as the stomach, intestines, and liver) to filter the blood. It works by putting a special fluid into the abdomen that absorbs waste products in your blood as it passes through small blood vessels in this lining. This fluid is then drained away. Peritoneal dialysis can often be done at home as a resident sleeps.

Neither form of dialysis can cure kidney failure; they are treatments to replace the function of the kidneys and may help a resident feel better and live longer.

Kidney transplant

Instead of dialysis, some people with kidney failure may be able to receive a kidney transplant. This treatment requires having a healthy kidney from another person surgically placed into the body. The donated kidney replaces the failed kidneys.

A donated kidney can come from:

- An anonymous donor who has recently died

- A living relative

- A living unrelated donor, including a spouse or friend

Unfortunately, due to the shortage of donated kidneys, residents on the waiting list for a donor kidney may have to wait many years.

It is important for residents to understand that a kidney transplantation is not a cure. Residents will need to be seen by a physician regularly and will need to take medications for as long as they have the transplant to suppress the immune system and limit the risk of the transplanted kidney being rejected by the body.

Age and kidney function

Kidneys may be significantly impacted by aging. As the kidneys age, there may be a decrease in the number of filtering units in each kidney, kidney tissue may decrease, and the blood vessels that supply the kidney may harden—all of which cause the kidneys to filter blood more slowly.

With a decrease in filtering function, a person may be more likely to have complications from certain medications and/or an unsafe buildup of medicines that, in a healthy person, would be removed from the blood by the kidneys.

Kidneys may also become more sensitive to certain medications. For example, nonsteroidal anti-inflammatory drugs (NSAIDs) and some antibiotics can cause acute kidney injury in some situations.

Additional conditions

Kidney disease can lead to other health problems. While working with residents who suffer from kidney disease, staff should be aware of the following related conditions.

- Depression

- Heart disease

- Bone disease

- Arthritis

- Nerve damage

- Malnutrition

To help keep residents safe and healthy, report any noticeable changes in a resident's condition to a supervisor.

Kidney disease is a difficult condition to diagnose in its early stages. Discuss the risk factors and prevention tips covered in this lesson with your residents and help kidney disease sufferers get the treatment they need before additional complications arise.

Figure 20.1 Kidney Disease BINGO Directions and Clues

Direction for teacher/leader of activity:

Gather some markers. These could be pennies, poker chips, candy, stickers, etc.
(Or have players mark their BINGO words with a pen or pencil).

Make copies of the following BINGO words, and cut each word square (or have players cut the squares). Give a set of these 25 words to each BINGO player, and have them create their own board using the blank BINGO sheet by placing the cut out words in random order on each square of the sheet. However they decide to create their BINGO sheet should not change once the game has begun.

To play the game, read out the clues. Whoever gets five in a row first wins, but keep playing until all clues are read and all players' BINGO sheets are totally covered.

BINGO Clues

- Bean-shaped organ about the size of a fist that filters blood. (kidney)

- This is a normal eGFR result. (≥60)

- This is one strategy to help prevent or slow kidney disease. (healthy diet)

- Kidney disease can be detected only by these. (tests)

- As part of the aging process, blood vessels that supply the kidneys may ____, which may cause the kidneys to filter blood more slowly. (harden)

- This is one of four main risk factors for developing kidney disease. (high blood pressure)

- These are filtering blood vessels in the kidneys. (glomeruli)

- This is treated by dialysis or kidney transplant. (kidney failure)

- This is a test that checks how much blood the kidneys filter each minute. (eGFR)

- This is a kidney tests that measures a protein in the urine. (urine albumin)

- This is the percentage of adults in the U.S. that likely have kidney disease. (10%)

- This is the medical term used to classify kidney disease that has progressed significantly. (ESRD)

- This is the medical term used to classify kidney disease that has progressed significantly. (ESRD)

- This uses the lining of a patient's abdominal cavity (the space that holds organs such as the stomach, intestines, and liver) to filter the blood. (peritoneal dialysis)

- This is the maximum amount of sodium, in milligrams, someone with any hint of kidney disease should consume daily. (1,500)

- This is one type of blood pressure medication that has been shown to slow down kidney disease and delay kidney failure. (ARBs)

- Kidney failure is when kidneys perform at less than what percentage of normal function? (15%)

- This is a urine albumin test result that may indicate kidney disease. (>30)

- This is another treatment option for end-stage renal failure other than dialysis. (transplant)

- Those who receive kidney transplants will have to take medications all their life to suppress what? (immune system)

- These are over-the-counter medications that can cause acute kidney injury in some situations when someone is aging and may have less than optimal kidney function. (NSAIDs)

- This is a treatment in which blood passes through a filter located outside of the body, where the blood is cleaned and returned to the body. (hemodialysis)

- This is a disease that often coincides to kidney disease. (depression)

- Kidney disease is known as the _____ disease because patients rarely suffer symptoms. (silent)

- This is an example of one source for a kidney for a kidney transplant. (living person)

Kidney Disease BINGO Words

kidney	urine albumin	10%	hemodialysis	transplant
ARBs	ESRD	tests	eGFR	harden
glomeruli	15%	FREE SPACE	depression	>30
immune system	kidney failure	high blood pressure	NSAIDs	living person
1,500	peritoneal dialysis	healthy diet	≥60	silent

Kidney Disease

Test

Name _____ Date _____ Score _____

Directions: Circle the correct answer.

1. Which of the following is not a main risk factor for developing kidney disease, as discussed in this lesson?

    a. Diabetes

    b. High blood pressure

    c. Cardiovascular disease

    d. Regular exercise

2. Every kidney contains around one million filtering units composed of blood vessels, known as _____.

    a. glomeruli

    b. villi

    c. white blood cells

    d. platelets

3. The gradual deterioration of kidney function over time is called _____ kidney disease.

    a. advanced

    b. slow

    c. chronic

    d. failing

4. Help residents at risk for kidney disease keep their kidneys healthy by _____.

    a. ensuring they are informed and educated about blood and urine testing for kidney disease

    b. monitoring and managing conditions such as diabetes, high blood pressure, high cholesterol, and heart disease

    c. encouraging a healthy diet with fresh fruits, vegetables, whole grains, low-fat dairy foods, and limited salt

    d. all of the above

5. Kidney disease is often called a "silent" disease, because with early kidney disease, most people have no symptoms. True or False

6. Estimate glomerular filtration rate (eGRF) is a measure of what?

    a. How quickly blood flows through the body

    b. How much blood the kidneys filter each minute

    c. How much urine a person produces hourly

    d. The level of angiotensin-converting enzyme (ACE) inhibitors in the blood

7. A urine albumin result below ___ is normal.

    a. 40

    b. 15

    c. 30

    d. 60

8. Which two types of medications below have been shown to slow down kidney disease and delay kidney failure? (choose two answers)

    a. Angiotensin-converting enzyme (ACE) inhibitors

    b. Nonsteroidal anti-inflammatory drugs (NSAIDs)

    c. Angiotensin receptor blockers (ARBs)

    d. Amoxicillin

9. In peritoneal dialysis, the blood passes through a filter located outside of the body, where the blood is cleaned and then returned to the body. True or False

10. Kidney failure is advanced kidney damage where kidneys perform at less than _____ of the normal function.

   a. 25%

   b. 10%

   c. 30%

   d. 15%

CERTIFICATE OF COMPLETION

I hereby certify that

_____

has successfully completed the in-Service

Kidney Disease

_____
Signature

21

Lifting and Transferring

Teaching Plan

To use this lesson for self-study, the learner should read the material, do the activity, and take the test. For group study, the leader may give each learner a copy of the learning guide and follow this teaching plan to conduct the lesson. Certificates may be copied for everyone who completes the lesson.

Learning objectives

After this lesson, participants should be able to:

- Demonstrate safe lifting and transferring techniques

- Practice skills that will prevent injuries

- Use devices to make tasks safer

Lesson activities

Have learners read the three stories in the activity in Figure 21.1 entitled "What Is Wrong in These Stories?" Ask them to identify the correct and incorrect things the staff did in the stories. After they have had a chance to find all of the problems, begin reviewing the material in the learner's guide.

As you talk about each item in the learning guide, give the participants an opportunity to practice the skill being covered. Use lightweight boxes or books to demonstrate proper body mechanics when lifting objects. Instruct learners to practice transferring one another from one chair to another chair using the correct posture and procedure.

After the learners have reviewed and practiced all the procedures in the learning guide, look at the stories in Figure 21.1 again and determine whether the learners can find any additional correct or incorrect actions. Be sure they identify everything before you conclude the lesson.

Include your facility's safe-lifting policies and equipment procedures as needed to ensure skill competence.

Conclusion

Have participants take the test. Review the answers together. Award certificates to those who answer 70% of the test questions correctly.

Test answers

1. job, worker	2. good posture, stretching and exercise, proper lifting and transferring skills, lifting equipment, teamwork	3. b, c, d	4. True	5. posture
6. Safety	7. True	8. True	9. False	10. True

Lifting and Transferring

Learning Guide

Contents:

- Introduction

- Ergonomics

- Posture and Work-Related Injuries

- Why Exercise?

- Lifting and Transferring Techniques

- Conclusion

Introduction

Caring for people who are not very mobile tends to involve a great deal of lifting. You may need to assist them from the bed to the chair or the wheelchair and back to bed, and, at times, you may need to help a person who has fallen onto the floor.

Improper lifting could injure your back and jeopardize your future ability to work. Do you know the correct techniques for lifting and transferring that might keep you from injuring yourself or the person you are assisting? Does your organization have a zero-lift policy and devices in place to prevent you from injuring yourself? You and your well-being are extremely important; be mindful to keep yourself safe during care and to learn all techniques to prevent unnecessary injuries to your body.

Practice preventive care, which includes:

- Good posture

- Stretching and exercise

- Lifting and transferring skills

- Proper lifting devices

- Teamwork

Ergonomics

Ergonomics is the science of fitting workplace conditions and job demands to the capabilities of workers. It is the science of fitting the job to the worker.

When the physical requirements of the job and the physical capacity of the worker do not match, then work-related injuries can result. Stress on the musculoskeletal system causes the majority of job injuries. Some of these muscular injuries have been linked to work habits that result in temporary or permanent disability.

Using ergonomic methods can mean:

- Using equipment that will take the strain out of lifting and transferring

- Organizing work in new ways, such as storing items that are used daily on easy-to-reach shelves rather than near the floor or above the shoulders

- Changing how tasks are done

Ergonomics can prevent injuries by helping us understand which tasks and body movements can hurt us and by finding new ways to do these tasks.

Keeping your back strong, stretched, and healthy is good. Good posture and mobility, proper lifting skills, and exercises are very important, but they are not enough to prevent injuries. Too much lifting and lifting in awkward ways can lead to injuries. Teamwork is important to ensure that you do not lift and transfer by yourself and do not get in awkward positions to do your tasks. Proper lifting devices also help prevent injuries.

Posture and Work-Related Injuries

Good posture means more than just sitting up straight, particularly when speaking of protecting workers from work-related musculoskeletal disorders. How does good posture affect the musculoskeletal system? Good posture ensures that muscles will receive a good blood supply, thereby allowing the muscles to eliminate waste, receive nourishment, and repair damage caused by stress. Good posture helps the body work more effectively and efficiently.

Since the body is designed to be in motion, standing or sitting in the same position for an extended period puts strain on the musculoskeletal system, as tendons are pulled and joints are compressed.

This leads to a reduction of the blood supply to the musculoskeletal areas, causing inflammation and pain.

Bad postures increase the risk of injury, so do not:

- Slouch

- Push the head forward beyond the plane of the shoulders

- Stand in an awkward position that unevenly distributes your weight

- Hold the head in an awkward or twisted position

Good postures decrease the risk of injury, so:

- Sit or stand tall

- Keep the ears over the shoulders

- Keep the shoulders over the hips

- Hold the head straight, not tilted

- Position the head over the neck

- Keep your abdomen and buttocks tucked in

The proper way to sit includes the following:

- Always sit all the way back on a chair.

- Your lower back can be supported with a pillow.

- Try to keep your knees at the same height as your hips. If necessary, elevate your knees by putting your feet on the rungs of a chair or stool, or support your feet on a phone book.

- You may need to raise the height of the seat in order to keep your knees at the same height as your hips. If possible, adjust the height of the chair, or sit on a phone book if necessary.

The proper way to stand includes the following:

- Spread your feet to shoulder width and put equal weight on each foot

- Put one foot up on something stable, such as the rung of a chair or stool

The proper way to sleep includes the following:

- Never sleep on your stomach

- Sleep on your side with the knees slightly bent and one pillow between the knees

- When sleeping on your side, pull your pillow down toward the shoulder to support the neck

- When sleeping on your back, place two pillows under the knees to reduce stress to the middle and lower back and the neck

- When on your back, support the neck with a pillow under the back of the head and neck

Poor posture can create problems by destroying the balance of the spine's natural curves. Strain on muscles adds stress to the spine that may harm the discs. Poor body mechanics upset the balance of the natural curves of the spine. Good body mechanics keep your spine balanced during movement.

Why Exercise?

Exercise relieves stress through activity. Stretching and strengthening exercises combine to balance the strength and tone of the muscles and ligaments. The muscles and ligaments are the supporting structure of the spine, so fitness benefits spinal health.

Lifting and Transferring Techniques

Serious back, shoulder, and neck injuries occur as a result of poor lifting and transferring habits. The following are some tips to reduce the strain on your back and the possibility of injuries. Protecting your back is working smarter, not harder. Be sure to follow your facility's policies for lifting and the procedures for your facility's lift equipment.

General tips for lifting and transferring include the following:

- When lifting and transferring, the most important consideration is safety for yourself and the resident.

- Ask for help and use teamwork. Talk to your helpers about what you plan to do, and talk to one another about what you are doing as you do it.

- When it is needed, use the right equipment.

- Plan the job. Move anything that is in the path.

- Maintain the correct posture: Keep your back straight and your knees bent. If you must bend from the waist, tighten your stomach muscles while bending and lifting. Bending your knees slightly will put the stress on your legs, not your back.

- Never twist when lifting, transferring, or reaching. Pick up your feet and pivot your whole body in the direction of the move. Move your torso as one unit. Twisting is one of the leading causes of injuries.

- Maintain a wide base of support. Keep your feet at least shoulder width apart or wider when lifting or moving.

- Hold the person or object you are lifting close to you, not at arm's length. Holding things close to your body can minimize the effects of the weight.

- Pushing is easier than pulling, because your own weight adds to the force.

- Use repeated small movements of large objects or people. For example, move a person in sections, by moving the upper trunk first and then the legs. Repeated small movements are easier than lifting things or people as a whole all at once.

- Always face the resident or object you are lifting or moving.

- Always tell a resident what you are planning to do, and find out how he or she prefers to be moved.

Take the following steps when transferring from the bed to a wheelchair or bedside chair:

- Plan the job and prepare to lift.

- Place the chair at a slight angle to the side of the bed.

- If using a wheelchair, lock both brakes. Fold up the foot pedals and remove the footrests.

- Stabilize the bed so it will not move.

- Put footwear on the resident.

- Lower the bed so the resident's feet will reach the floor.

- Move the person to the edge of the bed. First move the upper trunk and then the legs one at a time.

- Place the person's legs over the side of the bed.

- Place your arms around the person, circling the back in a sort of hug.

- Raise the person to a sitting position on the side of the bed.

- Place a gait belt around the resident's waist if desired (this is recommended).

- Gradually slide or "walk" the person's buttocks forward until his or her feet are flat on the floor. "Walk" the buttocks by grasping both legs together under the knees and swinging them gently back and forth as the buttocks move forward.

- Place your feet on both sides of the person's feet for support. Your feet should be far enough apart to give you a good base of support.

- Have the person lean forward and, if possible, place his or her arms around your shoulders. Do not allow the person's arms around your neck, as this can injure your neck.

- Allow the person to reach for the far wheelchair arm.

- Bend your hips and knees while keeping your back straight.

- Place your arms around the person's waist. If using a gait belt, grasp the belt at the sides of the back with both hands. Do not hold the person under the arms—this can cause injury to the resident.

- Keep the person's knees stabilized by holding your knees against his or hers.

- Pull up to lift the resident, straightening your knees and hips as you both stand.

- Keep the resident close to your body. Keep your knees and hips slightly bent.

- When the person is high enough to clear the armrest or chair surface, turn by taking small steps. Keep the person's knees blocked with your own knees.

- When you have turned, bend your hips and knees to squat, lowering the resident to the seat.

- Replace the footrests. Adjust the height of the foot pedals so the person will be sitting with a 90-degree angle at the hips and knees.

- When transporting a person in a wheelchair, pull it backward up steps or curbs.

- Follow the same principles to return the person to bed.

If a resident begins to fall, keep the following in mind:

- Once a resident has started to fall, it is almost impossible to stop the fall

- Instead of trying to stop the fall, try to guide the resident to the floor

- Once the resident is on the floor, get help to lift him or her

Take the following steps when lifting from the floor:

- You might find that someone has slipped to the floor but is not seriously injured. He or she may be able to assist you in getting up.

- Always get a coworker to help you get a resident up if the resident cannot assist you. Assistance of four to six people may be required. When appropriate, use a mechanical lift or hoist to raise a resident.

- Roll the resident onto a blanket or lift sheet.

- Have two or more people stand on each side. Each person should kneel on one knee and get a secure hold on the blanket. On the count of three, everyone should lift the resident and stand up, moving the resident onto a bed or stretcher.

Take the following steps when transferring in and out of a car:

- Put the front seat of the car as far back as possible.

- Position the wheelchair at a 90-degree angle to the car seat.

- Bend your knees and hips in a squat.

- Place your arms underneath the person's armpits and around the upper part of his or her back. The person may place his or her arms around your shoulders but not your neck. Grasp the person's upper back and do not pull under his or her arms. Hold the person close to you.

- Straighten your legs and hips slightly as you smoothly lift the person's torso into the car, placing his or her buttocks on the seat. Move your feet to turn; do not twist.

- Be sure the person's buttocks are as far back toward the driver's side as possible before lifting his or her legs into the car. When lifting the person's legs, keep your back straight.

Take the following steps when pulling a resident up in bed:

- Always get help when pulling a resident up.

- Place a draw or lift sheet under the resident.

- Remove the resident's pillow from under his or her head and place it against the head of the bed to provide a cushion between the resident's head and the headboard.

- Place the bed at a comfortable height for you and your coworker.

- Both you and the coworker should bend your knees and push with your feet.

- Grasp the draw or lift sheet firmly, holding the sheet close to the resident's body.

- Lean in the direction you want to move the resident.

- Instruct the resident to lower his or her chin to the chest if possible. If the resident cannot hold his or her head up, be sure the lift sheet is supporting the neck and head.

- Ask the resident to bend his or her knees so he or she can assist by pushing backward.

- On the count of three, lift the draw or lift sheet and pull the resident up.

Take the following steps when pulling a resident up in a chair:

- Have the resident fold his or her arms across the chest. Lock the wheelchair brakes.

- Stand behind the resident, bend your knees, and wrap your arms around him or her, hugging the torso securely by folding your arms just under his or hers in front.

- Straighten your legs, lifting the resident's torso up and back in the chair.

Take the following steps when turning a resident from side to side:

- Stand at one side of the bed, with the bed raised to waist height.

- Place your arms under the resident's shoulders and hips, or grasp the lift sheet.

- Pull the resident to the edge of the bed, trunk first and then legs.

- Cross the resident's leg closest to you over the other leg.

- Place your hands on the resident's shoulder and hip closest to you.

- Lean in toward the resident and push the resident's torso away from you.

- Place the top leg in front of the bottom leg.

- Support the resident's shoulders, back, and hips with pillows. Place a pillow between the resident's legs to support the top leg. Adjust for comfort.

Devices that can help you work smarter, not harder, include the following:

- **Draw sheets (or lift sheets)** make it easier to pull a person up in bed or move a person to the side. To place a draw sheet under a resident, turn the resident on his or her side and lay the draw sheet on the bed. Roll half of the draw sheet up against the resident. Turn the resident to the other side, rolling him or her over the rolled-up draw sheet, pull the rolled draw sheet out, and straighten it on the bed. The draw sheet should extend from above the shoulders to below the hips and should support the neck and head if the resident cannot do so.

- **Bed controls** raise or lower the bed to a comfortable and safe position for you, your coworker, and the resident.

- **Slide boards** help to reduce friction so the resident can slide from the bed to another surface.

- **Trapeze** over the bed can allow residents to help you move them. They can grasp the trapeze, pull themselves up, and assist as you move them.

- **Gait belt** is made from heavy canvas with a sturdy buckle. Place the belt around the resident's waist and use it to assist you in moving him or her.

- **Mechanical lifters/hoists** can lift a resident who is heavy or who has fallen. Ask your supervisor for instructions before using these devices.

Conclusion

Protect yourself:

- Work in teams

- Call for support to prevent unsafe transfers

- Use lifting equipment

- Exercise to maintain a strong, healthy back

- Use proper posture and body mechanics

Most companies have an ergonomic plan to prevent back sprain and strain injuries from happening. These plans should include:

- Regular inspections to discover hazards that might lead to strain and sprain injuries

- Training for everyone on how to prevent injuries

- Safe staffing levels so workers don't get hurt lifting heavy residents alone

- Useful and safe lifting devices

Your body has natural limits. Some tasks can lead to injuries when you go beyond these limits. Jobs should be designed to fit the worker. This is ergonomics. This is working smarter, not harder.

Figure 21.1: What Is Wrong with These Stories?

1. Sharon is helping Mr. Smith move from a chair into bed. She positions the chair close to the bed at a slight angle. She locks the brakes on both the bed and the wheelchair. She places her feet widely apart but does not block Mr. Smith's knees. She bends over, puts her hands under Mr. Smith's arms and instructs him to place his arms around her neck. She pulls Mr. Smith to a standing position, twists her body to pivot him so his back is to the bed and then sits him down on the bed. The bed's position is at the lowest level. Sharon lays Mr. Smith back on the bed and then bends over and lifts his legs onto the bed. As she straightens up, she feels a sharp pain in her back.

   Identify at least five things Sharon did that may have contributed to her injury and at least two things she did that could have harmed the client. What techniques did she do right? What steps did she incorrectly perform?

2. Mike sees that Mrs. Jones has slipped down in her chair. He leans over her from the back, grasps her under the arms and pulls her up. He keeps his feet close together and stands so the wheelchair will push against his legs as it rolls backward.

   What process did Mike do wrong? What process did he do right?

3. Patty is walking with Mr. Smith when he begins to fall. She tries to stop the fall, but instead he pulls her to the floor with him. What should she have done differently?

Answers to stories:

1. Sharon should have bent at the knees instead of the waist; she should not have let Mr. Smith put his arms around her neck; she should not have twisted her body; she should have raised the bed to the right height; and she should not have bent over to lift his legs. If she had raised the bed to waist height after sitting him on the bed, she could have moved his legs without bending. She could have injured the client by pulling him under his arms and by not blocking his knees. She correctly locked the brakes on the bed and wheelchair, kept her feet widely spaced, and placed the chair close to the bed.

2.	Mike should not have kept his feet close together, he should not have put his hands under Mrs. Jones' arms to pull her up, and he should have locked the wheelchair's brakes. He correctly approached the client from behind the chair, but he should have bent with his knees instead of bending at the waist.

3.	Patty should have tried to guide Mr. Smith to the floor instead of trying to stop his fall.

Lifting and Transferring

Test

Name _____ Date _____ Score _____

Directions: Fill in or circle the correct answer.

1. Ergonomics is fitting the _____ to the _____.

2. List five ways to practice preventive care for injuries. (five points)

   1._____

   2._____

   3._____

   4._____

   5._____

3. Putting ergonomics to work might include the following. Choose three. (three points)

   a. Making sure the worker is strong enough to handle a heavy resident

   b. Using appropriate equipment

   c. Changing how tasks are done

   d. Organizing work in new ways

4. As a rule, you should not sleep on your stomach. True or False

5. Good _____ helps the body work more effectively and efficiently.

6. _____ for yourself and the resident is the most important consideration when lifting and transferring.

7. When moving a person to the edge of the bed, you should move the upper trunk and then the legs one at a time. True or False

8. You should always face the resident when you are lifting and moving him or her. True or False

9. If a resident begins to fall, you should grab the resident and try to keep him or her from falling. True or False

10. Good standing posture includes spreading your feet to shoulder width and putting equal weight on each foot. True or False

CERTIFICATE OF COMPLETION

I hereby certify that

_____

has successfully completed the in-Service

Lifting and Transferring

_____

Signature

22

Malnutrition and Dehydration

Teaching Plan

To use this lesson for self-study, the learner should read the material, do the activity, and take the test. For group study, the leader may give each learner a copy of the learning guide and follow this teaching plan to conduct the lesson. Certificates may be copied for everyone who completes the lesson.

Learning objectives

After this lesson, participants should be able to:

- Explain physical and chemical changes in the ill and elderly that affect the way their bodies absorb nutrients from food

- Explain why the body needs fluids

- Recognize symptoms that may be caused by not getting enough nutrients or fluids

- Describe foods, nutrients, and fluids that are needed every day

- Describe ways to encourage healthful eating and drinking

Lesson activities

1. Before the lesson, share the history of elderly residents who for some reason are not getting their nutrients or calories as needed—perhaps someone with a poor appetite, or a senior who has poorly fitting dentures. Instruct learners to look for ideas for meeting these needs as they read the lesson.

2. After reviewing the lesson, do the learning activity "Solve the Problem" individually or as a group (Figure 22.1).

3. After the lesson, ask learners to share their ideas about meeting the nutritional and fluid needs of their residents, especially any residents that were discussed in the introductory activity. Discuss changes that might enable those residents to have their nutritional needs met.

Conclusion

Have participants take the test. Review the answers together. Award certificates to those who answer 70% of the test questions correctly.

Test answers

1. True	2. False	3. True	4. True	5. True
6. False	7. True	8. True	9. True	10. False

Malnutrition and Dehydration

Learning Guide

Contents:

- Physical and Chemical Changes That Influence Nutritional Needs

- Malnutrition

  - Signs and symptoms of malnutrition

- Dehydration

  - Preventing dehydration

  - Symptoms of dehydration

  - Treatment for dehydration

- A Healthful, Nutritious Diet

- Ways to Help People Get Needed Nutrients

Physical and Chemical Changes That Influence Nutritional Needs

People who are sick or elderly have different food requirements than young, healthy people. They are also more likely to suffer harm from not eating the right foods. After age 50, there are chemical and physical changes in the body that affect nutritional needs.

- The metabolic rate, or metabolism, slows down. The metabolic rate is the speed at which the body uses energy. Older bodies burn less fuel for daily operations. This means seniors need fewer calories for normal, everyday activities. This also applies to anyone who is not very active or is confined to bed.

- Lean tissue and muscle mass decrease. There is less bone mass. Body fat increases.

- Stomach acid may decrease and the stomach might not empty as fast. The intestine may absorb less nutrition from the food it gets.

- Tooth and gum problems increase, sometimes making it difficult to chew.

- Some people have trouble swallowing, especially those who have had a stroke.

- There is a loss of taste and smell. This causes people to be less interested in food.

- Sometimes people are too tired or weak to eat an entire meal.

- Appetite and thirst decrease. Many elderly or ill people eat and drink less than they should. This leads to fatigue, sadness, infections, skin breakdown, and lack of energy.

- Medications can affect appetite or thirst. Sometimes medicines upset the stomach or cause intestinal problems like diarrhea or constipation.

- Many diseases affect the way the body uses food or water. Someone with an illness usually needs more food and water because the body needs energy to heal. People with some conditions, however, must carefully control the amount and type of calories they take in. Diabetes is one example.

> Although the body may need fewer calories because of age or inactivity, it still needs the same amount of nutrients and fluid it always has—or more. It is important to eat foods that have a high nutritional value.

Malnutrition

Bodies will break down if they do not get the type and amount of fuel they need. Malnutrition means "badly nourished," another way of saying that the person isn't getting enough of the right nutrients the body needs to stay healthy. Malnutrition can be caused by not eating enough nutritious foods or by not adequately digesting and absorbing nutrients from food. Getting too much food is harmful and is also called malnutrition.

Someone who does or experiences one or more of the following things might be headed for malnutrition:

- Doesn't eat from the major food groups most of the time.

- Eats less than half of two or more meals per day.

- Eats less than one hot meal per day.

- Changes from solid foods to pureed foods, or other dietary changes.

- Drinks a lot of alcohol.

- Is socially isolated or depressed.

- Is poor or has difficulty obtaining or preparing food because of physical or mental disabilities. Someone with cognitive problems might not remember to eat.

- Uses laxatives excessively (which hinders digestion of nutrients by causing food to pass through the intestines too quickly).

- Has had recent surgery or illness or has chronic or multiple diseases.

Twenty-five percent to 30% of senior citizens are malnourished. Nearly two-thirds of people over age 60 are at risk for malnutrition.

Signs and symptoms of malnutrition

If a person shows any of these signs, he or she should be seen by a doctor. Taking care of someone with malnutrition means helping the person get enough of the right nutrients.

- Tiredness and lack of energy

- Loss of appetite

- Loss of (or gain in) weight

- Sore lips, tongue, or throat

- Infections or slow healing

- Diarrhea or constipation

- Easy bruising

- Depression or confusion

Older adults and those who are chronically ill should be weighed regularly to be sure they are getting enough calories and are not losing or gaining weight.

Unless a person is overweight and trying to lose weight, a loss of just 5% of body weight can be harmful. Any unintended weight loss or weight gain is a sign of possible malnutrition. Report a resident's changes in weight to a supervisor.

Dehydration

Dehydration is a serious, sometimes fatal condition. It means there are not enough body fluids and important blood salts in the body to carry on normal functions at the best level. This happens by loss of fluids, not drinking enough water, or a combination of both.

Water is essential in all the vital functions of the body. It is part of regulating temperature; building new cells; lubricating joints; and keeping the kidneys, brain, heart and other organs working.

Thirst is the warning signal that we should drink. However, just drinking when we are thirsty is not enough. Many people stay mildly dehydrated much of the time.

You are drinking enough water if your urine is always pale in color and you are urinating every two to three hours.

Preventing dehydration

- A healthy adult should drink at least 6–8 eight-ounce glasses of water per day.

- It is possible to get some of the necessary fluids from other drinks, but anything with caffeine in it does not count in the daily requirement. In fact, caffeinated drinks, such as coffee, tea, and cola, actually increase the daily requirement. Caffeine pulls water from the body, increasing the need for fluid intake. For every eight-ounce caffeinated drink, add an extra eight ounces of water to the daily requirement:

  - Consuming two eight-ounce cups of coffee increases the daily water need to at least 8–10 eight-ounce glasses per day

  - Consuming two 12-ounce cans of cola increases the daily water need to at least 9–11 eight-ounce glasses per day

Reasons people don't drink enough fluid:

- Loss of appetite

- Lack of thirst

- Don't like frequent bathroom trips

- Forget to drink

Reasons people lose fluid:

- Fever

- Vomiting

- Diarrhea

- Excessive urine output

- Excessive sweating; exercise

- Heat exhaustion

Symptoms of dehydration

Always pay attention to what residents drink and how much they urinate. The following symptoms could be signs of dehydration and must be reported immediately. Severe dehydration can result in seizures, permanent brain damage, heart and blood-vessel collapse, and death if not treated quickly.

Mild dehydration:

- Thirst; dry lips and tongue

- Dry membranes in the mouth

- Skin looks dry

Moderate dehydration:

- Skin is not very elastic, may sag, and doesn't bounce back quickly when lightly pinched and released

- Sunken eyes

- Decreased urine output

Severe dehydration:

- Small amounts of dark-colored urine

- Rapid, weak pulse over 100 (at rest)

- Rapid breathing

- Low blood pressure; dizziness

- Blue lips

- Cold hands and feet

- Confusion, lack of interest, difficult to arouse

- Shock

Pinch a fold of skin on the back of your hand and hold it for a few seconds. Let it go, and time how quickly the skin returns to normal. The skin should return to normal within a second or two. If it stays pinched for longer than that, you may be dehydrated.

Treatment for dehydration

For mild dehydration, giving fluids by mouth is usually enough. This is called oral rehydration:

- The physician may order an oral rehydrating solution (ORS) that replaces important blood salts and water in balanced amounts designed especially for dehydration in sick people. These solutions allow the intestines to absorb maximum amounts of water.

- Don't confuse ORS with sports drinks designed for concentrated energy and salt replacement in healthy, high-performance athletes. These drinks can cause vomiting and diarrhea and are so concentrated they can limit intestinal water absorption.

- IV fluids may be necessary for moderate to severe dehydration.

- Rapid recognition and treatment of dehydration results in a good outcome.

A Healthful, Nutritious Diet

Fruit (at least two servings daily) and vegetables (at least three servings daily)

- Everyone should eat a variety of fruits and vegetables every day

- Different fruits and vegetables are rich in different nutrients

- Vegetables and fruits contain fiber, vitamins, and minerals

Grain products (at least six servings daily)

- Give residents a variety of whole grain and refined breads, cereals, pasta, and rice

- Grains provide vitamins, minerals, carbohydrates, and fiber

- The high fiber content of whole grains promotes proper bowel function

Dairy (at least two servings daily)

- Low-fat dairy products are needed daily to provide calcium

- Adults over age 50 have an especially high need for calcium to maintain bone mass

Meat and beans group (at least two servings daily)

- Choose from the meat and beans group each day. Peanut butter, cheese, and eggs may substitute for meats.

- These foods provide protein to build and maintain healthy body tissues.

- People need more protein when they are dealing with illness, surgery, or trauma.

Fat

- Fats are highly concentrated sources of energy, and they provide fatty acids needed for good health.

- Monounsaturated oils (e.g., canola, olive) are believed to lower unhealthy cholesterol levels (LDL) and raise healthy cholesterol levels (HDL).

- Avoid saturated fat. Choose lean cuts of meat and remove the skin from poultry.

Water

- Water is the most important nutrient in the body. Oxygen is the only thing the body craves more. At least six to eight glasses of fluid are needed every day.

Ways to Help People Get Needed Nutrients

Care providers have a responsibility to ensure that residents' food needs are met. Take the following steps:

- Create person-centered menus, which fit the amount and the kinds of food to the individual.

- Serve tasty foods and foods you know that the person enjoys. Learn the person's life story, culture, and unique preferences.

- Increase fiber to help move food through the intestines and prevent constipation.

- Encourage people to eat with family and friends.

- Use a blender or food processor for those with chewing or swallowing problems. Be creative with plating of the foods if they are pureed. Find ways to reconstitute the meal items to still have the appearance they did before pureeing. There are food molds and other tools you can use to pipe puree foods to look much more appetizing.

- People with swallowing problems can choke on liquids that are too thin. A thickening agent can be added to liquids to help them drink. They may do best using a straw.

- Chop or mash meats and vegetables with a little gravy or broth.

- Use soft foods such as tuna, eggs, cheese, and peanut butter for meat substitutes.

- Small, frequent feedings and healthful snacks can encourage some people to eat. Have fruit, yogurt, or vegetables readily available.

- Adding nonfat dry milk powder to foods such as casseroles, cream soups, puddings, or gravy increases calcium and protein intake.

- Food that is served warm (not too hot or too cold) may seem tastier.

- For someone who can't eat a whole meal, try six small meals per day.

- Offer finger foods, such as sandwiches and fruits, to those who have difficulty managing utensils. Cut food into bite-sized pieces.

- If caring for a person with dementia who has difficulty bringing food to their mouth with a fork, or if the person has progressed in their dementia and require more assistance to dine, work with OT to learn how to use a hand-over-hand or a hand-under-hand approach to keep the person engaged with eating.

- No single food can supply all the nutrients in the amounts needed.

- The diet should include a variety of plant foods, including whole grains, fruits, vegetables, protein, dairy foods, and fats.

- Combining powdered meal mixes with milk, puddings, or fruit purees bolsters the nutrient content.

- Anyone with mouth or teeth problems will benefit from soft foods like yogurt, cottage cheese, applesauce, mashed potatoes, ice cream, puddings, milkshakes, or custards.

- Clear beef or chicken broth is a good way to get warm liquids in cold weather.

- Some people may need to take vitamins and minerals in a supplement. People who get little sunlight may need vitamin D.

- Fruit juices and milk provide fluid, nutrients, and calories, but they do not fulfill the need for six to eight glasses of water per day.

- Thirst decreases with age, so encourage older people to drink fluids throughout the day. Offer water often and keep it readily available.

Figure 22.1 Malnutrition Learning Activity

Learning Activity: Solve the Problem

Directions: Match the situation on the left with the best solution on the right.

Put the letter of the solution in the blank next to the problem.

1. Someone who has difficulty chewing. _____

2. Someone who has difficulty swallowing. _____

3. Someone with a dry mouth and dry skin. _____

4. Someone who can't eat an entire meal at one time. _____

5. Someone who doesn't like meat. _____

6. Someone who needs more protein but not more calories. _____

7. Someone who has trouble managing a fork, knife, and spoon. _____

8. Someone who is tired, has little energy, is depressed, and is losing weight. _____

9. Someone who is confused and has sunken eyes, rapid breathing and heart rate, and small amounts of dark urine. _____

10. Someone who doesn't like to eat. _____

    a. Add nonfat dry milk powder to foods.

    b. Offer water frequently.

    c. Serve six small meals a day.

    d. Offer soft foods like cottage cheese; chop food into small bits.

    e. Give peanut butter, cheese, eggs, and beans.

    f. This person is probably seriously dehydrated. Report the person's condition to a supervisor at once.

    g. Use finger foods; cut food into bite-sized pieces.

    h. This person may be malnourished. Report the person's condition to a supervisor.

    i. Give thickened liquids and soft foods.

    j. Encourage the person to eat with friends or family. Offer frequent snacks.

Answer key:

1. d	2 i	3. b	4. c	5. e	6. a	7. g	8. h	9. f	10. j

Malnutrition and Dehydration

Test

Name _____ Date _____ Score _____

Directions: Circle the correct answer.

1. There is a difference in nutritional needs in the elderly compared to younger adults.
   True or False

2. The elderly need fewer calories and also fewer vitamins and minerals in their food.
   True or False

3. Any weight loss or weight gain in a resident should be reported to a supervisor. True or False

4. Protein needs increase during acute illness or surgery. True or False

5. A diet that does not contain needed amounts of protein, vitamins, and minerals may slow the healing of a wound. True or False

6. Someone who cannot eat enough food at a meal because of fatigue or poor appetite must wait until the next meal to eat (it is healthier to eat only three meals per day). True or False

7. Signs of malnutrition include tiredness, weight loss, and slow healing of a wound or sore.
   True or False

8. In the elderly, decreased thirst and poor intake of fluids could lead to dehydration.
   True or False

9. A person whose body severely lacks fluid can suffer heart and blood-vessel collapse and even death if not treated quickly. True or False

10. When you pinch the skin on the back of someone's hand, it will spring back to normal quickly if the person is dehydrated. True or False

CERTIFICATE OF COMPLETION

I hereby certify that

_____

has successfully completed the in-Service

Malnutrition and Dehydration

_____

Signature

23
Mental Illness

Teaching Plan

To use this lesson for self-study, the learner should read the material, do the activity, and take the test. For group study, the leader may give each learner a copy of the learning guide and follow this teaching plan to conduct the lesson. Certificates may be copied for everyone who completes the lesson.

Learning objectives

After this lesson, participants should be able to:

- Recognize symptoms of mental illness

- Describe characteristics of mental illness

- List treatments and care measures for mental illness

- Discuss medicines used in the treatment of mental illnesses

Activity

Work through the learning guide with the participants, discussing the symptoms and characteristics of each type of mental disorder. Emphasize that participants should learn to recognize signs of mental illness and report them to a medical professional. If you have residents with any of these disorders, you might want to discuss their care at this time.

Review the treatment options and medications presented in the learning guide and discuss the care measures required for people who take medicines for mental illness.

Conclusion

Have participants take the test. Review the answers together. Award certificates to those who answer 70% of the test questions correctly.

Test answers

1. brain	2. d		3. True	4. False	5. depression
6. False	7. obsessive-compulsive		8. False	9. True	10. antipsychotic; schizophrenia

Mental Illness

Learning Guide

Contents:

- Introduction

- What Is Mental Illness?

- Types of Mental Disorders

    - Cognitive disorders

    - Dissociative disorders

    - Anxiety disorders

    - Personality disorders

    - Mood disorders

    - Psychotic disorders

- Treatment of Mental Illness

    - Medications

    - Psychotherapy

Introduction

Mental-health problems are common among the elderly, the chronically ill or disabled, and the poor. Since people with mental illness can demonstrate many different symptoms, we often do not recognize the signs. As a result, many people do not receive the medications or treatments that might help. Caregivers should learn how to recognize mental illness and how to care for the mentally ill.

What Is Mental Illness?

Mental illness is any brain disorder that causes abnormal ways of thinking, feeling, or acting.

Symptoms of abnormal thinking include:

- **Delusions.** This means believing things that are not true. A person might think someone wants to kill or hurt him or her.

- **Hallucinations.** This means seeing or hearing things that are not really there. A person who is hallucinating might hear people talking to him or her when no one is.

- **Confused thinking.** The person might be illogical or not understand things happening around him.

- **Suicidal thoughts.** Someone with a mental illness might have frequent or constant thoughts of killing himself or herself.

Symptoms of abnormal behavior include:

- Disruptive or antisocial behaviors

- Changes in sleeping routines

- Changes in eating habits

- Alcohol, drug, or medicine abuse

- Very slow or fast speech or movements

Symptoms of abnormal feelings include:

- Frequent mood changes

- Depression or sadness

- Anxiety, worry, or panic

- Irritability or anger

- Frequent crying, tearfulness

- Agitated behavior or fits of temper

- Changes in hygiene practices

- Unwillingness to cooperate

- Inability to pay attention, easily distracted

- Withdrawal from normal activities or from people

- Apathy, poor motivation

- Hopeless and/or helpless feelings

- Excessively low or high self-esteem

- Excessively energetic or euphoric

- Poor judgment, impulsiveness

Types of Mental Disorders

Many different things cause mental-health problems. Sometimes mental disorders are genetic, meaning they run in families. Mental illnesses can be caused by reactions to stressful events, by imbalances in the body's chemistry, or by a combination of several factors. The symptoms of mental illness occur because the brain is not functioning well. This affects the person's thought processes, emotions, and/or behavior. It is important to remember that people who are mentally ill usually cannot control the way they think, feel, or behave. Mental illness is not the person's fault. People with mental illness cannot help themselves.

The seven main types of mental disorders are cognitive, dissociative, anxiety, eating, mood, personality, and psychotic disorders.

Cognitive disorders

Cognitive impairment is a loss of mental abilities and awareness that occurs in varying degrees with a variety of underlying causes. In the elderly, it is usually caused by physical changes in the brain. Symptoms include loss of intellectual abilities, personality changes, forgetfulness, inability to concentrate, poor judgment, and verbal confusion. It can hinder a person's ability to do daily activities.

Dementia. This disorder involves the parts of the brain that control thought, memory, and language. Healthy brain tissue deteriorates, causing a steady loss in memory and mental abilities. Strokes or changes in the brain's blood supply may result in the death of brain tissue. Symptoms of dementia caused by problems with blood vessels can appear suddenly, whereas symptoms develop slowly in persons with Alzheimer's disease. Although dementia is found primarily in the elderly, 50% of people with AIDS develop dementia.

Alzheimer's disease. This is the most common form of dementia among people age 65 and older. It may begin with slight memory loss and confusion but eventually leads to a severe, permanent mental impairment that destroys the ability to remember, reason, learn, and imagine. On the average, people die within 10 years of developing Alzheimer's.

Dissociative disorders

These disorders come in many forms, all thought to stem from traumatic events. When an extremely stressful event occurs, the person is too overwhelmed to process it and tries to cope with the trauma by separating himself or herself from the experience. This can lead to loss of memory or the formation of separate personalities.

Dissociative identity disorder. This disorder is evidenced by two or more personalities or identities that control a person's consciousness at different times. It used to be called multiple-personality disorder.

Dissociative amnesia. In this disorder, the person forgets some or all personal information, such as who he or she is or where he or she lives.

Anxiety disorders

Anxiety causes physical symptoms such as rapid, shallow breathing, increased heart rate, sweating, and trembling. It can cause emotional symptoms, including alarm, dread, and apprehension. Treatment may include medication, therapy, or a combination of these options.

Panic disorder. This is a sudden onset of intense fear, apprehension, and impending doom that may last from minutes to hours. Approximately one in three people with panic disorder develop agoraphobia. Persons with agoraphobia are afraid of having attacks in public, so they avoid leaving the house.

Posttraumatic stress disorder. Persons with this disorder reexperience the anxiety associated with a previous traumatic event. Many times it is caused by exposure to an extremely stressful event, such as abuse or rape.

Phobias. A person with a phobia feels very anxious when exposed to a particular object or situation, such as a high place. The person fears and avoids whatever causes the anxiety.

Obsessive compulsive disorder (OCD). OCD is characterized by the need to maintain control, order, neatness, cleanliness, and/or perfection. People with OCD feel compelled to perform repetitive acts, such as hand washing or repeatedly checking to be sure a door is locked. Luvox is the drug used to treat this disorder.

Generalized anxiety disorder (GAD). This disorder may occur at any age. It is diagnosed after at least six months of persistent, excessive anxiety and worry. Drugs used to treat many forms of anxiety disorders include Tenormin, Tranxene, Valium, Xanax, Ativan, Centrax, Inderal, Serax, BuSpar, and Klonopin.

Personality disorders

Personality disorders are chronic conditions with biological and psychological causes. Psychotherapy is the treatment, sometimes along with medications.

Borderline personality disorder. This personality disorder is characterized by impulsive behavior, unstable social relationships, and intense anger. People with this disorder can have periods of psychotic thinking, paranoia, and hallucinations.

Obsessive-compulsive personality. People with this personality disorder tend to be high achievers. They are dependable and orderly but can't adjust to change and are intolerant of mistakes. They can be uncomfortable with relationships. This is not the same as obsessive-compulsive disorder.

Passive-aggressive personality. People with this personality disorder hide hostile feelings and try to control or punish others.

Narcissistic personality. Persons with this personality disorder feel superior to others and expect to be admired. They may be seen as self-centered and arrogant.

Antisocial personality, formerly called **psychopathic** or **sociopathic personality.** People with this personality disorder show no regard for the rights and feelings of others. They do not tolerate frustration and become hostile or violent when frustrated. They show no remorse or guilt, and they blame others for their own behavior. They are prone to addictions, sexual deviation, job failures, and abusive behavior. Most are male.

Mood disorders

Mood disorders usually involve chemical imbalances in the brain and are often treated with antidepressants and/or psychotherapy.

Depression. Depression causes severe, prolonged sadness. It can affect a person's thoughts, feelings, behavior, and physical health. It may develop at any age. Depressed people often look sad or expressionless and lose interest in normal activities. Depression is the leading cause of disability in the United States, affecting more women than men.

Older people often think sadness is part of aging, or that signs of depression such as forgetfulness, loss of appetite, and insomnia are symptoms of dementia. Depression is not a sign of old age. It is an illness and needs treatment like any other illness.

Drugs used in the treatment of depression include:

- Tricyclics: Anafranil, Elavil, Tofranil, Norpramin, Pamelor, Sinequan, Vivactil, Aventyl

- Selective serotonin reuptake inhibitors (SSRIs): Celexa, Paxil, Luvox, Zoloft, Prozac

- Monoamine oxidase inhibitors (MAOIs): Parnate, Nardil, Marplan

- Others: Desyrel, Effexor, Remeron, Serzone, Wellbutrin, Buspar, Zyban

Bipolar disorder, also called manic depression, causes episodes of severe mania (euphoria, increased energy and confidence) and depression (sadness, fatigue, poor concentration) that alternate with periods of normal mood. It occurs equally in men and women. This illness can be successfully treated with medications like Eskalith, Lithobid, Lithonate, Depakote, and Depakene.

Seasonal affective disorder (SAD). This disorder is characterized by recurrent bouts of depression in certain months of the year, usually fall and winter. Symptoms include oversleeping, carbohydrate craving, weight gain, lethargy, and social withdrawal. SAD is treated by bright fluorescent light, which alters the levels of brain chemicals. Sometimes antidepressants are used.

Psychotic disorders

In acute phases of psychosis, a person loses touch with reality and is unable to meet the ordinary demands of life. Most psychotic episodes are brief.

Schizophrenia. Schizophrenia is a severe and chronic brain disorder that impairs the ability to think clearly, make decisions, and relate to others. Persons with this disorder suffer frightening symptoms that leave them fearful and withdrawn. One out of every 100 people has this treatable illness, men and women alike. It involves problems with brain structure and chemistry.

People with schizophrenia do not have a "split personality." They may have delusions or hallucinations. They cannot tell what is real and what is not real. People with this disorder may talk to themselves, walk in circles, pace, and have difficulty carrying on conversations. There may be a lack of facial expression. They may be unable to follow through with activities they start.

Schizophrenia is manageable with medication and psychotherapy. Acute episodes are treated with hospitalization and antipsychotic drugs.

Treatment of Mental Illness

Mental-health disorders are treatable, and many people recover. Medications, psychotherapy, psychoeducation, electroconvulsive therapy, and self-help and support groups are used in the treatment of mental illnesses. Anything that improves a person's quality of life can help, such as pets, social events, activities, or reality-orientation classes. Many communities and facilities are affiliated with mental-health professionals that can screen for mental-health problems and conduct therapy sessions.

Medications

Many of the medicines used to treat mental illness cause unpleasant side effects. Some of the more common ones are dry mouth, constipation, blurred vision, appetite changes, loss of sexual function, drowsiness, and weight gain. Drinking eight glasses of water per day and eating fruits and vegetables can help with some of this.

Antipsychotic drugs can cause tremors, stiffness, muscle contraction and rigidity, restlessness, and loss of facial expression. Elderly people and those that have taken these medicines for years sometimes develop a condition called tardive dyskinesia. This causes uncontrolled facial movements and jerking or twisting movements of other body parts. This condition can be treated with medication.

Psychotherapy

Psychotherapy is the use of psychological techniques to change behaviors, feelings, thoughts, or habits. It is recommended for persons experiencing emotional distress.

- **Behavior management.** The aim of behavior management is to increase the occurrence of desirable behavior by rewarding the person for acting correctly. Unsuitable behavior is reduced by giving negative consequences.

- **Cognitive therapy.** Cognitive therapy emphasizes a rational and positive view. This therapy attempts to change destructive thought patterns that can lead to disappointment and frustration. It is effective with anxiety and depression.

- **Psychoeducation.** Psychoeducation is teaching people about their illness, treatment, and how to recognize a relapse. Teaching coping skills to the family will help them deal with an ill relative.

- **Electroconvulsive therapy.** This treatment is used only for delusions and hallucinations, major depression, or serious sleep and eating disorders that cannot be effectively treated with drugs. Sedatives are given, and then low doses of electric shock are applied to the brain. Most people show rapid improvement.

- **Self-help and support groups.** These groups help because members give one another ongoing support. It's comforting to know others have the same or similar problems. These groups can also help families work together for needed research, treatments, and community programs.

Mental Illness

Test

Name _____ Date _____ Score _____

Directions: Fill in or circle the correct answer.

1. Mental illnesses are disorders of the _____.

2. Mental illnesses may be caused by _____.

    a. genetic factors

    b. chemical imbalances

    c. reactions to stressful events

    d. all of the above

3. Anxiety may cause physical symptoms as well as emotional symptoms. True or False

4. Posttraumatic stress disorder is caused by overreacting to something mildly unpleasant.
    True or False

5. The leading cause of disability in the United States is _____.

6. Depression is a normal part of getting older.   True or False

7. If a person must have everything in order and in its place and is continually cleaning, you
    might suspect he or she has _____-_____ disorder.

8. A person with schizophrenia has a "split personality."   True or False

9. A person with schizophrenia may hear or see things that are not real.   True or False

10. Risperdal is a(n) _____ drug used in the treatment of _____.

CERTIFICATE OF COMPLETION

I hereby certify that

_____

has successfully completed the in-Service

Mental Illness

_____
Signature

24

■ Multiple Sclerosis

Teaching Plan

To use this lesson for self-study, the learner should read the material, do the activity, and take the test. For group study, the leader may give each learner a copy of the learning guide and follow this teaching plan to conduct the lesson. Certificates may be copied for everyone who completes the lesson.

Learning objectives

After this lesson, participants should be able to:

- Describe multiple sclerosis (MS) and how it affects the body

- Understand the most common physical, emotional, and cognitive problems of people with MS

- List ways to assist people with some of the problems of MS

Lesson activities

1. Use the crossword puzzle at the beginning of the session as a pretest to stimulate interest in the topic (Figure 24.1). Or, introduce the lesson by asking your learners to tell you what they know about MS. Even if you do not currently care for people with MS, the chances are good that you will eventually.

2. Using your board or flip chart, draw a large outline of the basic human central nervous system, similar to the example in Figure 24.2. Use this picture (it can be very rough) as you deliver a lecture based on the learning guide. Illustrate your talk by writing some of the terms and the signs and symptoms of MS on the board. If you prefer, copy the example illustration for your learners.

Figure 24.1: Multiple Sclerosis Crossword Puzzle Answer Key

	1. S		2. B							3. M				
	4. P	A	R	A	L	Y	5. S	I	S		6. S			
	A		A				W				E			
	S		I				A				N			
	M		N			7. S	C	L	E	R	O	S	I	S
							L				A			
8. S	P	I	N	A	L	C	O	R	D		T			
							W				I			
						9. H	I		10. M		O			
						O	N		Y		N			
					11. F	A	T	I	G	U	E			
									E		L			
						12. M	U	L	T	I	P	L	E	
							N							

Across:

4. Means the muscles are unable to move.

7. Hard scar tissue on the covering of the nerves.

8. This connects the brain to the nerves.

11. A symptom experienced by 90% of people with MS.

12. Means that many places in the nervous system are affected.

Down:

1. What happens when a muscle tightens up and can't relax.

2. This sends and receives messages to and from the nerves and muscles.

3. Initials that stand for a disease of the central nervous system.

5. When people with MS have trouble with this, it can be difficult to eat.

6. Feeling or awareness of conditions within or without the body.

9. If bath water is at this temperature, it can worsen MS symptoms temporarily.

10. The insulating sheath that covers the nerves.

3. If you did not use it as a pretest, use the crossword puzzle now as a learning activity. Review the answers together.

4. Lead your group to discuss the "Helping People With MS" section in the learning guide. If you currently have people with MS in your agency, ask if your staff members have any specific questions or problems with the people with MS that they are caring for. Work "together to suggest solutions based on what was learned in this lesson.

The lesson

Review the material in the lesson with participants. Allow for discussion.

Conclusion

Have participants take the test. Review the answers together. Award certificates to those who answer 70% of the test questions correctly.

Test answers

1. d	2. b	3. b	4. True	5. True
6. False	7. False	8. True	9. True	10. True

Multiple Sclerosis

Learning Guide

Contents:

- Overview

  - How does MS affect the body?

  - What happens to people with MS?

  - Common problems in MS

- Helping People With MS

  - Managing fatigue

  - Assisting with movement and muscle problems

  - Relieving painful and abnormal sensations

  - Managing cognitive and emotional difficulties

  - Helping people with depression and anxiety

  - Managing bowel and bladder problems

Overview

Multiple sclerosis (MS) is a disease that damages the body's central nervous system. There is no cure for MS, but while it is sometimes disabling, it is not fatal.

The central nervous system is composed of the brain and the spinal cord. It controls voluntary movements. When you move, the brain sends a message down the spinal cord to nerves that go throughout the body and to the muscles, telling the muscles what to do. The nerves send reports back to the brain about how you are moving and what you are feeling.

A protective substance called myelin covers the nerves in the brain and spinal cord. It works like the insulating cover on an electric wire, enabling electric impulses to travel to and from the brain.

MS causes the body to attack its own myelin, creating hard scar tissue on the damaged myelin and sometimes severing the nerve fiber itself. These damaged or destroyed areas interrupt the nerve impulses in their travels. The messages from brain to body and back again can get lost or distorted by these bumps in the road. The body may not work like it is supposed to because of lost or garbled messages.

The term sclerosis in the name of this disease refers to the scar formation, and multiple refers to the many areas of the central nervous system that are damaged.

How does MS affect the body?

Some common signs and symptoms of MS:

- Weakness

- Numbness and tingling

- Stiffness

- Tremors

- Difficulty walking

- Visual problems

- Speech problems (slurred or slow)

- Swallowing problems

- Pain (in face, body, legs, and arms)

- Bowel and bladder problems

- Sexual difficulties

- Fatigue

- Depression

- Difficulty remembering things

- Difficulty solving problems

What happens to people with MS?

MS is very unpredictable, and it follows a different course and causes different symptoms in every individual. Not knowing what will happen is very frustrating for the person with MS.

Many people with MS do well over their lifetime and do not need much help. Others become disabled and may need home care, assisted living, or skilled nursing care.

Usually, people with MS develop symptoms that may last a few days or several months, after which the symptoms may disappear or level off for a while (remission). The symptoms can appear again at any time (exacerbation). Some people may completely recover between exacerbations. Others may never have a remission. Some people continue to get worse, losing more functions with time.

Common problems in MS

Fatigue is experienced by 90% of people with MS. It often interferes with the ability to perform routine daily activities. The body is working extra hard, because nerve impulses have to struggle past scar tissue to get to their destination, creating overwhelming fatigue that can happen at any time, without warning or apparent cause. In addition, it takes more effort to do things because of other symptoms of MS, such as difficult movement or depression. Some things that may worsen MS fatigue are:

- Heat, fever, increased body temperature

- Stress

- Excessive physical activity

Problems with movement are often disabling and cause the individual with MS to need the help of others. When a person can't control arm or leg movements, he or she has difficulty doing everyday activities.

When messages from the brain to the limbs are interrupted or distorted, many different things can happen. The muscles might tighten up or spasm, or the hands may have tremors. Or, a message to move might get through only partially or not at all, resulting in weakness, paralysis, clumsiness, or falling. When the muscles around the mouth or throat are affected, the individual may have difficulty speaking or swallowing.

Stress, fatigue, and heat may temporarily worsen MS symptoms. Hot weather, or hot bath or shower water, may make it difficult for the person to see or move for a while.

Problems with sensation include difficulties with any of the five senses: hearing, sight, smell, taste, and touch. When messages from the nerves in the body cannot be properly sent back to the brain, the person may not be able to feel normal sensations, such as temperature, pressure, or position. The individual with MS might have poor vision, double vision, or see "holes" in the field of vision. Hearing, taste, and smell are rarely affected.

People with MS might have feelings of numbness, burning, or tingling. They may feel pain even when there is no injury. Muscle spasms can be very painful, as can the stabbing pains people with MS sometimes experience in the face. Injuries can result from sensory problems. For example, if someone with MS can't feel that bath water is too hot, he or she might get burned. Falls or foot damage can occur if the person cannot feel the ground under his or her feet.

Cognitive changes affect some, though not all, people with MS. Thought processes may be slowed. Common problems are:

- Difficulty remembering things

- Difficulty solving problems, which can lead to poor judgment

- Language problems, such as being unable to think of the right word

- Difficulty in concentrating or focusing

People who have these problems are not crazy or lazy. The symptoms may come and go and may get worse with depression, anxiety, fatigue, or stress.

Emotional discomfort, such as depression or anxiety, is a serious difficulty in people with MS. Many people with MS become depressed if they can't do things for themselves. Signs of depression include social withdrawal, altered sleeping or eating habits, and talk of hopeless feelings or suicide. Always report these signs to a supervisor.

Bowel and bladder problems, such as constipation, diarrhea, bowel incontinence, urinary incontinence, and urinary retention (inability to void) are common in people with MS because of the disrupted communication between the brain and the body.

Helping People With MS

There are many different ways to assist people with MS and to alleviate discomfort. Because MS symptoms are different in every person, guidance on how to help is listed by symptom.

Managing fatigue

The following guidelines can help people with MS manage their fatigue and maximize their activities:

- People with MS should stay in a comfortably cool, well-ventilated room

- Bath or shower water should not be too hot

- Activities and tasks should be planned ahead and spread throughout the day

- Activities and tasks should be paced, with periods of rest during the day

- Focus on activities and tasks that must be done or have the highest priority

When helping someone with MS, remember that fatigue has a big impact on an individual's ability to carry out activities of daily living. A person might be able to transfer with assistance in the morning but be so fatigued or weak by evening that they must be lifted. Even someone who can normally do certain things might need your help occasionally.

Assisting with movement and muscle problems

Because people with MS may have problems with movement, be sure to:

- Encourage as much independence in self-care as possible.

- Keep mobility aids such as walkers, canes, crutches, scooters, and wheelchairs maintained, and ensure they are used properly and safely.

- Keep the physical environment as safe and uncluttered as possible.

- Respect privacy for hygiene and dressing. Ask the person what he or she would like to wear.

- Remember that hot bath or shower water, or hot weather, may temporarily worsen symptoms.

- Help the individual stay well groomed. Put a magnifying mirror at eye level and style hair or assist with makeup as requested.

- Check that braces or splints worn by someone to support a leg or arm do not cause pressure sores or skin irritation.

- Follow the therapist's instructions if the individual with MS needs to have his or her arms and legs moved through a range of exercises and you are responsible for helping.

- Turn the person and ensure he or she changes positions at least every two hours to prevent pressure sores and skin breakdown if that person cannot move independently in bed or a chair must be used.

- Keep assistive devices within reach.

- Provide a straw, cut up tough foods, and open food containers at meals.

- Be very careful with hot food or liquids if the person's ability to feel is impaired.

- Ask what he or she would like to eat next if you are feeding someone.

- Allow plenty of time for chewing and swallowing, and watch for swallowing problems.

- Supervise the person constantly during eating to reduce the risk of choking. Also:

    – Have the person sit up while eating, and encourage the individual to eat slowly

    – Reduce distractions by turning off the TV or eliminating other noises

    – Be sure the food is the proper consistency for the person's needs (soft, pureed, etc.)

- Immediately report any choking or coughing problems associated with drinking or eating.

Relieving painful and abnormal sensations

To help a person who might be in pain or experience abnormal sensations, remember that wearing a glove or stocking may ease the burning or tingling in a hand or leg and that range-of-motion and stretching exercises may ease the discomfort caused by immobility.

Managing cognitive and emotional difficulties

The following are some strategies that can help manage cognitive problems:

- Organize the environment so that items used regularly remain in familiar places.

- Develop a consistent daily routine.

- Limit activities to a short time period.

- Conduct conversations in quiet places to minimize distractions.

- Repeat information and write down important points.

- Follow verbal instructions with written backup and visual aids when possible.

- Introduce change slowly, one step at a time. Work on one task at a time.

- Encourage the person to keep a notebook of important information.

- Provide a quiet environment for activities that require more mental activity.

Helping people with depression and anxiety

Encourage people who are feeling depressed or anxious to express their feelings, and listen without judging. Help them stay connected to others by phone and letters; support friendships. Assist with hobbies, interests, and activities.

Managing bowel and bladder problems

People with MS often experience issues with bowel and bladder function. The following guidelines can help you assist the person and ease discomfort.

Constipation

Observe how often the person has a bowel movement, and:

- How hard or soft the stool is and how much difficulty the person has passing the stool

- Any complaints of fullness in the stomach area

Report these signs to a supervisor. A high-fiber diet and plenty of fluids help with constipation.

Diarrhea and bowel incontinence

Diarrhea can occur if a person has been constipated and developed an impaction. Irritating foods, such as coffee and some spices, might also cause it. In people with MS, diarrhea might be due to other problems with the muscles and organs. Report diarrhea to your supervisor.

To help a person with bowel incontinence:

- Respond quickly when they need help going to the bathroom.

- Encourage a high-fiber diet and offer fluids often.

- Become familiar with the person's pattern of bowel elimination, and then offer opportunities for bathroom use as often as needed. Assist the individual to the bathroom and give sufficient time and privacy. Be sensitive to the embarrassment the person might feel.

- Use protective undergarments. Change them as soon as they become soiled.

- Wash affected areas with gentle soap and dry thoroughly after each bowel movement.

- Observe skin for moistness, redness, or breakdown.

Urinary incontinence

You may need to help the person control the amount and timing of fluid intake. If the person is incontinent at night or during a recreational activity, he or she might want to avoid fluids in the evening or before the activity, but remember that it is important to get at least eight glasses of liquid per day. Always be prompt in answering requests for assistance to get to the bathroom.

Urinary retention

Sometimes people with MS are unable to completely empty urine from the bladder because of nerve damage or medications. To help them, monitor voiding patterns so that you will notice if they are experiencing an inability to empty the bladder. Some people with MS insert a catheter into their bladder several times per day to drain the urine. You can help by gathering the necessary supplies. Sometimes a catheter must stay in all the time. Help by keeping the tubing and drainage bag as clean as possible.

Figure 24.2: Simple Diagram of Nervous System

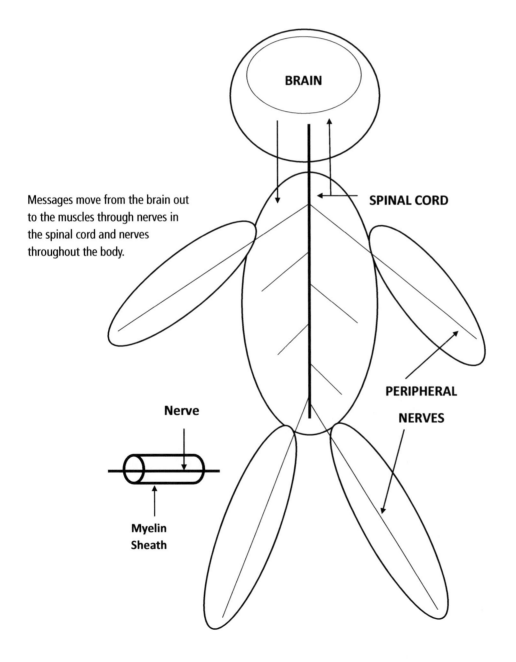

Messages move from the brain out to the muscles through nerves in the spinal cord and nerves throughout the body.

BRAIN

SPINAL CORD

PERIPHERAL

NERVES

Nerve

Myelin
Sheath

Multiple Sclerosis

Test

Name _____ Date _____ Score _____

Directions: Circle the correct answer.

1. Common symptoms of MS include all of the following *except*:

   a. Problems with vision

   b. Bladder problems

   c. Numbness

   d. Deafness

2. Which of the following is true about MS fatigue?

   a. Most people with MS never feel fatigued

   b. people with MS can get fatigued even without doing much

   c. There isn't much you can do to manage MS fatigue

   d. A hot tub would be good for someone with MS who is suffering from fatigue

3. Which of the following is true about cognitive changes in people with MS?

   a. MS never affects cognitive functions

   b. People with MS may have difficulty concentrating and solving problems

   c. Fatigue and emotional stress do not make cognitive functions worse

   d. If a person with MS has a memory problem, it is likely to become very severe

4. When myelin is damaged, messages traveling from the brain and spinal cord may be disrupted, causing weakness. True or False

5. Pressure sores can be caused by a tight splint or brace. True or False

6. Most people with MS have difficulty in understanding language. True or False

7. Hot baths and heat packs can alleviate MS symptoms. True or False

8. Sometimes people with MS get better for a while and then get worse again. True or False

9. A person with MS who has problems with sensation is at risk for burns. True or False

10. Wearing a stockings or gloves may relieve tingling or burning. True or False

CERTIFICATE OF COMPLETION

I hereby certify that

_____

has successfully completed the in-Service

Multiple Sclerosis

_____

Signature

25

Nutrition: Guidelines for Balanced Meals and Special Diets

Teaching Plan

To use this lesson for self-study, the learner should read the material, do the activity, and take the test. For group study, the leader may give each learner a copy of the learning guide and follow this teaching plan to conduct the lesson. Certificates may be copied for everyone who completes the lesson.

Learning objectives

After this lesson, participants should be able to:

- Relate the basic elements of good nutrition and why they are important

- Understand what makes up a balanced diet, including foods and portion sizes

- Be familiar with common special diets and how to prepare them

- State important factors in food safety and service

Lesson activities

Introduction:

- Ask your learners "Have any of you ever been on a diet?" Encourage some to talk about the types of diets they have tried and the results they obtained.

- Explain the content in the lesson overview and list the learning goals on a board if available.

Section 1: Basic elements of good nutrition

1. Explain "You are what you eat." Using the learning guide, deliver a lecture on the three elements of good nutrition. Emphasize that water is the most important element in the body.

2. Ask different learners to use the learning guide and teach the group about one of the five nutrients.

Section 2: The balanced diet

1. Use the picture of the plate at *www.choosemyplate.gov* to illustrate the content in the learning guide. Point to each food picture and ask the learners to tell you how many servings of each one are needed every day.

2. Emphasize that calorie needs vary by size, weight, age, and activity. A small female should use the smaller number of recommended servings.

3. Discuss the serving size examples listed in the learning guide. Point out that most fast-food hamburgers contain at least 4 oz. of meat, so that a small person who needs only two two-ounce servings of meat per day will receive the entire allotment with one hamburger.

4. Emphasize that elderly people have the same needs for nutrients, water, and fiber but have a decreased sense of taste. Everything they eat should have good nutrient value.

5. If time allows, ask the learners to use the balanced diet and serving sizes to write a one-day meal plan using foods they like. Discuss.

Section 3: Special diets

Review the six types of special diets in the learning guide, and add others that you use.

Section 4: Food safety and serving tips

Discuss the content in food safety and serving tips and allow time for questions.

Conclusion

Have participants take the test. Review the answers together. Award certificates to those who answer 70% of the test questions correctly.

Test answers

1. a	2. a	3. c	4. a	5. b
6. d	7. c	8. b	9. d	10. c

Nutrition: Guidelines for Balanced Meals and Special Diets

Learning Guide

Contents:

- Basic Elements of Good Nutrition

  - Fiber

  - The balanced diet

  - What's a serving?

- Special Diets

  - Low salt

  - Low fat (also low cholesterol)

  - Soft

  - Diabetic

  - High protein

  - Liquid diets

- Serving Tips

- Food Safety

Basic Elements of Good Nutrition

Everybody needs the right amount of nutrients. Nutrients are the elements of food used by the body for energy, maintenance, healing, and growth. They include:

- **Proteins** for growth of muscle and body tissue

  - Sources: meat, fish, eggs, milk, peas, beans, nuts

- **Carbohydrates** for energy

  - Sources: bread, grains, cereals, potatoes, peas, beans

- **Fats** for warmth, vitamin storage, and energy
  - Sources: meat, dairy products, vegetable oils, egg yolks
- **Vitamins** for healthy functioning of body systems
  - Sources: fruit, vegetables, meat, dairy products
- **Minerals** for growth, strength, healthy blood, bones, and body system functions
  - Sources: fruit, vegetables, meat, fish, dairy products, grains

Fiber

Fiber is important for digestion and waste elimination. Sources include cereals, grains, fruits, and vegetables.

> Fluid Needs
>
> Body weight = 2/3 water
>
> Daily need = 80 oz. fluid intake (8–10 glasses)
>
> Fluid intake should equal fluid output
>
> Too much water loss = dehydration
>
> Not enough water loss = edema
>
> Urine = 40% of fluid output
>
> Evaporation = 60% of fluid output

The balanced diet

The USDA recommends to fill plates ½ full of fruits and vegetables. The MyPlate icon is now used instead of the food pyramid (Figure 25.1).

Figure 25.1

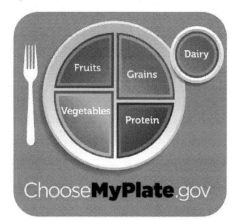

We all need balanced intake from six groups:

1. Breads, cereals, rice, pasta (6–11 servings)

2. Vegetables (3–5 servings)

3. Fruits (2–4 servings)

4. Meat, poultry, fish, beans, eggs, nuts (2–3 servings)

5. Milk, yogurt, cheese (2–3 servings)

AND

6. Limited intake of fats, oils, and sweets

Using a variety of different foods within these groups ensures balance and good nutrition.

What's in a serving?

- 1 serving of breads, cereals, rice, pasta (carbohydrates) = 1 slice bread or 1 tortilla, ½ cup cooked rice or pasta, 1 oz. dry cereal

- 1 serving of vegetables = 1 cup leafy vegetables (salad), 10 French fries, ½ cup cooked vegetables, ½ cup vegetable juice

- 1 serving of fruit = ½ cup canned, fresh, or frozen fruit, 1 medium (about the size of a baseball) apple, orange, or banana, ½ cup fruit juice

- 1 serving of protein meat, poultry, fish, beans, peanut butter, eggs (protein) = 2–3 oz. meat, poultry, fish, ½ cup dry beans or peas, 2 tablespoons peanut butter, 1 egg

- 1 serving of milk, yogurt, cheese = 1 cup milk, 8 oz. yogurt, 1.5 oz. cheddar cheese

> Calories are the amount of energy in food. Calorie need varies by size, weight, age, and activity. Body metabolism slows as we age, so the elderly require fewer calories. However, the need for water, fiber, and all nutrients remains the same in older people—so eating healthy food is more important!

Special Diets

Many people have special dietary needs because of illness, surgery, or ongoing conditions. Be sure you know the type of diet every resident is supposed to be eating. Mistakes on special diets can have serious results and cause many problems for the resident.

Low salt

Also called restricted sodium or low NA (the chemical abbreviation for salt or sodium). Many people with heart or kidney disease or high blood pressure must eat this way.

Guidelines:

- Little or no salt is used in preparing food

- No salt should be added by the resident

- Salty snacks are not allowed (e.g., potato chips, pretzels)

- Condiments that contain salt may be prohibited (e.g., ketchup, mustard, margarine)

Low fat (also low cholesterol)

Often recommended for people with heart disease or obesity.

Guidelines:

- Eat low-fat foods like chicken, vegetables, fruits, pasta, and cereal

- Do not eat fatty foods like ice cream, egg yolks, bacon, and sausage (or eat rarely and in very small amounts)

Soft

This diet helps people who have difficulty chewing or who suffer from certain kinds of stomach trouble. Eat cooked vegetables, ground meat, fish, and pureed foods.

Diabetic

It is important for people with diabetes to eat the right foods, whether or not they are taking insulin or other medicine to control their diabetes. A diabetic resident should have a diet plan designed especially for him or her by a doctor or nutritionist. It will specify certain amounts of carbohydrates, proteins, and fats.

High protein

A resident who has just had surgery or who has a wound often needs high protein to speed healing. To get protein, eat lots of meat, fish, eggs, beans, peas, and dairy products.

Liquid diets

Full liquid includes all liquids, such as strained soups, milk, and ice cream. Clear liquid includes only liquids you can see through, such as water, tea, apple juice, clear broth, and black coffee (no cream or milk).

Taste tip: Elderly people have a decreased sense of taste and often their stomachs can't handle spicy foods. Fresh, tasty foods with creative seasoning will help them get the nutrients they need.

Serving Tips

If a resident has impaired vision, identify the foods on his or her plate by using the clock face: "Your pork chop is at 3 o'clock, your mashed potatoes are at 6 o'clock, and your pudding is in a separate dish above the plate at 12 o'clock."

When assisting a resident, identify the foods and ask the resident what food he or she wants next. Offer seasonings if allowed. Offer liquids often, using a different straw for each liquid. Allow hot liquids to cool. Offer one bite at a time, using a spoon two-thirds full. Serve hot foods hot and cold foods cold!

Food Safety

To avoid food poisoning:

- Never undercook meat—cook until meat temperature is 165 degrees to kill the bacteria

- Refrigerated foods must be kept below 45 degrees

- Thaw frozen foods quickly and cook them before they reach room temperature

- Foods that will spoil at room temperature should be prepared last

- Keep fresh foods separate from one another and use different surfaces and utensils when preparing each one

- Cover unserved portions to prevent contamination

- Cool leftovers quickly and refrigerate in small containers

Nutrition: Guidelines for Balanced Meals and Special Diets

Test

Name _____ Date _____ Score _____

Directions: Circle the correct answer.

1. What do proteins do?

   a. Build muscle

   b. Nothing

   c. Build fat

   d. Provide an alkaline environment in the stomach

2. What are nutrients?

   a. The elements of food used by the body for energy, maintenance, healing, and growth

   b. The part of food that passes through the entire body

   c. People who provide nutritional advice

   d. None of the above

3. Which of the following stores vitamins?

   a. Protein

   b. Minerals

   c. Fats

   d. All of the above

4. What would be a serving of bread?

   a. 1 slice

   b. 2 slices

   c. A loaf

   d. 4 slices

5. Those on a low-salt diet should not be able to snack on _____.

   a. strawberries

   b. potato chips

   c. hard-boiled eggs

   d. carrots

6. Low-fat foods include _____.

   a. whole milk

   b. cheese

   c. bacon

   d. fruit

7. Someone with diabetes _____.

   a. cannot eat sugar

   b. should limit fluid intake

   c. usually has a plan that needs to be followed and includes a specified amount of fats, proteins, and carbohydrates

   d. needs soft foods

8. A high-protein diet is sometimes recommended to _____.

   a. lose weight

   b. speed up healing

   c. help with heartburn

   d. lower blood pressure

9. A clear-liquid diet can include _____.

   a. ice cream

   b. strained soup

   c. cookies

   d. tea

10. Which of the following follows food safety guidelines?

   a. After making a large beef stew, leave it on the stove to cool, and then put it in the refrigerator in the large pot you cooked it in.

   b. Leave your refrigerator at 57 degrees.

   c. Cover leftovers and put them in small containers, then put them in the fridge to cool them quickly.

   d. First, take out the ground beef from the refrigerator. Then, chop all your vegetables and other ingredients before you add the beef to the pan last.

CERTIFICATE OF COMPLETION

I hereby certify that

_____

has successfully completed the in-Service

Nutrition

_____

Signature _____

26

Oxygen Therapy

Teaching Plan

To use this lesson for self-study, the learner should read the material, do the activity, and take the test. For group study, the leader may give each learner a copy of the learning guide and follow this teaching plan to conduct the lesson. Certificates may be copied for everyone who completes the lesson.

Learning objectives

After this lesson, participants should be able to:

- Explain the body's normal mechanism for processing oxygen

- Describe conditions for which supplemental oxygen is used

- Recognize the different types of delivery systems for oxygen therapy

- Explain safety considerations for the use of oxygen

Lesson activities

Review the different delivery systems generally used for the delivery of oxygen therapy (oxygen concentrators, portable tanks, liquid oxygen). If possible, ask a local oxygen or medical-equipment supplier to bring different types of equipment to teach participants how to turn on the supply and set liter flow, allowing time for practice.

Conclusion

Have participants take the test. Review the answers together. Award certificates to those who answer 70% of the test questions correctly.

Test answers

1. oxygen	2. carbon dioxide	3. asthma, pneumonia, bronchitis, severe allergies
4. False	5. compressed gas, liquid oxygen, oxygen concentrator	6. True
7. True	8. headaches, slurred speech, sleepiness, or shallow, slow breathing	9. difficult, irregular breathing, restlessness or anxiety, tiredness or drowsiness, blue fingernail beds or lips, confusion, or the resident is easily distracted
10. True		

Oxygen Therapy

Learning Guide

Contents:

- Introduction

- How a Healthy Person Processes Oxygen

- When Things Don't Work Correctly

- Oxygen Therapy

  - Obtaining oxygen equipment

  - Types of oxygen delivery systems

  - Oxygen administration

  - General guidelines

- Safety Tips

  - When to notify your supervisor

Introduction

Oxygen is one component of the air that is all around us. It is a colorless, odorless, tasteless gas that forms 21% of our atmosphere. About two-thirds of the human body is composed of oxygen. About nine-tenths of all water is oxygen. It is absolutely essential to life on this planet. The human body must constantly take in fresh oxygen. We cannot survive longer than a few minutes without it.

How a Healthy Person Processes Oxygen

When we breathe in, or inhale, our respiratory system takes oxygen in through the nose, warming it as it moves down the trachea (windpipe), through the bronchial tree and into the lungs. Once in the lungs, the oxygen moves into the blood through special cells called alveoli. In the blood, red blood cells trade waste products (carbon dioxide) for oxygen and carry the fresh oxygen to the cells.

When everything is working properly, the oxygen goes into the blood and to every cell in our body, providing oxygen for energy, growth, and cell reproduction. When the demand for oxygen increases, as when we exercise, we take more air into the body to meet the needs of the cells. The body also uses the mechanism of breathing to release carbon dioxide, a waste product. As we breathe out, or exhale, the carbon dioxide leaves the body.

When Things Don't Work Correctly

When something goes wrong with the body's normal method for processing oxygen, medications and supplemental oxygen are used to help make sure the body gets the oxygen it needs.

If a resident has heart failure, he or she may have difficulty breathing. In this case, oxygen is often given along with special medications to make sure tissues in the heart and throughout the body receive needed oxygen.

If a resident has emphysema or chronic obstructive pulmonary disease (COPD), the alveoli become ineffective in exchanging oxygen for carbon dioxide. Supplemental oxygen therapy helps meet the resident's need for oxygen.

Residents with sleep disorders such as sleep apnea may also need oxygen therapy.

Other conditions, such as asthma, pneumonia, bronchitis, and severe allergies, may require short-term use of oxygen therapy. Usually, people with these conditions use extra oxygen for only a short time, until they are well.

Oxygen Therapy

Some people use supplemental oxygen only while exercising, others only while sleeping, and still others need oxygen continuously. A person's physician can do blood tests to help determine how much oxygen is needed and when. Oxygen therapy is a plan of oxygen supplementation prescribed by a doctor.

For people who do not get enough oxygen naturally, supplements of oxygen can have several benefits. Supplemental oxygen can improve their sleep and mood, increase their mental alertness and stamina, and allow their bodies to carry out normal functions. It also prevents heart failure in people with severe lung disease.

Oxygen at very high levels over a long period of time can be toxic and very harmful to one's health; therefore, a doctor's prescription is required. Oxygen used to treat medical conditions is a drug. We administer and document oxygen therapy according to the rules that govern medication administration.

The doctor's prescription will spell out the flow rate in liters per minute (LPM or L/M). This is how much oxygen the person for whom the prescription was written needs per minute, and it should not be changed without a doctor's order.

Obtaining oxygen equipment

Medical-equipment suppliers provide oxygen and an oxygen delivery system as ordered by a physician. When a resident obtains an oxygen system from the medical-equipment supplier, you'll learn how to assist the resident to set it up, store it, check for problems, and clean it. Keep the supplier's phone number handy in case of problems.

Types of oxygen delivery systems

The purpose of oxygen delivery systems is to get extra oxygen into the person's respiratory system and blood. Oxygen is available from three different delivery systems, each with advantages and disadvantages:

- **Compressed gas.** Oxygen gas can be compressed and stored in tanks or cylinders of steel or aluminum. These tanks come in many sizes; larger ones usually stay in one place, and people take the smaller ones with them when they want to move around. The tanks must be refilled with oxygen when the oxygen in them is gone.

- **Liquid oxygen.** When oxygen gas is cooled, it changes to a liquid form. People who are more active often use liquid oxygen, because larger amounts of oxygen can be stored in smaller, more-convenient containers than compressed oxygen. The disadvantage is that liquid oxygen cannot be kept for a long time, because it will evaporate. The containers must be refilled with liquid oxygen.

- **Oxygen concentrators.** Oxygen concentrators deliver oxygen directly from the air, but in higher concentrations. An oxygen concentrator is an electric device about the size of an end table. It produces oxygen by concentrating the oxygen that is already in the air and eliminating other gases. Compared to compressed gas and liquid oxygen, this method is less expensive, is easier to maintain, and doesn't require refilling, but it is not portable. Some oxygen concentrators give off heat and are noisy. The electric bill may rise with the use of these devices, and backup methods are necessary in case of a power failure. Oxygen concentrators may not deliver enough oxygen for some people. An oxygen concentrator will usually include a humidifier to warm and add moisture to the prescribed oxygen.

- **Large tanks and portable tanks.** Skilled-care facilities sometimes have a system for delivering oxygen directly into the person's room or apartment. Individuals living in any setting may have large tanks to store large amounts of liquid oxygen or compressed oxygen gas. In either case, the resident may need small, portable tanks of liquid or compressed oxygen for brief periods—a few hours—outside his or her room or apartment. Portable tanks are a backup system suitable to use in an emergency or when the resident leaves the room or apartment for meals or outings.

Oxygen administration

Oxygen is usually administered with continuous flow through a two-pronged nasal tube called a nasal cannula, even though this system wastes oxygen. To improve efficiency and increase the person's ability to move around, there are other devices. These include face masks, reservoir cannulas, and demand-type systems. Usually, a respiratory therapist, medical-equipment specialist, nurse, or physician instructs the person about proper oxygen use.

General guidelines

When assisting with an oxygen tank, an oxygen concentrator, or liquid oxygen, follow these important guidelines:

- Always stabilize the oxygen tank (using a special stand) and store it in an area that is out of the way, so it will not fall.

- Close the oxygen tank tightly when not in use.

- Because oxygen can cause an explosion, keep the oxygen tank away from any flammable source, such as matches, heaters, or hair dryers.

- Check the water level in the humidifier bottle (if one is provided) often. If it is near or below the refill line, pour out any remaining water and refill it with sterile or distilled water.

- If the resident complains of his or her nose "drying out," ask your supervisor about obtaining a water-soluble lubricant like K-Y Jelly to help keep nasal passages moist. Do not use petroleum-based products.

- If the oxygen tubing irritates the resident's skin (on sides of face or behind ears), ask your supervisor about using cotton balls or getting special moleskin protectors to protect skin from the tubing.

- If the resident's supply of oxygen is getting low (for portable tanks), advise him or her to reorder, or check with your supervisor about reordering. Oxygen should be ordered at least two or three days in advance to allow time for delivery.

- Maintain the oxygen flow at the prescribed rate. If you're not sure whether oxygen is flowing, check the tubing for kinks, blockages, or disconnection. Then make sure the system is on. If you're still unsure, submerge the nasal cannula in a glass of water, with the prongs pointing down. If bubbles appear, oxygen is flowing through the system. Shake off extra water before reinserting the cannula in the resident's nose.

Safety Tips

- Oxygen is highly combustible and may explode. It should not be used near electrical equipment or while using an electric appliance, such as an electric razor.

- A sign is usually placed on or near the apartment or room door to alert visitors that oxygen is in use. In a care facility, your supervisor will notify the local fire department that oxygen is in use in the building.

- Familiarize yourself with the location of fire extinguishers in the facility. If a fire does occur, turn off the oxygen immediately.

- Don't smoke—and don't allow others to smoke—near the oxygen system. Keep the system away from direct sunlight, space heaters and other sources of heat, and open flames, such as gas stoves.

- Don't run oxygen tubing under clothing, bed covers, furniture, or carpets.

- Keep the oxygen system upright.

- Make sure the oxygen is turned off and stored appropriately when not in use.

- Keep oxygen concentrators away from the wall to allow air to circulate.

When to notify your supervisor

The resident may not be getting enough oxygen if you notice the following signs:

- The resident has difficult, irregular breathing

- The resident is restless or anxious

- The resident is tired or drowsy

- The resident has blue fingernail beds or lips

- The resident is confused

- The resident is easily distracted

The resident may be getting too much oxygen if you notice these signs:

- The resident has headaches

- The resident has slurred speech

- The resident is sleepy or has difficulty waking up

- The resident has shallow, slow breathing

If any of these signs develop, call your supervisor or a nurse immediately. And—above all—never change the oxygen flow rate unless a licensed medical professional tells you to do so.

Oxygen Therapy

Test

Name _____ Date _____ Score _____

Directions: Fill in or circle the correct answer.

1. When breathing is normal, inhaling causes _____ to be drawn into the lungs.

2. Exhaling releases _____ _____ from the lungs.

3. People may need short-term oxygen therapy for _____,

   _____, _____, and _____.

4. It is safe to use electric razors and hair dryers in areas where oxygen is in use.   True or False

5. Three types of oxygen delivery systems are used. They are: _____,

   _____, and _____.

6. You should not adjust the rate of oxygen flow unless the nurse and/or doctor directs you to do

   so.   True or False

7. If a fire occurs, oxygen should be turned off immediately.   True or False

8. If a resident is getting too much oxygen, these signs may be noticed (name three):

   _____, _____, and _____.

9. If a resident is not getting enough oxygen, these signs may be noticed (name three):

   _____, _____, and _____.

10. You should report signs or symptoms of too little or too much oxygen immediately.
    True   or   False

CERTIFICATE OF COMPLETION

I hereby certify that

_____

has successfully completed the in-Service

Oxygen Therapy

_____
Signature

Pain Management

Teaching Plan

To use this lesson for self-study, the learner should read the material, do the activity, and take the test. For group study, the leader may give each learner a copy of the learning guide and follow this teaching plan to conduct the lesson. Certificates may be copied for everyone who completes the lesson.

Learning objectives

After this lesson, participants should be able to:

- Recognize the right to pain management

- Understand pain as the fifth vital sign

- Pay attention to residents' reports of pain and recognize nonverbal signs

- Know about different kinds of pain

- Know basic pain management concepts

Lesson activities

1. Before reviewing the lesson, ask your learners to read each of the conversations from the "What's Wrong Here?" section. As each one is read aloud, ask the group if anyone can tell you what is wrong with the conversation. Determine whether they have any ideas about how the conversation should be handled. Don't give them any answers or clarifications at this time; just have them share their ideas. Explain that we will learn more about pain in this lesson.

2. Explain to your workers that many people misunderstand pain and how we should respond to it. Ask them to look at the list of common misconceptions in the lesson. Tell them that all these things are incorrect. Refer them back to the conversations in "What's Wrong Here?" and ask them to identify the misconceptions in those conversations. Discuss this and allow for questions. The answers are on the test key.

3. Ask if any of your workers have ever experienced an illness that caused them pain. Did they find out that sometimes people or doctors didn't believe they were having pain or didn't think there was anything wrong? Emphasize that all complaints of pain should be investigated, and that only the resident knows the type and amount of pain he or she has. Review the section in the learning guide, "Pain: The Fifth Vital Sign." Review the nonverbal symptoms of pain and the importance of reporting a resident's pain to a supervisor.

4. Help staff go over the information about reporting and treating pain in the lesson. You may want to have them read it aloud. Discuss any policies and procedures you have in your facility about reporting pain, applying warm or cold compresses, exercise, or massage. Emphasize the importance of support, which is something all caregivers can give. Allow time for discussion and questions.

Conclusion

Have participants take the test. Review the answers together. Award certificates to those who answer 70% of the test questions correctly.

Test answers

1. d	2. b	3. e	4. a	5. c
6. True	7. False	8. False	9. False	10. False

Pain Management

Learning Guide

Contents:

- Introduction

- Common Misconceptions About Pain

    - How do you know if someone is in pain and can't or won't tell you?

- Types of Pain

    - Acute pain

    - Chronic pain

    - Major types of chronic pain

- Major Types of Pain Management

Introduction

The following are four conversations that were overheard while taking care of a resident. Each one demonstrates a misunderstanding about pain. Can you identify the problem or suggest a better way to think and talk about pain? Don't worry if you don't recognize the problem, because in this lesson you will learn about pain and how to deal with it in your work.

Scenario 1:

Mrs. Flynn: "My hands are really hurting today. That medicine the doctor gave me doesn't help very much."

Care partner: "I know how you feel. I have arthritis in my knees and they really hurt sometimes with all the walking I have to do. I guess it just gets worse the older you get, so we might as well get used to it and not complain about it."

Scenario 2:

Care partner Mary: "That Mrs. Garrett is always complaining about her pain. She takes way too much of her pain medicine if you ask me. I think she's addicted to it."

Care partner Alex: "You're probably right. Anyway, I don't think she really hurts all that bad. She's just lonely and wants some attention."

Scenario 3:

Care partner Joan: "Poor Mr. Howard. He's so confused, he doesn't even recognize his own daughter sometimes."

Care partner Jerry: "Well, one good thing, at least he doesn't complain about anything. Even when he fell and hurt his leg, he didn't ever say it bothered him. I heard that when your mind goes you don't feel pain."

Scenario 4:

Care partner: "Good morning, Mrs. Moore. How are you feeling today?"

Mrs. Moore: "I don't like to complain."

Care partner: "Is something wrong?"

Mrs. Moore: "Yes, my back is killing me and it hurts to walk, but please don't tell anyone. If my daughter or my doctor hear about it, they'll start doing a lot of painful tests on me and put me in a nursing home. Just help me get up and I'll be okay."

Common Misconceptions About Pain

Residents and workers may think that:

- Pain is a sign of aging

- Nothing can be done about some kinds of pain

- Pain is a punishment for past actions

- Pain is a sign of serious illness or impending death

- Complaining of pain is a sign of weakness

- Complaining of pain will lead to unpleasant medical tests

- Complaining of pain will result in losing one's independence

- Elderly and disabled people have a higher pain tolerance

- Confused people have a higher pain tolerance

- People who complain of pain are just trying to get attention

- Elderly and disabled people are likely to get addicted to painkillers

In the conversations you read, which of these misconceptions about pain can you find? Write the number of the matching misconception(s) beside the conversations on the preceding page.

All these ideas are wrong. Pain is a sign that something is wrong with our bodies, and it doesn't occur just because we get older. Healthy older people should not have pain. If something hurts, a physician should investigate to determine whether the pain is caused by a treatable condition. If the pain is caused by a condition that cannot be improved with treatment, then the doctor should prescribe medications that will allow the person to live without constant pain.

Everyone has the right to try to live without pain if it is possible to do so and the right to receive appropriate pain management when necessary. No one should suffer unnecessarily when treatment or relief is available.

Pain: The fifth vital sign

Pain is defined as an unpleasant sensory and emotional experience; however, it's important to realize that with pain, it's whatever the experiencing person says it is, and existing whenever they say it does.

To find out whether a person is healthy or not, we often check the four major vital signs: blood pressure, temperature, pulse, and respirations. In addition, we should check to determine whether the person is experiencing any pain. This is now being called "the fifth vital sign," because we know that the presence of pain is an indication of a health problem that should be investigated. When residents tell you they are having pain, or you see nonverbal signs of pain, you should always report this to your supervisor.

In addition, we must remember that only the resident really knows how he or she is feeling or how much pain he or she is experiencing. The person having pain is the only expert on this subject, and no one else has the right to make a judgment about the type or amount of pain an individual has.

We must always believe a person's self-report of pain. When we care for people with dementia, we may see that they exhibit their pain in nonverbal communication, such as pacing, moaning, aggression, anxiety, changes in usual behaviors, or withdrawal.

How do you know if someone is in pain and can't or won't tell you?

Watch for these nonverbal signs of pain:

- Guarded movements

- Facial grimacing

- Rapid heartbeat

- Rapid breathing

- Sadness or depression

- Elevated blood pressure

- Restlessness or sleeplessness

- Moaning, groaning, or sighing

- Bracing, or tensing the muscles

Any of these symptoms should be reported to your supervisor.

Types of Pain

Acute pain

Acute pain is severe and usually signals an injury or illness that must be treated. Kidney stones and heart attacks cause acute pain. When the cause of the pain is cured, the pain goes away.

Acute pain can be a symptom of serious problems that require emergency treatment. Acute pain is generally too intense to ignore and will often cause people to clutch the part of the body that is in pain. This type of pain indicates that medical attention is needed.

Chronic pain

Chronic pain is a persistent, ongoing pain that lasts for weeks, months, or years. Sometimes the pain was originally caused by an injury or illness that was cured, but for unknown reasons the pain continues. There may be an incurable disease causing the pain, such as cancer. Chronic pain can even occur without any known injury or illness causing it. The best that can be done in these situations is to treat the pain, without curing the underlying disease.

Chronic pain is not always constant and continuous but can come and go. Sometimes chronic pain becomes very sharp or severe for a time and then subsides. It can be very disabling to live with chronic pain, because the pain makes it too painful or tiring to perform everyday activities.

Chronic pain is caused when the nervous system keeps sending out pain signals repeatedly. It can cause loss of appetite, depression, irritability, and sleeplessness. Chronic-pain sufferers get caught in a vicious cycle of exhaustion and depression that can make the pain worse.

New medicines and treatments make it possible to relieve even the most severe pain. No one today should have to live with untreated chronic pain.

Major types of chronic pain

The following are some of the common kinds of chronic pain. Each has a variety of causes.

- Headache.

- Low back pain.

- Cancer pain.

- Arthritis pain.

- Angina—the chest pain caused by restricted blood flow to the heart.

- Neurogenic pain—this kind of pain comes from the nerve tissues and includes such painful conditions as trigeminal neuralgia, a disease that causes severe pain in the face.

- Psychogenic pain—this kind of pain is not due to any known disease or injury, but seems to come from the brain or mind.

- Persistent pain—this type defines pain that lasts for a prolonged period (usually more than three to six months) and is associated with chronic disease or injury. Persistent pain is not always time dependent, but can be characterized as pain that lasts longer than the anticipated healing time. Autonomic activity is usually absent, but persistent pain is often associated with functional loss, mood disruptions, behavior changes, and reduced quality of life. One example of persistent pain is osteoarthritis.

- Nociceptive pain—this type of pain refers to pain caused by stimulation of specific peripheral or visceral pain receptors. It results from disease processes (e.g., osteoarthritis), soft-tissue injuries (e.g., falls), and medical treatment (e.g., surgery, venipuncture, etc.). It is usually localized and responsive to treatment.

- Neuropathic pain—neuropathic type refers to pain caused by damage to the peripheral or central nervous system. This type of pain is associated with diabetic neuropathies, post-herpetic and trigeminal neuralgias, stroke, and chemotherapy treatment for cancer. It is usually more diffuse and less responsive to analgesic medications.

Major Types of Pain Management

Medication prescribed by a doctor is the best treatment for pain. There are also nondrug treatments that caregivers can use.

Mild exercise helps to increase flexibility and strength, relieving muscle stress that can cause backaches, headaches, and fatigue. Exercising in warm water is particularly good for arthritis sufferers, because the water relaxes and supports the muscles, making exercises easier to perform.

Warm or cool compresses applied to a painful area can bring temporary relief for headache, backache, and arthritis.

Massage is useful for back pain, but any painful area that is red or swollen should not be massaged until a doctor has evaluated the problem.

Sometimes a sympathetic listening ear and a caring attitude are the best medicine for people with chronic pain.

Pain Management

Test

Name _____ Date _____ Score _____

Directions (1–5): Fill in the blank by using the answer options that follow.

1. This kind of pain is severe and goes away when the underlying problem is cured. _____

2. This is a nonverbal sign of pain that should be reported to a nurse or doctor. _____

3. This is a common type of chronic pain. _____

4. This can be a helpful treatment for back pain, headaches, and arthritis. _____

5. This kind of pain is persistent and ongoing and sometimes occurs without a known cause.

_____

Answer options:

a. Mild exercise

b. Guarded movements

c. Chronic pain

d. Acute pain

e. Arthritis

Directions (6–10): Circle the correct answer: True or False.

6. We should always believe what a resident tells us about his or her pain. True or False

7. Warm or cold compresses aren't helpful in relieving pain. True or False

8. Confused people and the elderly have a higher pain tolerance. True or False

9. Nothing can be done to relieve certain types of pain. True or False

10. Elderly and disabled people are likely to get addicted to painkillers. True or False

CERTIFICATE OF COMPLETION

I hereby certify that

_____

has successfully completed the in-Service

Pain Management

_____

_____
Signature

28

Parkinson's Disease

Teaching Plan

To use this lesson for self-study, the learner should read the material, do the activity, and take the test. For group study, the leader may give each learner a copy of the learning guide and follow this teaching plan to conduct the lesson. Certificates may be copied for everyone who completes the lesson.

Learning objectives

After this lesson, a participant should be able to:

- State the cause and symptoms of Parkinson's disease

- List the main ways Parkinson's disease is treated

- Recognize ways to help a person with Parkinson's disease with mobility, swallowing, speech, and stomach problems

Lesson activities

1. Have participants do the word search puzzle in Figure 28.1 to familiarize them with terms and concepts related to Parkinson's disease. Then, review the learning guide with them and discuss any questions or concerns that may arise.

2. Ask the learners to close their eyes and try to imagine what it would feel like to suddenly lose control of their muscles. Ask them to imagine that the following things start to happen:

- Their hands shake uncontrollably

- They drool on themselves and can't make it stop

- Their face becomes a blank mask that is incapable of showing either anger or happiness

- They can't blink their eyes

- Their limbs and body are stiff and rigid

- They shuffle as they walk, and they can't help it or make it better

- They are unbalanced, leaning to one side

- They can't speak well enough to be understood

Conclude the exercise by explaining the cause and symptoms of Parkinson's disease as discussed in the learning guide.

3. Emphasize that there is no cure for Parkinson's disease. Briefly review the following ways to deal with the symptoms, as presented here and in the learning guide:

   - **Medications.** The most common side effects of the main drugs for Parkinson's disease are nausea and low blood pressure. Medication dosages often have to be adjusted as they become less effective.

   - **Surgery.** Most surgeries for Parkinson's disease are still experimental.

   - **Exercise.** This is an important treatment that your learners can help with by encouraging as many safe exercise activities as possible.

4. Review the four main complications of Parkinson's disease and allow for questions or comments. Have the learners complete the word search activity to review what they have learned.

5. Divide the learners into four groups, or ask four different people to assist you. Ask each group or person to review one of the "Ways to Help" sections on the second page of the learning guide. After they have had time to review, ask each group or person to tell the rest of the learners what they learned from the section. Allow time for learners to share other helpful techniques for assisting residents with Parkinson's disease

The lesson

Review the material in the lesson with participants. Allow for discussion.

Conclusion

Have participants take the test. Review the answers together. Award certificates to those who answer 70% of the test questions correctly.

Test answers

1. orders/commands	2. exercises	3. muscles	4. tremors, rigidity, slowness, balance
5. thinking	6. exercise	7. Constipation	8. count, music
9. tongue	10. encouraging		

Parkinson's Disease

Learning Guide

Contents:

- Understanding Parkinson's Disease

- Treating Parkinson's Disease

- Problems of Parkinson's Disease

- Helping Those With Parkinson's Disease

    - Improving mobility

    - Swallowing difficulties

    - Stomach problems

    - Speech difficulties

Understanding Parkinson's Disease

Imagine for a minute what would happen if the computers in the air traffic control tower at an airport began malfunctioning, shutting down and then working again at random, or giving the wrong information to the controllers. Airplanes would be flying without proper coordination or direction. The result would be chaos, confusion, and probably many accidents.

This is similar to what happens when a person has Parkinson's disease. This disorder is the result of the death or impairment of brain cells that produce the chemical dopamine. Dopamine helps direct muscle activity, so when the cells that produce it are lost, the brain can't correctly coordinate the body's muscle movements. It's as if the body's control tower computers are malfunctioning, and the muscles are left without direction. The result is disorganized movement and sometimes a complete inability to move at all.

Parkinson's disease is one form (the most common) of a group of disorders called Parkinsonism. These disorders all share the same main symptoms and are the result of the loss of dopamine-producing brain cells, but the disorders may have different causes and treatments. These disorders affect the motor, or movement, systems of the body. There are four main symptoms, which are:

1. Tremor or trembling in hands, arms, legs, jaw, and face

2. Rigidity or stiffness of limbs and trunk

3. Slowness of movement

4. Impaired balance and coordination

Parkinson's disease has the following characteristics:

- It is chronic, persisting over a long time

- It is progressive, growing worse over time

- It is not contagious or directly inherited

- It does not affect the thinking or feeling parts of the brain, so a person is aware of his or her disabilities and is often depressed by them

Symptoms of Parkinson's disease include:

- **Tremor.** Tremor, or shaking, usually begins in an extremity. The resident may notice a back-and-forth rubbing of their thumb and forefinger, known as a pill-rolling tremor. One characteristic of Parkinson's disease is a tremor in the hand when it is relaxed.

- **Slowed movement (bradykinesia).** Parkinson's disease may reduce the ability to move and slow the resident's overall movement, making simple tasks difficult and time-consuming. The person's steps may become shorter when he or she walks, or the person may find it difficult to get out of a chair. Also, the person may drag the feet as he or she tries to walk, making it difficult to move.

- **Rigid muscles.** Muscle stiffness may occur in any part of the body. The stiff muscles can limit the resident's range of motion and cause pain.

- **Impaired posture and balance.** The posture may become stooped and/or balance problems may result from Parkinson's disease.

- **Loss of automatic movements.** In Parkinson's disease, there may be a decreased ability to perform unconscious movements, including blinking, smiling, or swinging of the arms when walking.

- **Speech changes.** There may be speech problems as a result of Parkinson's disease. The person may speak softly or quickly, or he or she may slur or hesitate before talking. The speech may be more monotone rather than with the usual inflections.

- **Writing changes.** Writing may appear small and become difficult.

Treating Parkinson's Disease

There is no cure for Parkinson's disease, but some of these treatments may help control the symptoms of the disease or delay the progressive worsening of the symptoms:

- **Medications.** There are many different kinds of medications that can help with some of the symptoms of this disease, and new ones are being developed. No medication exists to cure the disease, and many of the medications become less effective over time.

- **Surgery.** Surgery is sometimes indicated to destroy parts of the brain that produce some of the symptoms, such as tremors and rigidity.

- **Exercise.** Physical therapy or muscle-strengthening exercises can tone muscles and put rigid muscles through a full range of motion. Exercises can improve balance, gait, strength, and speaking and swallowing ability. Exercise may also help with depression. It can postpone the worsening of the disability and enable the affected person to be able to continue more activities of daily living for a longer time.

- **Diet.** Although research has not found any nutrients or special diets that have any therapeutic value for this condition, adequate fluid and calorie intake are important to prevent dehydration and weight loss.

Problems of Parkinson's Disease

Parkinson's disease presents many problems to those affected, mainly:

- **Impaired mobility,** including a halting or shuffling gait and freezing or slowing when trying to move.

- **Slowing of the stomach and intestinal muscles,** causing constipation, loss of appetite, and weight loss.

- **Inability to control the muscles in the mouth, face, jaw, and throat.** This leads to drooling and swallowing difficulties, causing dehydration and weight loss. It also creates difficulties with speech and is a factor in respiratory infections and pneumonia.

- **Falls** caused by impaired mobility. Often people with Parkinson's disease need to use ambulatory aids (e.g., rails, canes, walkers) and fall-prevention techniques.

Helping Those With Parkinson's Disease

The best way to help people with Parkinson's disease is to understand their struggles with different areas of life. The following are some tips in each of those areas.

Improving mobility

Maintaining a rhythmic stride—this is the key to smooth mobility and gait but is very difficult for someone with Parkinson's disease. Try this:

1. Teach the resident to look ahead to anticipate changes in the flooring, such as a change from carpet to tile. Anticipating these changes in advance gives the brain a longer time to coordinate the change and may help prevent the freezing or slowing that can occur when an adjustment to the stride is required.

2. Teach the resident to count while he walks, counting "1, 2, 3, 4" over and over again. Another way is to listen to strongly rhythmical music in a headset (such as marching music). This provides cues to the brain, stimulating regular movement.

3. If the resident freezes in place:

   – Never pull him or her forward by the arms—this can cause a fall.

   – Have the resident take a step backward or sideways, which can stimulate a return of movement so the resident can again move forward.

   – Have the resident give orders to his or her body. The person should say, "Right foot up, right foot down," etc., while starting to walk. This prompts the brain to send the right signals to the muscles.

Swallowing difficulties

To help a resident with swallowing difficulties:

- Use thick liquids, not thin, for the resident who has trouble swallowing. Give soft and semisoft foods.

- Teach the resident to think of swallowing as a sequence of small events:

   – Put food on the tongue

   – Close the lips

   – Chew the food

- Lift the tongue up and back

- Swallow

- Teach the resident to alternate chewing on one side of the mouth and then the other.

Stomach problems

Constipation can be a very serious problem for these residents. Be sure to:

- Provide a diet high in fiber—vegetables, fruits, and whole-grain breads are good.

- Encourage fluid intake—make sure the resident has cups and utensils that he or she can easily manipulate. Straws often help.

- Encourage exercise, such as a daily walk.

- Weight loss caused by a loss of appetite and by swallowing difficulties leads to poor health. It can help to:

  - Weigh the resident weekly

  - Offer smaller, more frequent meals, which can be easier to swallow and digest

  - Offer high-calorie liquids like instant breakfast drinks

Speech difficulties

Teach deep breathing exercises to build strength in the respiratory muscles:

- Take five deep breaths, expanding the stomach muscles on inhalation

- Exhale while speaking the sounds "ah" and "oh" aloud

- Deeply inhale, then exhale while saying the days of the week with pronounced facial motions

Also, remember to:

- Have patience. Don't rush the resident who is trying to talk. Be sure your body language is relaxed and that you are patient and encouraging. If the resident becomes frustrated when trying to speak, phrase questions that require only a yes or no answer. Offer to provide a word or phrase, or offer to return later.

- Encourage the resident to sing and to read or speak aloud. This provides exercise, stimulation, and practice.

Figure 28.1 Parkinson's Disease Word Search

```
E   D   I   R   T   S   C   I   M   H   T   Y   H   R
P   N   E   U   M   O   N   I   A   P   G   C   G   M
Q   L   D   E   H   Y   D   R   A   T   I   O   N   O
W   Z   D   E   P   R   E   S   S   I   O   N   I   B
I   N   S   T   A   B   I   L   I   T   Y   S   W   I
E   V   I   S   S   E   R   G   O   R   P   T   O   L
M   B   S   O   R   D   S   E   A   H   U   I   L   I
U   A   S   F   C   O   O   L   A   I   T   P   L   T
S   L   E   T   I   S   M   P   L   T   T   A   A   Y
C   A   N   F   N   U   O   E   A   A   H   T   W   I
L   N   W   O   O   F   H   H   R   M   F   I   S   T
E   C   O   O   R   D   I   N   A   T   I   O   N   R
S   E   L   D   H   F   R   E   E   Z   I   N   G   G
W   Z   S   S   C   E   X   E   R   C   I   S   E   Y
Y   T   I   D   I   G   I   R   H   C   E   E   P   S
```

Balance	Exercise	Progressive
Chronic	Falls	Rhythmic stride
Constipation	Freezing	Rigidity
Coordination	Gait	Slowness
Deep breathing	Instability	Soft foods
Dehydration	Mobility	Speech
Depression	Muscles	Swallowing
Dopamine	Pneumonia	Tremors

Parkinson's Disease

Test

Name _____ Date _____ Score _____

1. If a person with Parkinson's disease freezes in place while trying to move, have him or her give _____ aloud to his or her body.

2. Singing, reading aloud, and speaking aloud are good _____ for the muscles of the mouth, face, and throat.

3. Parkinson's disease is the result of the death or impairment of brain cells that produce dopamine, which is a chemical that helps direct _____ activity.

4. What are the four main symptoms of Parkinson's disease?

    a. _____ in hands, arms, legs, jaw, and face

    b. _____ or stiffness of limbs and trunk

    c. _____ of movement

    d. Impaired _____ and coordination

5. Parkinson's disease does not affect the _____ or feeling parts of the brain.

6. Three things that are used to treat the symptoms of Parkinson's disease are medications, surgery, and _____.

7. _____ and loss of appetite are problems for Parkinson's disease sufferers because the stomach and intestinal muscles slow down and do not work properly.

8. You can teach a resident to use cues to stimulate his or her brain to keep a regular stride when walking. Two ways to do this are: (1) teach the resident to _____ while walking and (2) have the resident listen to strongly rhythmic _____ in a headset.

9. It is useful for a resident who has difficulty swallowing to think of the process as a series of small events. As you teach the resident to do one thing at a time, use this sequence:

    a. Put food on the tongue

    b. Close the lips

    c. Chew the food (alternate chewing on one side of the mouth and then the other)

    d. Lift the _____ up and back

    e. Swallow

10. When a resident with speech difficulties is trying to talk, you should not rush him or her and you should be patient and _____.

CERTIFICATE OF COMPLETION

I hereby certify that

_____

has successfully completed the in-Service

Parkinson's Disease

_____

Signature

29

Resident Education

Teaching Plan

To use this lesson for self-study, the learner should read the material, do the activity, and take the test. For group study, the leader may give each learner a copy of the learning guide and follow this teaching plan to conduct the lesson. Certificates may be copied for everyone who completes the lesson.

Learning objectives

After this lesson, participants should be able to:

- Understand adult education principles

- State the three pillars of resident safety

- Recognize three core concepts of resident-centered care

- Identify how a resident's culture might affect care

- Implement strategies to correct potentially unsafe practices in a culturally sensitive way

Lesson activities

After reviewing the lesson, have participants read the worksheet "Figure 29.1: How Would You Change These Resident Education Scenarios?" out loud and then discuss whether they think the resident actually learned in a way that will improve their care and understanding. If they don't think so, have them brainstorm why and discuss education strategies that would prevent the patient's confusion and lack of compliance.

The lesson

Review the material in the lesson with participants. Allow for discussion.

Conclusion

Have participants take the test. Review the answers together. Award certificates to those who answer 70% of the test questions correctly.

Test answers

1. a	2. (1) health literacy, (2) resident-centered care, (3) culture	3. d	4. b	5. True
6. b	7. b	8. d	9. b	10. True

Resident Education

Learning Guide

Contents:

- Education Leads to Better Care

- Adult Education Principles

- Three Pillars of Resident Education

- Choose the Right Time

- Listen to the Resident

- Education Outcomes

Education Leads to Better Care

Resident education is important to ensure proper care of your resident. The more your residents can understand about their care, the better they can take care of themselves in between your visits. Education increases safety in care and is likely to increase satisfaction in your residents and also in you!

Adult Education Principles

General adult education principles suggest that adults learn best when you address the following:

- Make them feel like they have control of their learning and the method for acquiring new knowledge

- Make them feel respected for their life experiences and other knowledge they bring to the "classroom"

- Provide educational experiences that build on previous experiences and have relevance to staff members' daily work and/or life

Three Pillars of Resident Education

1. **Health literacy: the ability to read, understand, and act on health information.** Giving a resident a handout or even verbal instruction and simply asking "Do you understand?" is not effective in terms of evaluating resident understanding. This is the critical difference between providing resident education and receiving resident education.

It's important to remember that even educated residents are often confronted with unfamiliar health terms. The resident may not be feeling well, may be quite sick, and/or may be worried about his or her health status, and in such cases, even very literate residents benefit from and appreciate simple communication (Figure 29.1).

It's helpful, especially on an initial assessment, to evaluate health literacy. Unfortunately, this becomes trickier for those who have difficulty reading (and who often have low health literacy as a result) because they usually have spent their lives actively hiding their affliction from just about everyone they come into contact with. Not being able to read, particularly as an adult, can create very embarrassing situations, and such residents will not tell anyone, let alone their care provider, that they cannot read. These residents have learned how to cope with not being able to read and have become skilled in hiding their problem. However, certain "red flag" behaviors indicate that a person may have difficulty reading and thus is prone to low health literacy. These are:

- Opening pill bottles to identify medication, as opposed to reading the label

- Eyes wandering over the page

- Taking a long time to complete forms

- Wanting friends/family members in the room during resident education interactions

Although it can be useful to try to gain an understanding of resident literacy level, a good practice is to use the same effective education strategies for everyone, similar to the use of universal precautions for all residents. For example, we do not actively screen all residents for infections before putting on gloves when providing direct resident care, yet we assume that all residents are potentially infectious, and to stop the spread of infection we don gloves. Even educated residents can have a difficult time comprehending their own health and care.

Figure 29.1 Examples of Clear Communication Techniques

Principle	Explanation	Example
Use a personal, conversational writing style.	Use second person as opposed to third person.	Use "you" or "your doctor" as opposed to "the doctor."
Use *active voice*. Passive voice is harder to comprehend.	Writing in active voice means the agent or doer of the action is the subject. Active sentences follow the agent-verb-receiver format.	*Active:* "Wash your hands before each meal." *Passive:* "Hands should be washed before each meal."
Be consistent in the terminology used.	Avoid confusing the reader by using several different terms for the same thing. Pick one and use it throughout.	Pick one term—for example, pills, medicine, or medication—rather than using all three in the same document.
Use common, one- and two-syllable words; define all medical terms.	Using one- and two-syllable words helps bring down the reading level.	Use "doctor" instead of "physician" and "pills" instead of "medication."
Engage the reader.	Documents that engage the reader are more likely to be read entirely and remembered.	Use a question-and-answer format or leave spaces for patients to fill in their responses on what they need to do.

2. **Resident-centered care:** Care that is collaborated with residents and their families, in which providers treat them holistically (i.e., viewing the resident as a whole and complete person, with specific fears, worries, issues, needs, and wants, instead of as a generic resident). Providers must also actively involve residents and their families in all aspects of care.

In addition, the Institute of Medicine has defined the core concepts of resident-/family-centered care to be as follows:

- **Dignity and respect:** Providers listen to and honor the resident's and his or her family's perspectives and choices. The knowledge, values, beliefs, and cultural backgrounds of the resident and his or her family are incorporated into the planning and delivery of care.

- **Information sharing:** Providers communicate and share complete and unbiased information with residents and their families in ways that are affirming and useful. Residents and their families receive timely, complete, and accurate information to effectively participate in care and decision-making.

- **Participation:** Residents and their families are encouraged and supported in participating in care and decision-making at the level they choose.

Not only is resident education woven into all of the core concepts, but providing resident education in a collaborative partnership is paramount to ensuring that residents and their families understand their care and what they need to do and know to stay healthy. Communicating in a way in which residents and their families can understand what is being discussed is the essence of utilizing resident-centered communication techniques. When we speak in medical terms, use jargon or complex approaches, or provide information that we feel the resident should know, we are taking a medical-centered (or practitioner-centered) approach.

3. **Culture:** The specific customs and beliefs given in a collective group of people. Everyone is influenced by his or her culture. Whether this influence is related to how holidays are celebrated, how foods are prepared, or what world view is held, culture impacts the daily life of every person. Not to be forgotten in the circle of influence are medical care and health belief systems. All cultures and different ethnic groups have beliefs related to healthcare, such as conceptualizations of health and illness, the nature of the disease, and the nature of the cause and effect. As a result, healthcare—in particular, resident education—has an obligation to provide information that is culturally sensitive and relevant.

There can be a distinction between illness and disease. Illness can be seen as the personal experience, unique to each individual, of what is currently happening to him or her and his or her body. Disease, in contrast, is the providers' interpretation of what is happening in the same context. This explains why residents perceive the same diagnosis in very different ways.

At times, the answers to these questions may uncover a potentially unsafe practice, such as usage of herbs or alternative therapies that may prove harmful. It's important to address this issue in a sensitive way, by:

- Listening to the resident, attempting to find out why the harmful practice is important to the resident.

- Explaining why the practice is harmful in a biological and medical way and why the provider is concerned about the resident's health and well-being if the practice continues. It's important to not make any disparaging remarks or otherwise offend the resident's preferred practice, but to approach the subject as objectively as possible.

> Example: "Mr. Smith, I understand that you like to use nightshade as a way to combat your asthma and that you find it helps. I am concerned about your use of nightshade because it can interfere with your heart rate and potentially cause you to have a heart attack. Nightshade often overexcites your heart."

- Acknowledge the differences but understand the shared purpose of reaching a state of health and well-being for the resident. This should be emphasized, while respectfully acknowledging each other's differences.

- Recommend a plan that is as mutually acceptable as possible. By starting with the resident's cultural norm, the nurse respects the resident's cultural needs and still alters the practice that is harmful.

- Negotiate the plan with the resident in a mutual relationship of partnership and involvement.

The answers to the earlier list of questions provide insight into how the resident views his or her condition and primary modes of treating it in his or her culture and may reveal complementary therapies that the resident utilizes for healthcare. This may also provide the resident educator with an opportunity to use and offer complementary/alternative healing practices.

Choose the Right Time

If a resident is worried about chapped lips or a scab on the arm, and you are providing education about nutrition, it might not quite get through. It's important to realize that residents' needs need to be addressed before they are likely to listen and comprehend care education. If it's not possible to meet their needs at that specific time, let residents know that you heard them and understand the importance of the problem and ask if you can change the subject for just a short while.

Listen to the Resident

Ensure that you listen to the resident before and during education. If the resident has asked about whether he or she can still eat spicy food as you are discussing nutrition, answer the question before moving on.

Education Outcomes

Any provider can offer stellar education strategies to teach a resident, but if the resident did not learn despite these strategies, the education has failed. It's important to take time to ensure that the resident understands what has just been taught.

To check whether residents understand what you have said, or given them to read, a golden rule is to ask them to repeat the education in their own words, and ask them to give some examples.

For example, if you have given some pamphlets with pictures of breathing exercises, ask for the resident to try an exercise with you. Or, if you have a resident with diabetes and have reviewed good nutrition, ask him or her to think of a day's worth of meals and snacks that would be beneficial to him or her. Or, if you're discussing monitoring, ask the resident "At what number is your glucose too low?"

Simply asking "Do you understand?" is not the best way to ensure someone understands. Asking the person to repeat you in his or her own words, give you examples of what has been taught, or mimic you are better ways to ensure the person is learning.

How Would You Change These Patient Education Scenarios?

Scenario 1:

A 64-year-old man who was recently told by his physician that he needed to begin taking insulin for his diabetes is afraid of needles. He has had diabetes for 20 years and doesn't think this new plan is necessary. He is very concerned about administering his own injections. The provider responds by instructing the patient on the physiology, because she believes the foundation for diabetes education is to understand how the illness works.

Scenario 2:

Mary is a 76-year-old former English literature professor with chronic obstructive pulmonary disease (COPD) and is underweight and malnourished. At one of her first visits, her nurse gives her an educational pamphlet on breathing exercises that includes text and pictures. The nurse also emphasizes the importance of eating more and gives her another pamphlet on nutrition. Mary barely glances over the pamphlets and puts them aside.

Scenario 3:

The provider visits an 80-year-old patient and asks if anything new has been bothering her. She says she has been having pain from her upper stomach and esophagus every night and gets slightly nauseous. She is Chinese and has been using her specially made peppermint tea to calm her stomach after dinner and before bed. Peppermint herbal tea has been used in her family as long as she can remember to calm the stomach. The nurse recognizes that this might be heartburn and acid reflux pain and tells her that peppermint will make it worse and to never drink peppermint or any other kind of tea before bedtime.

Suggestion for Improvement

Scenario 1: Although the provider offers education, she does not address the patient's fear of needles nor assessed his understanding. It's likely he didn't listen to anything she said. Instead, she could have explained to him why insulin is important, why it needs to be injected, assured him that needles don't hurt that much and that anyone can learn to inject themselves, and that he will get used to it. The provider could possibly go over injection techniques and have him mimic them and have him explain in his own words what has changed with his diabetes and why he now must take insulin.

Scenario 2: The provider here has likely taken the patient's background and former career as a sign of immediate comprehension, but the patient has not read the pamphlets and the provider did not assess her comprehension of them. Instead, it would have been useful to ask the patient to practice some of the breathing exercises with the provider and also to perhaps give some examples of what she might eat in a day that would help her gain nourishment.

Scenario 3: Although the provider may likely be correct that the peppermint tea is causing heartburn and acid reflux, he did not take the patient's culture into account. Instead of bewildering the patient by telling her to go against this decades-old family cure, he should explain that peppermint is known to help with nausea, but he thinks that her specific nausea might be caused by heartburn/acid reflux and might be caused by what she's eating, and that, unfortunately, the peppermint in the tea often makes heartburn/acid reflux much worse, especially right before lying down for the night. If she is adamant about drinking tea, discuss other herbal teas she might have earlier in the day.

Resident Education

Test

Name _____ Date _____ Score _____

Directions: Fill in or circle the correct answer.

1. Which of the following is an adult education principle?

    a. Make them feel like they have control of their learning and the method for acquiring new knowledge

    b. Always use technical and medical terminology, as they are adults

    c. Unless told otherwise, assume adult residents comprehend your education

    d. Only give them literature to read so they can learn on their own time

2. The three pillars of resident education are:

    1) _____

    2) _____

    3) _____

3. What is a sign that the resident cannot read or see well?

    a. Looking at pills, instead of at the label on the pill bottle, to determine what the pills are

    b. Eyes wandering over the page

    c. Wanting friends/family members in the room during resident education interactions

    d. All of the above

4. Which of the following is a core concept of resident-/family-centered care?

    a. Pamphlets

    b. Participation

    c. Exclusion

    d. Only seeing the resident as a disease to treat

5. Culture is defined as the specific customs and beliefs given in a collective group of people. True   or   False

6. The best way to handle a resident who might be performing an unsafe practice is to _____.

    a. yell at them

    b. listen to the resident explain why the practice is being performed and then explain why the practice is harmful, and then discuss together a new practice that can be a substitute

    c. assume the person is illiterate or deaf

    d. let the resident continue his or her harmful practice without saying anything, as you don't want to upset or offend him or her

7. You are providing nutritional guidance and your resident asks whether he can eat popcorn. You _____.

    a. ignore him because you don't want to interrupt the education

    b. answer him and then continue on with the education

    c. give him popcorn

    d. stop the education completely, as he is not paying attention

8. After you provide education, you _____.

    a. are done

    b. should ask whether the resident understands what you've reviewed

    c. should repeat it

    d. should ask the resident to tell you what you just said in his or her own words, or ask a specific question about the education to see whether he or she understands

9. Educating the resident:

    a. Is not important

    b. Can help ensure the resident receives better care and performs better self-care

    c. Is the resident's job

    d. All of the above

10. Dignity and respect are core principles of resident-centered care.   True   or   False

CERTIFICATE OF COMPLETION

I hereby certify that

_____

has successfully completed the in-Service

Resident Education

_____

Signature

30

Personal Care

Teaching Plan

To use this lesson for self-study, the learner should read the material, do the activity, and take the test. For group study, the leader may give each learner a copy of the learning guide and follow this teaching plan to conduct the lesson. Certificates may be copied for everyone who completes the lesson.

Learning objectives

After this lesson, participants should be able to:

- Create approaches for care that are person-centered and reflective of the wishes or unique needs of the resident

- Respect the rights and privacy and maintain the comfort, independence, and safety of a resident during the personal-care process

- Provide and assist with all major aspects of personal care and grooming in an approach that is person-centered

Lesson activities

Ask the learners to imagine for a minute that they are unable to take care of themselves and must have someone else help them with their personal cleanliness and grooming. As they think about this, ask them to say what they think their greatest need is in this situation. What is important to them as someone else provides their personal care?

After a few minutes of discussion, suggest the following three important rules of person-centered care assistance:

- Respect privacy, dignity, and choices

- Maintain safety, independence, and comfort

- Observe condition and report problems

Instruct the learners to write these rules down on the learning guide. Explain that you will now discuss specific personal care procedures.

Section 1: Dressing

1. Bring a large jogging suit or scrub suit to the classroom. Ask for a volunteer to come up and be "dressed." Demonstrate the way to dress and undress a resident by putting the jogging suit or scrubs on over the volunteer's clothes. Follow the learning guide procedure.

2. Ask why it is important to put pants on the resident when he or she is either sitting down or lying down. Be sure your learners understand that this procedure is the only safe way to assist with dressing the lower body.

Section 2: Bathing and shaving

1. Ask each learner to read one of the seven steps of bathing assistance in turn until all seven have been read aloud. Then ask the learners to cover up the learning guide and say the seven steps from memory, either working as a group or individually. Continue working on this until they are able to recite the steps in order. The learners do not need to recite each step in the exact words given but should be able to state the main idea.

2. Review the definitions of partial bath and soaks with the learners. Clarify your facility's bathing policies and procedures as needed.

3. Repeat the exercise in step 1 above, this time using the procedure for shaving. Learners should practice until they can say the six steps of the shaving procedure from memory.

Section 3: Other personal care assistance

1. Review the procedures for hair and nail care with the learners, encouraging discussion.

2. Clarify your facility's policies regarding fingernail and toenail care. Discuss the procedures for oral care.

3. If desired, review bedbound care procedures.

Conclusion

Have participants take the test. Review the answers together. Award certificates to those who answer 70% of the test questions correctly.

Test answers

1. b	2. c, d	3. 105; 110	4. brushed	5. a
6. 4, 3, 1, 7, 5, 2, 6	7. b	8. b	9. privacy; condition; comfort	10. b

Personal Care

Learning Guide

Contents:

- Dressing Assistance

- Bathing Assistance

  - Definitions of partial bath and soaks

- Procedure for Shaving

- Hair and Nail Care Assistance

- Oral Care Assistance

- Bathing the Bedbound Resident

Write the three basic rules for providing or assisting with personal care (your teacher will tell you, or look on the teaching plan for self-study):

1. _____

2. _____

3. _____

Dressing Assistance

Encourage the resident to select the clothing if possible. Make sure it is clean and neat. As you assist, watch for signs of dizziness or unsteadiness and be sure the resident is properly supported. As you assist the resident, make sure the resident can safely perform these dressing tasks.

1. Dress and undress the upper body first

2. If the resident has a weak side because of a stroke or other disability, dress that side first

3. Put the resident's footwear on before he or she gets out of bed

To put on pants:

1. Have the resident sit down

2. Put on underwear, socks, and pants, pulling the underwear and pants as high as the thighs

3. Put on shoes and help the resident stand up, and then pull the underwear and pants all the way up

4. If the resident cannot sit up, ask him or her to raise the hips off the bed while you pull the pants up

To remove pants:

1. Remove shoes and help the resident lie down

2. Unfasten pants, and pull pants off while the resident raises hips off bed by pushing with the feet

Bathing Assistance

When assisting a resident with a tub bath or shower, be alert to slippery floors, overly hot water, drafts, or dizziness. As you assist the resident, make sure the resident can safely perform these bathing tasks. Procedure for tub or shower bath:

1. Assemble soap, washcloth, towel, and gloves. Clean the floor of the shower if resident is taking a shower.

2. Place a rubber mat on the shower floor and a towel or mat on the tub bottom. Put a bath mat in front of the tub or shower.

3. Fill tub or get shower water to a comfortable 105–110 degrees.

4. Assist the resident to remove clothing and carefully enter the tub or shower.

5. Let the resident wash as much as possible, and then wash any areas the resident cannot reach.

6. Assist the resident out of the tub or shower and assist to pat dry (pat, don't rub) and dress.

7. Clean the tub or shower.

Definitions of partial bath and soaks

- **Soak:** Place a body part in water for a period of time—usually warm water between 105 and 110 degrees.

- **Sitz:** Soak the perineal area in warm water.

- **Partial bath:** Bathe only certain parts of the body. Residents may need you to assist only with parts they can't reach, such as the back, or they may prefer to wash only certain areas on some days to prevent the dry skin that can be caused by daily all-over bathing. Often this term refers to washing only the following areas: the face, the armpits, the perineum (private parts), the hands, and the feet.

Procedure for Shaving

1. Resident should be sitting up if possible. Assemble razor, soap, shaving cream/lotion, towel, washcloth.

2. Cover the chest and neck with a towel. Have warm (105–110 degrees) water handy in a basin or sink.

3. Wash the face and neck to soften the beard.

4. Rub shaving cream over the beard, or use shaving lotion for an electric razor if appropriate.

5. Hold head steady with one hand and shave with the other, using smooth downward strokes on the face and upward strokes on the neck and under the chin.

6. Wipe clean.

If you cut a resident's skin with a razor, apply direct pressure to the cut with your gloved finger until the bleeding stops.

Hair and Nail Care Assistance
Brushing hair:

1. Place resident in a sitting position

2. Cover the resident's shoulders (and pillow, if in bed) with a towel

3. Remove glasses, hairpins, and clips

4. Brush gently in sections

5. Remove tangles without pulling or tugging

6. Style in the manner the resident requests

Clean hair is necessary for good grooming. You may need to assist the resident in the tub or shower, or you may need to wash the hair in bed.

Washing hair:

1. Water temperature must be 105–110 degrees.

2. Hair should be brushed before washing.

3. Give the resident a towel to cover the eyes while washing the hair.

4. Wet hair thoroughly before applying shampoo. Warm the shampoo in your hands before putting it on the resident's head.

5. Massage the resident's scalp as you lather the shampoo.

6. Rinse the hair and wrap it in a towel. Dry the resident's face.

7. Comb the hair and dry it with a hair dryer or put it in rollers, styling as the resident requests.

When washing hair in bed, follow the same steps given above, with the following differences:

- Have the resident lie down without a pillow, with the head and shoulders on the side of the bed nearest you (but don't have the resident too close to the edge of the bed).

- Use a shampoo trough under the resident's head, with a basin on a chair next to the bed so the water flows from the trough into the basin. Remove the trough when finished.

Nail care:

Soak, clean, and shape fingernails and toenails with an emery board. Only trim nails if you have your supervisor's permission.

Oral Care Assistance

Procedure for handling dentures:

1. Handle with gauze so you have a good grip on the dentures.

2. Use only cold water to wash and soak dentures. Hot water can warp them.

3. Use denture cleaner to brush the dentures. Only store in the resident's personal holder.

Procedure for brushing teeth:

1. Everyone should brush the teeth at the beginning and end of every day and after meals if possible. If you assist with oral care, be sure to wear gloves.

2. Cover clothing and linens with a towel.

3. Use a wet toothbrush and toothpaste.

4. Use a gentle horizontal back-and-forth motion for brushing the inside and outside of the teeth.

5. When brushing the inside of the front teeth, hold the brush at an angle and use a side-to-side motion.

6. Be careful not to cause choking or gagging by putting the brush too far into the mouth.

7. Allow resident to rinse with a glass of water and spit it out and then wipe his or her mouth.

Oral care in bed:

1. When assisting a bedbound resident, raise the resident to a sitting position if possible, or place the resident on his or her side. Follow the steps given above, using a basin for spitting.

Procedure for flossing teeth:

1. Take about 18 inches of dental floss and wrap the ends around the middle finger of each hand. Wind around one finger until fingers are about eight inches apart.

2. Use your thumbs and index fingers to position the floss between each tooth. Gently move the floss up and down against the teeth, moving from tooth to tooth.

3. Unwind new floss about every other tooth, winding the used floss around the other finger.

4. Let the resident rinse.

Bathing the Bedbound Resident

Bed baths are given to residents who can't get out of bed for reasons that may be either temporary or permanent. The resident's entire body is washed one part at a time. The bath is usually given after elimination has occurred and is given along with oral care and a change of bed linens. *To avoid irritating the resident's skin, always pat with the washcloth and towel; don't rub.* Procedure for bed bath:

1. Place the resident in a supine (lying down) position and cover with a blanket.

2. Remove the resident's clothing, keeping him or her covered with the blanket.

3. Assemble equipment (basin, washcloth, soap, gloves, towel) and fill the basin with warm water. The water temperature should be between 105 and 110 degrees.

4. Put on disposable gloves. Place a towel over the resident's chest and blanket.

5. Wet the washcloth in the basin and form a mitt around your hand with the washcloth.

6. Wipe the resident's eyes with the washcloth and clear water, using a different corner of the mitt for each eye so you don't spread infection. Wipe each eye gently from the inside corner out.

7. Apply soap to your washcloth mitt. Wash the face, neck, ears, and behind the ears with the soapy mitt, and then rinse and pat dry.

8. Place a towel under the resident's far arm and wash the arm, shoulder, and underarm with a soapy mitt. Support the resident's elbow as you wash the arm. Rinse and pat dry.

9. Put the basin on the bed and place the resident's hand in the water. Wash the hands and between the fingers with soap and water. Clean under the fingernails carefully. Dry the hand and cover the arm with the blanket. Repeat steps 8 and 9 for the near arm and hand.

10. Pull the blanket back to the waist and cover the resident's chest with the towel. Lift the towel to wash the chest with a soapy mitt. Rinse and pat dry. Wash, rinse, and dry thoroughly under the female breast.

11. Repeat for the abdomen, keeping the resident covered everywhere besides the abdomen.

12. Place a towel under the far leg. Support the leg under the knee while washing, rinsing, and drying.

13. Wash the foot and between the toes in the basin, dry thoroughly, and cover the leg with the blanket. Repeat steps 12 and 13 for the near leg and foot.

14. Change the bath water. Turn resident on side, facing away from you. Put a towel on the bed beside the back. Uncover the back and buttocks and wash, rinse, and dry from neck to buttocks.

15. Provide perineal care last. Perineal care involves cleaning the private parts, or the genitals and anus.

Perineal care

1. Protect the bed with a waterproof pad under the resident's hips.

2. Lift the knees so the resident's feet are flat on the bed.

For females:

Spread the folds of genital skin (labia) apart and wipe each side from the front toward the back in one motion. Use a clean part of the cloth for each side. Replace the cloth as necessary. Repeat until clean, and then rinse and pat dry.

For males:

Lift the penis and wipe around the tip in a circular motion, and then rinse. Wash the shaft of the penis by wiping from the tip to the base and rinsing. Wash and rinse each side of the scrotum (testicles) and the inside of the thighs. Pat everything dry.

Anal area (sometimes called the rectum or rectal area): Turn resident on side, facing away from you. Wipe the anal area from the front of the genitals toward the back in one motion. Wipe first with toilet paper, and then wash one side at a time with a clean area of the washcloth. Replace the washcloth as needed.

Personal Care

Test

Name _____ Date _____ Score _____

Directions: Fill in or circle the correct answer.

1. To wash, rinse, and soak dentures, use only: _____

   a. hot water

   b. cold water

2. Follow these steps and techniques when shaving a man's face (circle two; worth 2 points):

   a. Apply shaving cream, shave face, and then wash face

   b. Wash face, apply shaving cream, shave face, wipe clean

   c. Cover chest and neck, wash face, apply shaving cream, shave face, wipe clean

   d. Use downward strokes on the face and upward strokes on the neck

   e. Use upward strokes on the face and downward strokes on the neck

3. Water temperature for personal care (showering, bathing, shampooing) should be between _____ degrees and _____ degrees (worth 2 points).

4. Before washing a resident's hair, the hair should be _____.

5. A partial bath means bathing _____.

   a. only certain parts of the body

   b. without soap

   c. once per week

6. You are assisting a resident with a shower. Put the following procedures in the correct order by placing the numbers 1–7 in front of the appropriate procedure.

_____ Help the resident undress and get into the shower

_____ Get the shower water to the right temperature

_____ Assemble equipment and clean the floor of the shower

_____ Clean the shower

_____ Let the resident wash, and then wash any areas he or she can't reach

_____ Put a rubber mat on the shower floor and a bath mat in front of the shower

_____ Help the resident out of the shower and assist with drying and dressing

7. When assisting with dressing or undressing, the _____ should be dressed and undressed first.

   a. lower half

   b. upper half

8. The correct procedure for assisting a resident in removing pants is _____.

   a. have the resident stand up while you pull the pants down and he steps out of them

   b. have the resident lie down and push his hips off the bed with his feet while you pull the pants off

   c. pull the pants off the bottom of one leg while the resident stands on the other leg

9. Write the three rules to remember when providing personal care (worth four points):

   1. Respect _____, dignity, and choices.

   2. Observe _____ and report problems.

   3. Maintain safety and _____.

10. When toweling a resident dry, _____.

   a. rub well to ensure the skin is dry

   b. pat dry

   c. use only hand towels

CERTIFICATE OF COMPLETION

I hereby certify that

_____

has successfully completed the in-Service

Personal Care

_____

Signature

31

■ Professionalism and Accountability

Teaching Plan

To use this lesson for self-study, the learner should read the material, do the activity, and take the test. For group study, the leader may give each learner a copy of the learning guide and follow this teaching plan to conduct the lesson. Certificates may be copied for everyone who completes the lesson.

Learning objectives

After this lesson, participants should be able to:

- List professional quality desired in skilled nursing staff

- Identify unprofessional behavior

- Define accountability

- Understand how accountability affects workplace culture

- List communication strategies to improve professionalism and accountability

Lesson activities

Review Figure 31.1 Case Study and then review the learning guide. Allow both to prompt discussion, and then discuss the following questions:

1. Take on the role of Heidi in taking note of Tina's behaviors and apply the personal accountability questions to Tina (e.g., does it appear that others—residents as well as supervisors—feel they can count on Tina?). In so doing, would you classify Tina as accountable?

2. Cite specific examples of Tina's behavior during her visit with Mr. Cortland that you believe showcased her accountability or professionalism. Which professional qualities did Tina exhibit? Did she conduct herself in an unprofessional manner in any way?

3. Cite specific instances of Tina's behavior during her visit with Mrs. Putnam that you believe showcased her accountability or professionalism. Which professional qualities did Tina exhibit? Did she conduct herself in an unprofessional manner in any way?

4. What lessons should Heidi incorporate into her own work as a new staff member based on Tina's conduct?

The lesson

Review the material in the lesson with participants. Allow for discussion.

Conclusion

Have participants take the test. Review the answers together. Award certificates to those who answer 70% of the test questions correctly.

Test answers

| 1. d | 2. c | 3. a | 4. b | 5. c |
| 6. b | 7. c | 8. a | 9. d | 10. b |

Professionalism and Accountability

Learning Guide

Contents:

- Professionalism

  - Professional qualities

  - Avoiding unprofessional behavior

- Accountability

  - Accountability and organizational roles

  - An accountability culture

  - Personal accountability

  - Identify sore spots

  - Your communication style

  - Holding peers accountable

  - Having the conversation

Professionalism

By understanding what accountability means in the skilled nursing setting, how to maintain personal accountability, and when to work with peers to achieve accountability, staff have the opportunity to improve the culture of accountability within a facility. Additionally, they display what it means, in part, to be a professional.

In a clinical, team-oriented setting where the shared goal is to provide the residents with the best possible care, professionalism among team members is critical. Professionalism entails consistent, appropriate, and respectful behavior on the part of an employee. It includes dressing properly, speaking in an appropriate fashion with peers, superiors, residents, and families, being punctual on a regular basis, and remaining accountable for all choices and behavior.

Those who act in a professional manner follow the golden rule: Treat others as you would like to be treated. If your loved one received care in your facility, how would you want to be addressed by staff and nurses? If you served as the facility's administrator, how would you want your clinicians to carry themselves? We can also use the platinum rule: treat others as they want to be treated. What you may want for yourself or your family might not be what the other person in your care wants; learn his or her unique needs and approach in a person-centered way.

Acting in a professional manner can be thought of as a skill that you can learn, and it is something that improves with practice. Knowing how to act and putting those skills into practice will ensure professionalism on the job. Professional behavior includes skills varying from how you greet residents to how you handle conflict. For example, how you treat residents' family and the level of respect you show for their ethnicity or traditions are both part of acting professionally.

Most facilities have a formal code of conduct or code of ethics that outlines acceptable, professional behavior. Depending on the level of detail, however, staff may face situations in which they will have to decide quickly how to act professionally in order to represent their agency and care for their residents successfully. When faced with such a decision, it helps to have a basic understanding of some behaviors that are part of acting professionally.

Professional qualities

Professionalism is a learned behavior. It must be practiced to seem natural. Professional behavior helps your residents and their families feel comfortable with you. This increases their trust in the care you give. There are some basic, common characteristics of professional behavior in the workplace. Some of the characteristics are especially important when working in the nursing and patient-care fields. Being pleasant and polite, treating others with respect, being honest, having a good work ethic, and doing your job to the best of your ability are qualities that all professionals try to achieve.

Think about the following qualities and descriptions. Do they apply to you and your work?

- Integrity:

  - Consistently honest and able to be trusted with the property and personal information of others

- Compassion:

  - Able to sense others' experiences and concerns and appreciates the experience of illness, including the suffering and fear

- Respect for others:

    - Maintains attitudes and behaviors that communicate concern for others, including consideration of values and the dignity of all feelings, beliefs, and experiences of different social and cultural groups; personal property and information are held confidential

- Self-motivation/time management:

    - Takes initiative to complete assignments and improve skills, accepts feedback and learning opportunities, and is punctual and completes tasks on time

- Personal grooming:

    - Maintains appropriate, neat, clean, and well-maintained clothing and uses little or no makeup and perfumes; nails are neat and meet infection-control standards

- Resident advocacy:

    - Does not allow personal beliefs or feelings to interfere with resident care, places the needs of residents above self-interest, protects and respects resident confidentiality and dignity, and encourages the residents to be as independent in his or her care as possible

- Service delivery:

    - Provides care in a safe, competent manner, does only the tasks assigned, and explains the care that will be given

Avoiding unprofessional behavior

Most employers consider certain behaviors unprofessional. Arriving to work late or discussing your personal problems with residents or their families are among those. Additionally, some actions are so serious that they can result in legal or disciplinary action. Those include:

- Verbal, physical, emotional, or sexual abuse of residents

- Not protecting resident confidentiality and violating rights

- Being negligent in performance of duties

- Destroying property

- Stealing from the residents' personal belongings

- Working while under the influence of alcohol

- Using illegal drugs

- Using your mobile phone or making personal calls during care

- Taking control of the financial or personal affairs of the residents

- Being absent from work without notifying supervisor and/or agency

- Showing disrespect to supervisors, managers, and/or coworkers

- Refusing to work where assigned

Remember to perform only tasks that you have been trained to do and are permitted within your job description. If you are not sure how to do something, ask your supervisor for direction. Demonstrate professional behavior at all times. Being respectful and sensitive when working with your residents lets them know that you truly care about them.

Find out about your facility's policy regarding accepting tips or gifts from residents or their families. Sometimes residents are so happy to receive care that they want to give gifts to staff. However, there can be problems associated with this, so know what your facility expects you to do when confronted with such a situation.

Figure 31.1: Case Study

Heidi recently began a new job as a CNA at Pinnacle Nursing Facility. Tina is one of the most experienced and respected CNAs in the facility and she will be Heidi's preceptor for her first week of clinical orientation. During this time Heidi will be able to observe Tina's interactions with residents, learn about routines and meet other team members.

On the first morning of clinical orientation Tina finds Heidi at the nurses station and they begin their shift by listening to the charge nurse share report updates about the residents. Tina introduces Heidi to the other CNAs and the charge nurse. She asks Heidi if she has any questions before they visit their first resident. Tina can see that the call light is on in Mr. Courtland's room. The first thing Heidi notices when they enter Mr. Cortland's room is how happy he is to see Tina. Sitting in his chair, he grabbed Tina's hand and said, "Good morning Tina, I am so happy to see you!" Tina said hello, introduced Heidi to Mr. Cortland, and explained that Heidi was a new CNA who would be helping her today. Mr. Cortland said hello to Heidi, who noticed that before providing any physical care, and before she turned off the call bell light Tina asked Mr. Cortland if there was something he needed, how he was feeling and if he had anything to report.

Later that morning, before they entered Mrs. Putnam's room, Tina shared with Heidi that at times Mrs. Putnam could be in distress or upset due to the pain she experienced as a result of end-stage renal disease. As they entered the room, Mrs. Putnam would not make eye contact with Tina or Heidi as she lay in her bed. Like she did with Mr. Cortland, Tina said hello to Mrs. Putnam, introduced Heidi and explained her presence, and asked Mrs. Putnam how she was doing. Tina told Heidi that she could tell Mrs. Putnam looked nervous by their standing in front of her. Tina sat down in an adjacent chair and asked Heidi to sit in the other chair in Mrs. Putnam's bedroom. Once they did, Mrs. Putnam seemed to relax but quickly spoke up and admonished Tina for taking so long to answer her call light. Heidi knew that Tina had been "running" all morning, but Tina avoided sharing the details with Mrs. Putnam and instead apologized for it taking a long time and assured Mrs. Putnam that she was there for her now and happy to help. After caring for Mrs. Putnam Tina shared with Heidi that if she had observed any indications that Mrs. Putnam was in pain or discomfort she would report them to the nurse.

Accountability

Accountability is a word we often hear in discussions about leadership. But what does accountability mean? And what do we mean when we talk about accountability in relation to the skilled nursing environment?

Accountability is a commitment—a promise to deliver a result by a given time. It is a word we use often in nursing and residents care. And just as often, it is a condition we find difficult to establish.

Simply put, accountability is about commitment: getting people to commit to doing something and then knowing they will follow through. It is always a challenge. You may say that you are committed to your residents and their positive outcomes or goals, but are you accountable in your care? Do you communicate with others to ensure all that can be done gets done? Being accountable will help your residents receive better care in the long run.

What people say they will do can be very different from what they actually do, and what we think they have committed to is often worlds apart from what they think they committed to. Yet accountability is critical when providing quality care and maintaining good working relationships with coworkers.

In this lesson, you will learn the basics of an accountability culture, the key elements of personal accountability, and how to improve communication to maintain peer accountability.

Before you can work toward achieving accountability, you need to ensure that you understand what the term means. We frequently hear the terms responsibility and accountability used interchangeably, but they do not mean the same thing.

A powerful distinction can exist between accountability and responsibility. An effective way to distinguish them is as follows:

- Accountability: a commitment to others to deliver and account for a result by a given date

- Responsibility: an authority over people to have them respond to one's direction

Accountability is about the results to be delivered. A result is a desired outcome that can be described. It is measurable, observable, and time limited—for example, "I will have the infection report completed by Friday."

Responsibility is about things that will respond to you. Think of responsibility as what is included in a job description. Your job responsibilities include the things you need to do to perform your job.

Accountability and organizational roles

Professionals in any organization often find themselves assuming three different roles at different times: supervisor, manager, and leader. Just because those specific words aren't part of your title doesn't mean you never take on these roles at work. Each role requires a different kind of work that calls for distinct skills:

- **Supervisors** are responsible for a well-defined set of activities to be carried out in a prescribed way. They know the work to be done and can tell someone else what to do and how to do it. However, supervisors are not held accountable for another professional's actions and results.

- **Managers** are responsible for how their teams run and the care that is provided. Managers have to produce results with those resources. A manager has all of the resources needed to deliver a well-defined set of expected results. A manager organizes, oversees, and responds to produce results. A manager needs to influence others to achieve expected results with available resources.

- **Leaders** appear when a person has intent that far exceeds his or her reach. The intent, expressed as a vision or goal, cannot be achieved with the resources the person is responsible for. A leader envisions exciting possibilities and enlists others in a shared vision. This person has accepted accountability for an outcome that is beyond his or her ability to produce independently.

An accountability culture

Being accountable is a choice people make. To have a culture that promotes accountability, facilities need a culture that encourages and celebrates people making choices, celebrates success, and celebrates the learning that occurs with every mistake.

In an accountability culture, there is no punishment. Punishment causes people to be risk averse and avoid accountability. Instead, an accountability culture promotes learning, performing, and improving. What does accountability look like in such a culture?

With accountability, you are seeking a result; you need someone to be accountable for the result. As a staff member, others may call on you to perform particular tasks with each residents, such as reporting vital signs that are outside of the normal range. With every task that is assigned, you accept accountability for that assignment. Based on your performance over time, staff members will gauge whether you are accountable.

Personal accountability

Accountability is about making and keeping commitments, and it starts with you. To demonstrate that you are accountable, you need to ask yourself what it will take for you to make a commitment. Start with yourself:

- Do you practice accountability?

- Do you do what you say you will do?

- Do others believe they can count on you?

It is unrealistic to expect accountability of others if you don't expect it of yourself. Accountability exists in all facets of your life, and in every relationship. It is about expectations and commitments. If you do not understand what is expected of you, you will not be successful in meeting commitments, even though you may work very hard to be accountable. It starts with clearly understanding what the other person is expecting.

Take time to assess your ability to be accountable with the following questions:

- When you say you are going to do something, do you mean it?

- Are your commitments realistic?

- Do you ensure that you understand what is expected of you?

- If you realize that you cannot keep a commitment, do you communicate this in a timely manner?

- Do you ask for help when making commitments and working on them?

Accountability often means you have to engage others to help you keep your commitments. Some people find this—depending on others—to be the most challenging part of accountability. Many times, we need others' help to be accountable. Approaching others for help demonstrates that you are holding yourself accountable to understanding your assignments and providing the best care possible to residents.

Identify sore spots

It is important to understand what prevents you from meeting expectations, making a commitment, and keeping a commitment. You need to understand your sore spots: the situations, individuals, or groups that threaten your ability to be accountable.

When someone of authority asks you to do something, do you say yes regardless of whether you mean it because of the position of the person who is asking you? Is there an individual who you have a hard time saying no to? You don't want to let this person down, so you say yes, but you may not be willing or able to do what this person is requesting. When you are not clear on what is expected of you, ask questions—make requests—until you understand what is expected, how it will be measured, and when it is expected to be completed.

Your communication style

How effectively do you communicate? Your accountability language can help you be an effective communicator. It will help you to clearly communicate your expectations. Consider the following:

- **Your actions and communication during a challenging situation.** When you are faced with challenges, it is easy to fall into the trap of blame and excuses. In an accountability culture, there is no blame or punishment. These create negative energy and cause you to lose focus on the goal. When you are in a difficult situation and are tempted to break into blame and negativity, remember that accountability is about clear expectations and making and keeping commitments. When commitments are not met, you need to understand what happened. What went well? The answer to this question is meant to create positive energy to generate more new ideas.

- **Your language and behavior.** Being accountable does not mean you can always do what is being requested. You may not be able to say yes to a request. The important part of accountability is that you commit to something. It is your job to make a commitment that you understand and can keep. If you cannot, you need to adjust the commitment to what you can achieve. Remember, use your accountability language to help you make and keep commitments. If you are unsure how to do something, you should not only ask but become accountability for learning and understanding the task.

- **Nonverbal communication.** Watch your nonverbal communication, too. Sometimes what you don't say reveals much more about your accountability. Take, for instance, a meeting you are in where everyone seems to be committing to doing something: Heads are nodding, people are smiling, and everyone seems to be engaged. In reality, the people walking out of the room may be saying to themselves, "I have no idea what they were talking about. I just said yes so that we could get out of there." Pay attention to whether you are behaving in the same way.

Holding peers accountable

The nature of an accountability culture and the dynamics of an effective accountability conversation are clearest when peers are involved. Here there is no clear line of authority to provide you with context. You might be trying to get another person to help you when the person doesn't have to, or perhaps someone is trying to get your support when you do not have to be involved.

The fact that all parties are equal puts the focus on the nature of the relationship you are creating. Most accountability conversations are about building relationships. Trust has to be built and communication has to be effective. Accountability is relationship driven; it's about relationships without fear of blame or punishment.

Think about who your team members are. As a care team member, you could work directly with your peers or you might work indirectly, but if you're working on the same community with the same residents, these are in fact your team members. Whether you communicate in person, by phone, or through documentation, you find yourself interacting with them, often on matters that affect your performance or your residents' care and outcome.

Having the conversation

You need to make sure the environment around you is free of punishment and blame and allows people to take risks. You need to make requests and offers. You need to ask your team members to make commitments and find out what it may take for them to keep their commitments.

Remember, commitments need to be defined, measurable, and time limited. When you are dealing with other people, you need to make sure you understand what the expectations are, the person you are working with understands what the expectations are, and you do your part to create an environment that supports and demands accountability.

The next time you want to achieve accountability, try using language that produces it. The following speech techniques can be very useful when having an accountability conversation:

- **Framing.** Turn on the listening you need by asking your audience to listen and process what they are hearing in a positive way.

- **Effective questions.** Turn on the creative power of the listeners by prompting them to consider positive questions during a discussion (e.g., "In what ways does this contribute to our goals?")

- **Active listening.** Make sure your team members understand the conversation by having them restate what is said in their own words.

- **Requests and offers.** How many times have you talked about what you needed but not received a response from the listener? We are good at describing and explaining, but we are not good at asking. This is how you generate commitments. Most meetings do not end with a clear understanding of who has promised to do what; often, it is just assumed that everyone knew what to do.

- **Hear yes/no.** When you are talking to someone about accountability, you want to know whether the person is committed to achieving the result under discussion. Too often, we hear what we want to, rather than what was said (e.g., "Yes, but …"). Verify what is being said.

- **Acknowledgment.** If someone makes a commitment and, more importantly, keeps that commitment, acknowledge it.

By understanding what accountability means in the clinical setting, how to maintain personal accountability, and when to work with peers to achieve accountability, you have the opportunity to improve the culture of accountability within an agency.

Accountability and Professionalism

Test

Name _____ Date _____ Score _____

Directions: Circle the best answer.

1. Accountability is _____.

    a. a commitment to others to deliver and stand by a specified result

    b. measurable, observable, and time limited

    c. distinguishable from responsibility

    d. all of the above

2. In an accountability culture, there is _____ punishment, because it causes people to be risk averse.

    a. limited

    b. frequent

    c. no

    d. sporadic

3. Which of the following is *not* one of the questions staff should ask themselves in attempting to determine whether they practice personal accountability?

    a. Do others seem to like you?

    b. Does your work meet your facility's established standards of timeliness and quality?

    c. Do others believe they can count on you?

    d. Do you regularly do what you say you will?

4. Commitments need to be all of the following *except*:

    a. Defined

    b. Measurable

    c. Ambiguous

    d. Time limited

5. Your accountability language can help you be an effective communicator. True or False

6. Professionalism entails consistent, appropriate, and respectful behavior and includes
    _____.

    a. avoiding the use of sick days

    b. being punctual on a regular basis

    c. relying on yourself and rarely on others

    d. changing jobs every few years to stay fresh and motivated

7. If a staff member maintains appropriate, clean, and well-maintained clothing, uses little or no makeup and perfumes, keeps his or her fingernails neat, and meets infection control standards, the staff member exhibits the _____ quality associated with professionalism.

    a. integrity

    b. compassion

    c. personal grooming

    d. resident advocacy

8. Which of the following behaviors is not professional conduct?

    a. Talking or texting on your phone during care

    b. Being on time

    c. Stating what you hope to achieve during care

    d. Respecting your resident's culture

9. To do well as a collective group of accountable professionals, a clinical team must have
   _____.

   a. clear goals

   b. trust

   c. a willingness to assist one another

   d. All of the above

10. It is nearly impossible to adhere to a collective plan, so team members should work according
    to their own individual concerns and needs. True or False

CERTIFICATE OF COMPLETION

I hereby certify that

has successfully completed the in-Service

Professionalism and Accountability

Signature

32

Psychosocial Care

Teaching Plan

To use this lesson for self-study, the learner should read the material, do the activity, and take the test. For group study, the leader may give each learner a copy of the learning guide and follow this teaching plan to conduct the lesson. Certificates may be copied for everyone who completes the lesson.

Learning objectives

After this lesson, participants should be able to:

- Define psychosocial care and recognize opportunities to provide it

- Practice good communication skills with residents

- Assist residents in fulfilling psychosocial needs

Lesson activities

Ask your participants to make a list of all the important people in their lives, such as family members, friends, and coworkers. Now ask them to look at the list and try to imagine what their lives would be like if they couldn't see some or all of those people anymore. Remind them that many of the residents we care for are lonely or have limited numbers of social interactions. Often, caregivers are the only people they interact with on a regular basis, so we are very important people in their lives.

Divide your participants into small groups of two or three. Assign each group one of the sections in the learning guide: self-esteem, adjustment to age or disability, coping mechanisms, communication, social relationships, intellectual stimulation, and sexuality. Give each group more than one topic if necessary, or make your groups larger to accommodate the number of participants. Ask each group to read the material on their topic in the learning guide and prepare to explain it to the rest of the participants.

After allowing enough time for the group work, bring everyone together and ask each group to present their material. Allow time for discussion and questions.

Discuss things the participants can do to meet the psychosocial needs of their residents. Ask each of the participants to look for opportunities to do these things. Plan to review their progress at some future date, and reward those who excel at good communication or other psychosocial care.

Conclusion

Have participants take the test. Review the answers together. Award certificates to those who answer 70% of the test questions correctly.

Test answers

1. False	2. True	3. d	4. True	5. False
6. b	7. False	8. True	9. False	10. True

Psychosocial Care

Learning Guide

Contents:

- Introduction

- Issues of Self-Esteem

- Adjustment to Illness, Disability, and Age

  - Anxiety and depression

  - The dying resident

- Coping Mechanisms

  - Faith

  - Stress management and relaxation techniques

  - Change of scenery

  - Communication

  - Social functioning and relationships

  - Intellectual stimulation

  - Sexuality

- Methods of Meeting Psychosocial Needs of Residents and Families

  - Education

  - Activities

  - Enjoying pets

  - Social workers

  - Education of healthcare workers

Introduction

Psychosocial care is care that enhances quality of life through the mental, social, spiritual, and emotional well-being of residents, families, and caregivers.

What does psychosocial care involve?

- Issues of self-esteem

- Adjustment to illness or disability

- Intellectual stimulation

- Social functioning and relationships

- Communication

- Sexuality

Issues of Self-Esteem

Anyone having contact with residents and their families provides psychosocial care. You can do your job in a way that helps your residents feel good about themselves, enhancing their self-esteem.

It is important to meet every resident's basic needs for acceptance, social opportunities, food, clothing, rest, activity, comfort, and safety. The way routine care is carried out affects a resident's mood, self-esteem, dignity, self-respect, and feelings of independence.

> Encourage and praise residents whenever possible, and remember that all physical care is an opportunity to provide good psychosocial care.

Physical care includes helping with daily activities. Paying attention to a resident's appearance, such as by shaving a man or fixing a woman's hair, is a practical way to enhance self-esteem. Look for small ways to make a difference.

Residents who are confined to bed or dealing with illness often experience tremendous emotional upset brought on by inactivity and dependence. Help the person express his or her feelings. High levels of emotional distress can make illness worse and can slow recovery.

Every resident should be encouraged to do as much of his or her personal care as possible. This gives many residents a real sense of dignity and accomplishment. Of course, always follow the plan of care.

Adjusting to Illness, Disability, and Age

Whether it happens suddenly or gradually, losing one's independence and finding it necessary to rely on others is a big adjustment that can create great emotional distress. Residents may feel the loss of friends and family as they become more dependent or isolated from their social network. In addition, family members often feel the stress of caregiving. Both residents and families may experience anxiety and/or depression.

Anxiety and depression

When a resident exhibits signs of anxiety or depression or says he or she feels anxious or depressed, pay attention. Anxiety and depression can be caused by some medicines, by withdrawal from medicines, or by a mental illness. Medications may be used to treat both conditions.

Cognitive loss or dementia can cause anxiety or depression or can be made worse by either condition. Anxiety and depression that go untreated may lead to physical problems or an increased risk of accidental injuries. Treatment can improve the person's quality of life.

Anxiety or depression may cause a decrease in daily functioning, behavior problems, or lapses in judgment.

The dying resident

Supporting a resident and family through death is important. Sometimes a dying person feels lonely and depressed. He or she may feel abandoned or hopeless and become resentful or withdrawn.

Many people are uncomfortable with the thought of death and prefer to withdraw and leave a dying person alone. Usually the sick and the dying need company. Sometimes there is nothing to do but hold the person's hand. If the dying person wants to talk about dying, listen and respond appropriately and honestly. If you do not know how to respond, simply assure the person that you care and encourage the person to talk about his or her feelings while you listen.

When you see that a resident is in pain or is uncomfortable, tell your supervisor. If appropriate, bring fresh pillows or sheets, remove wrinkles from the bed, or help the resident change position. Restlessness, tension, and discomfort may be relieved by a change in position. Determine whether the resident is thirsty or hungry, and ask if the temperature in the room is all right. Encourage the person to tell you what is causing his or her distress. Excitement, anxiety, and depression can contribute to pain—not all pain is physical.

When in a resident's presence, always speak directly to, not about or around, him or her. Since hearing is thought to be the last of the senses to fade, an unconscious person may hear and be hurt by careless conversations.

Coping Mechanisms

Faith

There is a difference between religion and spirituality. Religion may be based on traditional activities at church. Spirituality involves personal thoughts, feelings, characteristics, and experiences based on a supreme being. People may think of themselves as spiritual even when they are not involved with a church.

A hopeful, positive attitude about life and illness improves physical and mental health outcomes. People who use religious coping skills (praying, reading a sacred book, etc.) are less likely to develop depression and anxiety. Persons with a strong personal faith and many social contacts are better able to cope with health problems and remain more motivated to recover and to stay well. Caregivers who maintain social contacts and faith are better able to cope with the stresses of caregiving.

Workers can enhance the coping skills of both the resident and the family. Interventions include praying with residents, reading sacred books to them, and seeing that they have the religious materials they need, such as audiotapes and large-print books. Spiritual health should be included as part of the physical, mental, emotional, and social needs addressed in psychosocial care.

Stress management and relaxation techniques

Help residents use the following techniques when they are feeling anxious or depressed. As simple as these techniques are, they can be very calming and cheering.

Imaging

- Get comfortable

- Imagine a favorite scene (beach, mountain, etc.)

- Feel the body relax, enjoy the warmth of the sun, the smells of the beach, or the gentle breeze and cool crisp air in the mountains

- Continue until the body feels totally relaxed

Abdominal breathing

- Relax (either sitting or lying)

- Place right hand on chest and left hand on abdomen

- Breathe in slowly through the nose

- Hold breath and slowly count to five

- Purse lips and exhale slowly

- Relax

- Repeat

Change of scenery

Everyone needs a change of scenery from time to time. Residents that are able should be assisted to go on outings with friends and family. Those who cannot go out need visits from friends and family or from staff and volunteers if others don't come. Room decorations can be changed, plants or flowers added, pictures hung, or new curtains put in place. Sometimes a simple rearrangement of the furniture, if safe and possible, can improve a person's emotional outlook.

Communication

Good communication between workers, residents, and families is essential. Workers should be able to recognize the difference between a resident who just needs a listening ear and a resident who should be referred for formal counseling.

Communication takes place on two levels—verbal and nonverbal. Verbal is what is said. Nonverbal is expressed through body movements, gestures, facial expressions, posture, tone of voice, or touch.

Communication includes both speaking and listening. Ask yourself how the resident is thinking and feeling. Listen to both the verbal and the nonverbal messages. Pay attention to your verbal and nonverbal messages.

Listening means to both understand and accept what a person says about his situation and his feelings. Empathy means understanding what the person says so well that you can identify. When you show you care, residents feel safe and will share concerns with you. This is therapeutic communication.

Active listening tells the resident that you have respect. When you look into the eyes of the person speaking, you show by your facial expressions that you are following. This encourages him or her to continue. A person can tell if you are distracted and not listening.

Ask questions to clarify what the resident is saying. This will encourage him or her to talk more. Avoid questions that require only a "yes" or "no" answer. Use open-ended questions like "Can you tell me about the problems you are having?" Don't ask questions that might steer the conversation in another direction.

Don't brush off the resident's concerns by saying "Don't worry about it, it will be okay." This makes the resident's concerns seem trivial. Try not to either agree or disagree with a resident's statements. You should not judge the things he or she says. You must leave room for the person to change his or her mind. Don't give advice. If the resident asks for advice, reply, "What do you think you should do?"

While listening:

- Don't plan your reply

- Don't daydream or think about your next task

- Don't change the subject

- Don't laugh if the resident is serious

- Don't interrupt

Say back to the resident what you heard. Don't use the exact words, but briefly rephrase or paraphrase his or her statements. This gives the resident a chance to restate what was meant or to clarify thoughts. It is important to make comments indicating that you understand what has been said. If you don't comment for a few minutes, the resident may think you have lost interest, you don't understand, or you disapprove. Short silences are good, however, to give the resident time to think.

Sometimes a good listener may understand what the resident is feeling before the resident has recognized or expressed his or her own emotion. If you ask the resident if he or she might be feeling a certain way, the resident might recognize an underlying emotion. A listener might say, "I wonder if …" or "Could it be that …." Try not to appear to be interpreting the feelings or the situation too quickly.

Social functioning and relationships

Social contact is a basic human need. People who are isolated from others have a higher risk of depression, anxiety, low self-esteem, mental disorders, and physical illnesses. Giving residents opportunities to maintain existing social relationships and develop new ones may be the most important thing we can do to meet psychosocial needs. It is our responsibility to provide social activities and to encourage residents to participate.

The following are some suggestions for encouraging social relationships:

- Find out if the resident has a hobby or activity he or she enjoys or used to enjoy. If so, help the resident obtain whatever is needed to be involved in that hobby or interest. Assistive devices or special accommodations may be necessary, so work with an occupational therapist to find ways the resident can do this activity.

- Help residents get to know others who like the same activities.

- Provide ample time and opportunity for social visits with family and friends. Do not let your routines or schedules interfere with social interactions.

- Find ways for residents to communicate with others. Make sure they have easy access to a telephone that is equipped for their use. They may need a volume booster on the phone so they can hear, or they might want help dialing. If possible, program numbers into a phone so they can speed-dial friends and family. Another good form of communication is electronic mail (email). Residents will need a computer, a phone line, and an Internet service provider (ISP) to use email. If the resident cannot type, he or she could use a voice recognition program that listens to spoken words and produces email or letters without typing.

- If the resident builds, makes, cooks, or otherwise creates something, be sure to praise the effort and admire the product. Provide the resident with books or videos that might be of interest on the subject. Encourage additional projects.

- Involving residents with younger people can make the residents feel valued, useful, and important. Give residents an opportunity to share knowledge and skills with others with similar interests or with students and young people.

- People like to feel successful. Everyone enjoys being recognized by others. Make every effort to recognize and validate residents. Encourage families to display pictures, awards, and diplomas. Be generous with praise and verbal rewards.

Intellectual stimulation

People also enjoy solitary pursuits that engage their minds. Audio books on tape, books with large print, videotapes, television programs, movies, music, and the Internet are all good sources of intellectual stimulation. Talk to residents about setting new learning goals for themselves and working to achieve them. People who are always learning new things strengthen their mental abilities and may slow or halt cognitive decline.

Sexuality

The fact that a resident is ill, disabled, or elderly does not necessarily mean he or she no longer has a need for sexual expression. Adults have the right to determine their sexual activities within the limits of polite behavior. Adults of any age or physical condition that choose to be in a consensual sexual relationship must be given appropriate privacy, protection, and support to fulfill this need.

Methods of Meeting Psychosocial Needs of Residents and Families

Education

Group education and discussion, social interaction, activity programs, support groups, and training classes for both family members and residents can improve resident/family relationships and attitudes. These programs enhance quality of life for both residents and families.

Accurate information about the aging process, illnesses, disabilities, and the specific problems of the resident can help caregivers understand their own reactions and feelings. They can be taught how to take better care of themselves and their loved ones.

Activities

Regular physical activity and social interactions must be encouraged. Programs should promote well-being and enjoyment and must be tailored to the abilities of the participants.

Enjoying pets

Having animals around for companionship has proven to improve people's quality of life. Encourage residents to have pets only if someone is capable of caring for the animal.

Social workers

Social workers help residents deal with illness, loss, and end-of-life issues. They may work with residents and/or families to help them cope with the psychosocial effects of these events.

Education of healthcare workers

Healthcare workers must be educated in order to provide the necessary care and services to attain or maintain the highest possible physical, mental, and psychosocial well-being of residents. Everyone should be aware of cultural diversity and be committed to antidiscriminatory practices.

Psychosocial Care

Test

Name _____ Date _____ Score _____

Directions: Circle the correct answer.

1. Assisting someone with personal care or giving physical care is not the time to worry about giving psychosocial care. True   or   False

2. High levels of emotional distress can make illness worse and slow recovery. True   or   False

3. Untreated anxiety or depression may cause which of the following effects?

    a. Decrease in daily functioning

    b. Increased risk of accidents

    c. Behavior problems

    d. All of the above

4. Some medications can induce anxiety or depression.   True   or   False

5. An unconscious resident cannot hear, so you may talk about him or her freely with others in the room.   True   or   False

6. Which of these statements gives a good example of active listening?

    a. The worker stands in the doorway with one foot out the door while the resident talks

    b. The worker sits down and looks at the resident while he or she talks

    c. The worker tells the resident not to worry about it, everything will be okay

    d. he worker listens and then says, "Now here's what you should do …"

7. Animals should not be kept around elderly, sick, or disabled people. True   or   False

8. Persons with a strong personal faith and many social contacts are better able to cope with health problems and more motivated to recover. True   or   False

9. Elderly, disabled, or sick people should not be allowed to have sexual relationships. True   or   False

10. Social contact is a basic human need. True   or   False

CERTIFICATE OF COMPLETION

I hereby certify that

_____

has successfully completed the in-Service

Psychosocial Care

_____
Signature

33

Range of Motion and Positioning

Teaching Plan

To use this lesson for self-study, the learner should read the material, do the activity, and take the test. For group study, the leader may give each learner a copy of the learning guide and follow this teaching plan to conduct the lesson. Certificates may be copied for everyone who completes the lesson.

Learning objectives

After this lesson, participants should be able to:

- Explain the importance of range of motion (ROM) exercises and proper positioning

- Demonstrate ROM exercises

- Use positioning skills to assist residents with limited mobility

Lesson activities

1. Ask participants to think about residents that would be able to function more independently if they had more strength and flexibility.

2. Use the learning guide to present the techniques for doing ROM exercises and proper positioning. Review the vocabulary in the "Know These Terms" section.

3. Have participants pair up. Assign them to perform active ROM exercises and then to do passive ROM exercises on each other, using the exercises in the learning guide. If time and space allow, demonstrate positioning techniques and have participants practice on each other.

Conclusion

Have participants take the test. Review the answers together. Award certificates to those who answer 70% of the test questions correctly.

Test answers

1. heart disease, diabetes, stroke	2. 4%, 10%	3. True	4. True	5. Range of motion
6. True	7. Exercise	8. True	9. Two	10. False

Range of Motion and Positioning

Learning Guide

Contents:

- Why Is Motion Important?

  - What kinds of motion are best?

- Getting Started

- Passive Range of Motion Exercises

- Positioning

  - Some basic rules of positioning

  - Bed positioning tips

  - Positions

Why Is Motion Important?

Most people take free, comfortable movement for granted. Motion is meant to be smooth and painless. The ligaments, tendons, muscles, and joint capsules that surround each joint in the body work best if they are used regularly.

As people get older, however, muscles gradually lose their strength, endurance, and flexibility. We experience a progressive loss of muscle mass at an average rate of 4% per decade from 25 to 50 years and 10% per decade thereafter. In addition, the joints in older people change, often becoming stiff and difficult or painful to move. Tissues in the joints sometimes become swollen or inflamed, hindering movement and making the joints more prone to injury.

As a result, people tend to move less as they age. This is the worst thing people can do. Lack of activity worsens the changes that occur with aging. Research confirms that regular exercise can slow or reverse many changes associated with the age-related loss of strength, endurance, and flexibility.

When people are not physically active, every cell and system in the body is affected. The body's cells and systems begin to lose the ability to perform their specialized functions.

When movement is difficult, people experience a general decline in quality of life. Self-image often suffers.

Lack of activity and exercise can lead to heart disease, diabetes, stroke, and other health problems. Decreased mobility hinders one's ability to feed and clothe oneself, to grocery shop, and to attend to personal hygiene. It promotes mental deterioration and loss of independence.

In addition, when muscles are not used, they continue to weaken. Muscle weakness increases the risk of falls and, therefore, of fractures. The risk of falling increases with age. Falls are the leading cause of injury and death for people age 65 and older.

What kinds of motion are best?

There are four types of exercise. They are:

- Strength

- Stretching

- Endurance (also known as cardiovascular)

- ROM

Exercise benefits people of all ages. Regular exercise can slow or reverse decreased mobility that contributes to disease and disability in the elderly.

Strength

Even a small change in muscle size can make a big difference in strength. That's why strength exercises are so important. Improving muscle size by lifting small weights helps people build their capacity to do such things as walk, climb stairs, and carry a package. These kinds of activities can mean the difference between keeping one's independence and relying on others.

Stretching

Stretching exercises that gently stretch the muscles and tendons help ensure flexibility. Stretching exercises do not build strength or endurance. Clinical research has demonstrated that most elderly, even the frail, benefit from a combination of flexibility and strengthening exercises. It helps them maintain function and mobility, prolong independence, and improve their quality of life.

Endurance

Walking, running, bicycling, and swimming are examples of endurance exercise. By spending time in motion, the body and muscles become able to endure for longer periods of time, and the heart and lungs become stronger.

Range of motion

ROM exercises are designed to increase flexibility. ROM is the normal amount a person's joints can be moved in certain directions or the range in which you can move a body part around a joint. Limited ROM is a reduction in the normal distance and direction through which a joint can move.

When a joint is not fully extended on a regular basis, over time it will become permanently unable to extend beyond a certain fixed position. To keep the joints, tendons, ligaments, and muscles loose and flexible, ROM exercises are used. These exercises move the joints through a full ROM, helping to prevent stiffening.

Getting Started

By doing a little exercise regularly, even in small 10-minute increments several times per week, it's possible to offset a variety of health problems. Exercise can help produce new red blood cells, strengthen the immune system, and improve bone density. Physical activity, even at low intensity in short sessions, may reduce the risk for certain chronic diseases. Exercise also helps relieve depression.

Older adults need to be up and moving seven days per week. They should spend time three to five days per week doing flexibility exercises or walking. Daily activities do not move joints through their full ROM.

Caregivers can help residents improve their health by encouraging them to exercise.

Exercise tips:

- Move joints through their full ROM one to two times per day.

- Do each exercise three times to 10 times.

- Move slowly. Do not bounce.

- Breathe while you exercise. Count aloud.

- Begin exercises slowly, doing each exercise a few times and gradually building up.

- Try to achieve full ROM by moving until you feel a slight stretch, but don't force a movement.

- Stop exercising if you have severe pain.

- Encourage residents with limited mobility to bear weight during transfers from bed to chair and to walk whenever possible.

ROM exercises that can be done while seated:

- Neck (breathe with the movements, breathing out when the head moves down, breathing in when it moves up; don't let shoulders or upper body sway to the side):

  - Turn head slowly to the right and then to the left. Repeat three to four times.

  - Tilt head toward one shoulder and then toward the other shoulder. Repeat three to four times.

- Arms and shoulders:

  - Raise shoulders up toward ears and hold. Make full circles: up, forward, down, and back.

  - Take a deep breath, extend arms overhead. Exhale slowly, dropping arms.

- Hands and fingers:

  - Massage each hand, one at a time. Take your time; go in between each finger.

  - Raise hands up and back. Slowly rotate hands down and around in circles.

  - Close hand in a fist. Open hands fully, stretching fingers and thumbs out wide.

- Chest and upper body:

  - With hands on waist, tilt to the right, return to center, and then tilt to the left and return to center. Exhale as the movement goes down; inhale as the movement comes up. Don't allow upper body to tilt forward. Don't try to hold head up; instead, let it relax to the side.

  - Sit straight in chair with hands on your hips. Gently rock hips from side to side.

- Legs:

  - Raise right leg up and forward. Repeat with left leg.

  - Sit up straight, knees together, with legs extended forward as far as possible, keeping feet on floor. Slowly stretch forward, sliding both hands down to ankles. Hold 10–15 counts.

  - Grasp one knee with both arms, pull to chest, and hold for five counts. Repeat with opposite leg.

- Ankle and foot:

    - Point toes toward floor. Point toes toward ceiling. Slowly rotate feet in circles.

    - Cross right leg over left knee. Rotate foot slowly, making large complete circles—
      10 rotations to the right, 10 to the left. Repeat for left leg.

Passive Range-of-Motion Exercises

When an individual is able to perform ROM exercises with minimal assistance, the person is doing active ROM. When an individual is unable to perform ROM exercises, a caregiver should move the person's joints in passive ROM exercises at least once or twice per day.

Guide every joint in the body through its full ROM. Go slowly and be very gentle. Do not force any body part to move in any way that creates resistance or causes discomfort. See Figure 33.1 for more ROM techniques.

Know These Terms

- Flexion: forward bending

- Extension: straighten out

- Hyperextension: backward bending

- Lateral flexion: sideways bending

- Internal rotation: turn toward the body

- External rotation: turn away from the body

- Circumduction: move in a circle

- Abduction: move away from the body (think of "abduct," or "take away")

- Adduction: move toward and/or across the body (think "add to the body")

- Inversion: move or twist inward

- Eversion: move or twist outward

- Supination: turn or lie upward; face up

- Pronation: turn or lie downward; face down

Positioning

Everyone positions himself or herslef when sitting, standing, moving, and lying down. The position used for these activities affects circulation, joint pressure, and muscle use.

People with limited mobility who sit or lie down for long periods of time are prone to skin breakdown and deterioration of muscles or nerves. Using correct positioning can prevent these problems. It is important to limit pressure over bony parts of the body by changing positions. Use pillows to keep knees and/or ankles from touching each other. Residents who are bedridden should avoid lying directly on their hipbones when on their sides. Assist residents to use positions that spread weight and pressure evenly, with pillows placed to provide support and comfort.

A person in a chair or wheelchair should use a cushion. Avoid donut-shaped cushions because they reduce blood flow and cause tissue to swell. People sitting in chairs or wheelchairs should change positions every hour. Good posture and comfort are both important.

Some basic rules of positioning

- Always be familiar with a resident's plan of care. Specific issues such as fractures, skin integrity, and health condition will determine the type of positioning that should be done.

- Turn individuals who cannot turn themselves at least every two hours when in bed. A person in a wheelchair should change positions at least every hour. External pressure from staying in one position compresses the skin's blood vessels and obstructs circulation, especially over the bones, leading to skin breakdown.

- When moving a resident, lift rather than drag. Dragging creates friction and heat, which can lead to skin breakdown.

- Straighten sheets and clothing to remove wrinkles.

Bed positioning tips

- Position the spine in alignment

- Position the hips straight without leg rotation

- Position the upper extremities away from the body

- Support the arms when the resident is lying on his side

- Keep the knee joints flexed 15 degrees when the resident is supine (lying on the back)

- Turn the resident from side to side and prone (lying face down) on a scheduled basis

- Keep the head in a straight, midline position

Positions

- Supine (on back)

    - Place a pillow under the head.

    - Place pillows under both arms. When bedridden residents lie on their back with forearms and palms facing down, pressure can damage wrist nerves.

    - Place pillows under legs from midcalf to ankle to keep heels off the bed. Do not put a pillow under the knees only, as this will cause the heel to rub against the bed.

    - Hand rolls (roll washcloths and place in hands to prevent freezing of finger joints).

    - Use foot-positioning devices such as shoes, boots, and footboards.

- Lying on side

    - Position resident up in bed if needed.

    - Position resident to one side of bed. Turn resident by sliding arm under the shoulders and head; lift upper body over, and then move hips and legs.

    - Cross the resident's top ankle over the bottom ankle, or flex top knee.

    - Turn the resident by placing one hand on the shoulder and one hand on the hip.

    - Place pillow under head and another behind resident's back.

    - Support flexed extremities with pillows and positioning devices.

    - Ensure proper body alignment.

- Prone (on stomach)

    - Lift resident toward you

    - Bend arm up around head

    - Place other arm at side

    - Place pillow under abdominal muscles

    - Roll resident on stomach

    - Support ankles with pillows

- Positioning while seated

- – Seat resident in a chair that supports the back

- – Keep ears in line with the hips

- – Support the curve of the lower back with a rolled up towel or lumbar roll

- – Knees should be level with the hips

- – Feet should be flat on the floor or on a footrest

- Positioning while standing (to help residents learn balance when using walkers or canes)

  - – Position the feet a few inches apart

  - – Position the hips in front of the ankles

  - – Position the shoulders over the hips

  - – Keep the head balanced over the hips

  - – Keep the spine straight

ROM exercises and proper positioning can help prevent the permanent disabilities and life-threatening complications that often result from immobility. Caregivers need to intervene to prevent physical decline and deterioration. We can accomplish this by keeping residents moving.

Range of Motion and Positioning

Test

Name _____ Date _____ Score _____

Directions: Fill in or circle the correct answer.

1. Name three health problems that can occur because of lack of activity and exercise.

   _____ _____, _____, _____

2. Progressive loss of muscle mass occurs at an average rate of _____ percent per decade from 25–50 years and _____ percent per decade thereafter.

3. Older persons' muscles, joints, and ligaments are more prone to injury.   True   or   False

4. Research confirms that regular exercise can slow or reverse many changes associated with the age-related loss of strength, endurance, and flexibility.   True   or   False

5. _____ _____ _____ exercises are used to keep joints, muscles, ligaments, and tendons loose and flexible.

6. Even a small change in muscle size can make a difference in strength.   True   or   False

7. _____ benefits people of all ages.

8. Regular exercise, even in short sessions several times per week, can help to offset a variety of health problems.   True   or   False

9. When confined to bed, residents should change positions at least every _____ hours.

10. Daily activities move joints through their full range of motion.   True   or   False

CERTIFICATE OF COMPLETION

I hereby certify that

has successfully completed the in-Service

Range of Motion and Positioning

Signature

34

Preventing Readmission to Hospitals

Teaching Plan

To use this lesson for self-study, the learner should read the material, do the activity, and take the test. For group study, the leader may give each learner a copy of the learning guide and follow this teaching plan to conduct the lesson. Certificates may be copied for everyone who completes the lesson.

Learning objectives

After this lesson, participants should be able to:

- Understand the importance of avoiding readmissions

- Identify strategies to avoid readmissions

- Recognize how proper medication compliance can affect readmission rates

- Recognize the role of resident, staff, and family education in reducing readmissions

- Identify red flags of care that indicate action is needed

- Understand the team approach to resident care to avoid complications

Lesson activities

1. Brainstorm reasons a resident might need to go back to the hospital. Come up with a few scenarios where proper identification of a change in condition earlier on may possibly have prevented the resident from going back to the hospital.

2. Read "Overcoming Obstacles: Case Study" and discuss the questions that follow it.

The lesson

Review the material in the lesson with participants. Allow for discussion.

Conclusion

Have participants take the test. Review the answers together. Award certificates to those who answer 70% of the test questions correctly.

Test answers

1. b	2. d	3. a	4. d	5. d	6. c

Preventing Readmission to Hospitals

Learning Guide

Contents:

- Introduction

- Understanding Readmissions

  - Relocation stress syndrome

- Strategies for Prevention

  - Recognize red flags

  - Engage the resident in self-care

  - Enroll the family caregiver or advocate

  - Resident education

Introduction

The need for containing and reducing healthcare costs has been in the news for quite some time. A significant cause of high healthcare costs is hospital readmissions. **Readmissions**, also called rehospitalizations, refers to residents who are discharged from an acute care hospital and are hospitalized again within 30 days of discharge.

Readmissions may have a financial impact on facilities; it may also have a significant impact on how partnering hospitals and—most importantly—beneficiaries view the safety and quality of care provided both in the hospital and at the skilled nursing facility.

Staff play a key role in preventing readmissions. Proper observation, monitoring, and documentation of residents' conditions will help limit the risk of complications.

Understanding Readmissions

Readmissions are classified as unanticipated, unscheduled readmissions to the hospital that are clinically related to the initial admission. Although the person is typically returned to the original admitting hospital, a readmission occurs when the person is being admitted to any hospital for treatment of the original condition. This phenomenon is sometimes called bounce back. A newer term is **complicated (or complex) transition**.

Very few people want to return to the hospital. Likewise, hospitals do not want their discharged residents to return. It is usually a lose-lose situation for both parties. In 2012, nearly 2 million Medicare beneficiaries were readmitted within 30 days of release, costing Medicare $17.5 billion in additional hospital bills. According to a 2013 Robert Wood Johnson Foundation study, residents admitted from larger, urban academic teaching hospitals are readmitted more than their counterparts. However, the vast majority of hospitals struggle with readmission rates.

In 2010, the surgical 30-day readmission rate was about 12%; the medical 30-day readmission rate was about 16%. Readmission rates for congestive heart failure were about 21%, acute myocardial infarctions 18%, and pneumonia 15%.The report also found that many residents feel they are discharged too soon and often do not understand discharge instructions they often found too general.

With the fragmentation of care and chaos of having multiple providers for one resident, the skilled nursing facility often remains the anchor in a sea of chaos for many residents transitioning after a hospital episode of care. Clinical staff can help residents understand their conditions, assist with medication regimes, and recognize problems before they become more severe.

Relocation stress syndrome

Transitioning from one setting to another has the potential for causing or increasing confusion and traumatizing an elderly or sick resident. Signs and symptoms include:

- Increased dependence
- Delirium
- Depression
- Anger
- Withdrawal
- Changes in behavior
- Changes in sleeping habits
- Feelings of insecurity, loss of trust
- Weight loss (or, less commonly, gain)
- Falls

This is the phenomena known as relocation stress syndrome. Older terms that may still be used are transfer trauma and relocation shock. Transfer trauma is a consequence of the stress and emotional shock caused by an abrupt relocation of a resident from one location or hospital to another, including the home. Unless a proposed transfer is emergent, involve the resident in planning for transfer.

Evidence suggests that ensuring continuity of care of elderly or sick people during care transitions improves resident outcomes, reducing the rate of avoidable readmissions.

Strategies for Prevention

Because skilled nursing can have an effect on readmission rates, it's import to implement strategies to prevent avoidable readmissions. The following are a series of strategies to help care for residents with the goal to prevent readmissions.

Recognize red flags

Obtain information from the discharging agency of key points for residents/families and clinical staff to monitor. This should include a written list of specific symptoms to watch for and what to do if they occur (Figure 34.1). This will help you know who to call and when.

Figure 34.1 Sample of Red Flag Instructions

Medical problem	Call RN (phone number)	Call 911
Heart failure	• Increased shortness of breath especially when lying flat • Increased fatigue/weakness • Weight gain of 3 pounds in a day or 5 pounds in a week • Swelling in ankles • Irregular heartbeat	• Severe shortness of breath (unable to breath) • Chest pain unrelieved with medication • Frothy sputum
Diabetes (low blood sugar)	• Dizziness, shakiness • Increased hunger • Headache • Changes in vision	• Loss of consciousness • Seizures
Respiratory (COPD)	• Increased shortness of breath • Increasing cough • Change in color, thickness, or amount of sputum • Loss of appetite • Fever greater than 101 degrees Fahrenheit	• Severe shortness of breath that does not respond to bronchodilator treatments • Changes in skin color to bluish or grayish tone • Increasing confusion

A red flag would be several treating providers (e.g., the resident sees a nephrologist, cardiologist, geripsychiatrist and internal medicine physician). It is important in this instance to pick the "captain of the ship," which is often the referring physician who oversees the medications and reviews and approves any changes. However, situations arise where an underlying condition is out of control; therefore, the primary physician becomes the one who is likely to change the medications because of the effect they are having. For example, a physician treating a resident with liver failure may request notification of any new medications the resident is given and require his approval of the medication prior to administration because of the effect it might have on the liver disease.

There are many red flags with which you are familiar. What is important is that the care team identifies those that are specific to the resident in order to be alert to potential problems so he or she will be aware of when to contact the physician if problems arise. Elevated blood pressure, elevated pulse, difficulty breathing, symptoms of wound infection or digoxin toxicity, and a bladder infection that affects residents with a Foley catheter are some examples.

Engage the resident in self-care

Engaging the resident in his or her care can be achieved in a number of ways. For example:

Ask open-ended questions during the interview process, which will help collect the resident's information.

- Provide the resident with information about his or her medications; this always seems to stimulate attention. In addition, stories about the medication help too and may also serve as a memory aid.

- Encourage the resident to ask questions, especially if new medications are ordered or if the dosage is changed on a medication.

- Provide the resident with handouts discussing his or her disease and the medications used to combat it.

- Use plain and simple terms to help the resident understand and feel more in control of his or her care. Use words that the resident can pronounce.

- Create a supportive atmosphere for the resident so he or she feels at ease in stating what is not understood or what is confusing.

- A resident may feel more engaged during treatment if there is an easy and comfortable way for him or her to report discrepancies or errors.

- Be sure to include potential risk to residents in your care plan and then list evaluation methods that are quick and easy for the other healthcare team members to follow.

> Residents with **diabetes, heart disease, and respiratory problems are at a high risk for readmissions** and remain a target population for intense monitoring of health status, self-care skill, and self-care knowledge. **Any discharged resident with four or five comorbid conditions requires a focused approach** with specified care guidelines, triggers for readmission, and resident-centered goals.

Enroll the family caregiver or advocate

Effective disease control requires that the resident and their family and the care team staff are active participants in the resident's care planning. The role of the family caregiver varies according to the individual's ability to participate in their own care.

Education and communication provide the caregiver with a better understanding of the disease and the disease process. The knowledge empowers the caregiver to feel supported in decisions.

Teaching the signs and symptoms of the disease and the disease process and the measures to take should there be a complication will help and decrease the frivolous rehospitalizations in chronic care residents.

Resident education

Educate the resident and the family to make them aware of a high-risk situation if that is what is present. Provide them with the signs and symptoms of complications and provide them with physician's orders that clearly state when to call and the parameters to follow for complications in the resident's disease or illness. For example, in cases of CHF, a daily weight gain of five pounds may cause a physician or pharmacist to order to take an extra furosemide dose or draw digoxin levels. Create an environment for the resident with chronic illness that is supportive and reassuring so anxiety is decreased (knowing what to do in an emergency is empowering to the resident).

Preventing Readmission to Hospitals

Test

Name _____ Date _____ Score _____

Directions: Circle the correct answer.

1. Delirium, depression, and changes in sleeping habits may be signs of _____.

    a. rehospitalization

    b. relocation stress syndrome

    c. proper discharge planning

    d. irregular respirations

2. Which of the following is a high-risk condition for readmission?

    a. Diabetes

    b. Heart disease

    c. Respiratory problems

    d. All of the above

3. A rehospitalization occurs when the person is being admitted to any hospital for treatment of the original condition. True or False

4. About _____ Medicare beneficiaries are readmitted within 30 days every year.

    a. 5 million

    b. 100

    c. 10 million

    d. 20 million

5. The specific roles and responsibilities that home health staff play in preventing rehospitalizations _____.

    a. ensure they are ready to go back to the hospital

    b. include keeping the resident at the care facility at all costs

    c. play no role in preventing readmissions

    d. include recognizing and reporting condition changes

6. A readmission or rehospitalization occurs when _____.

    a. a resident is transferred from one hospital to another

    b. a resident is admitted back to the hospital within the following year

    c. a resident who was discharged from a hospital and is hospitalized again within 30 days of discharge

    d. a resident is admitted to a hospital after an outresident procedure

CERTIFICATE OF COMPLETION

I hereby certify that

_____

has successfully completed the in-Service

Preventing Readmission to Hospitals

_____

Signature

35

Respiratory Disorders

Teaching Plan

To use this lesson for self-study, the learner should read the material, do the activity, and take the test. For group study, the leader may give each learner a copy of the learning guide and follow this teaching plan to conduct the lesson. Certificates may be copied for everyone who completes the lesson.

Learning objectives

After this lesson, participants should be able to:

- Explain the breathing process

- Recognize and report symptoms of respiratory disease

- Use knowledge of respiratory disorders to provide care for affected individuals

Lesson activities

Lesson preparation

Before class, tape a piece of paper under each chair participants will sit in. Write one of these words on some of the pieces of paper: nose, sinuses, pharynx, epiglottis, larynx, trachea, bronchi, bronchioles, lungs, alveoli, pleura, and diaphragm. Use each word once.

1. Ask participants to find the piece of paper taped to their chairs. Ask those who have a word to look in the first two pages of the learning guide and prepare to explain what the word means and what role it plays in respiration. Give participants time to look up the words, and then ask them to tell the group what they know. Participants without words should spend the time reading the first two pages of the learning guide.

2. Go over the material about different respiratory disorders in the learning guide with the participants. If any of them care for residents with a respiratory disorder, ask them to share what they know. Remind workers that they should not wear perfume because it irritates

sensitive lungs. Discuss care measures such as quick showers to reduce humidity, fans to circulate air, and techniques to conserve a resident's energy.

3. Have the participants practice each of the techniques on the last page of the learning guide: pursed-lip breathing, controlled coughing, the orthopneic position, and the relaxation and visualization exercise.

4. Discuss the behavior problems that sometimes occur with residents with respiratory disorders. Emphasize that these residents often feel very uncomfortable and unhappy and need lots of compliments, support, encouragement, and understanding.

5. Have the learners take the test, and then grade the test together.

Conclusion

Have participants take the test. Review the answers together. Award certificates to those who answer 70% of the test questions correctly.

Test answers

1. 12–20	2. True	3. True	4. False	5. hand washing
6. False	7. a	8. b	9. d	10. c

Respiratory Disorders

Learning Guide

Contents:

- Introduction

- The Upper Respiratory Tract

- The Lower Respiratory Tract

- How the Respiratory System Works

  - Problems that develop in the respiratory tract

- Common Symptoms of Respiratory Problems

- Chronic Obstructive Pulmonary Disease

- Breathing Techniques and Relaxation Exercises That Help Those Who Feel Breathless

Introduction

Respiration means breathing. In this lesson, you will learn about the respiratory tract, also called the respiratory system. This is the passage that air goes through as we breathe in and out. The respiratory tract contains these important parts.

The Upper Respiratory Tract

- **Nose**—warms the air breathed and filters out bacteria and debris. Nasal breathing is important for best lung function.

- **Sinuses**—cavities (holes) in the skull. They connect to the nasal passage and are lined with nasal tissue.

- **Pharynx**—passageway that conducts air from the nose to the voice box. The pharynx also conducts food from the mouth to the esophagus, the tube that leads to the stomach.

- **Epiglottis**—flap that covers the entrance to the voice box when we swallow. It prevents food and liquids from getting into the lungs.

- **Larynx**—the voice box, located between the pharynx and the windpipe (trachea).

- **Trachea**—windpipe. This is the airway connecting the larynx to the tubes leading to the lungs (bronchi).

The Lower Respiratory Tract

- **Bronchi**—two tubes that lead from the trachea to the lungs. The bronchi divide into many smaller airways, called bronchioles.

- **Lungs**—pair of large spongy organs that take oxygen out of the air we breathe and exchange it for carbon dioxide in our blood.

- **Alveoli**—millions of tiny air sacs in the lungs, surrounded by tiny blood vessels called capillaries. This is where the exchange of oxygen and carbon dioxide takes place. These sacs look like bunches of grapes.

- **Pleura**—a membrane that covers the lungs and helps them move freely.

How the Respiratory System Works

The respiratory tract inhales oxygen into the lungs, transfers the oxygen to the blood, and exhales carbon dioxide. Breathing is usually automatic, controlled subconsciously by the respiratory center at the base of the brain. The brain senses when oxygen levels are too low or carbon dioxide levels are too high and increases the speed and depth of breathing. Normal respiration occurs 12–20 times per minute.

All cells in the body need oxygen. They get oxygen when the body breathes in air that the blood can circulate to all parts of the body. Breathing is accomplished with the help of the diaphragm, a set of muscles lying across the bottom of the chest cavity. Oxygen is pulled into the lungs when the diaphragm contracts. Carbon dioxide is pumped out when the diaphragm relaxes.

Air inhaled through the nose is filtered, moistened, and warmed in the nasal passages. Air goes down the pharynx, into the trachea, through the larynx, and into the two large bronchi. The bronchi branch into smaller airways that conduct the air into the lungs. The inhaled oxygen diffuses into the blood through the many capillaries. The blood exchanges carbon dioxide for oxygen. The carbon dioxide is then exhaled.

Oxygenated blood travels from the lungs through the pulmonary veins and into the left side of the heart, which pumps the blood to the rest of the body.

The blood delivers its oxygen to the tissues and picks up and distributes nutrients and waste products and then returns to the heart and gets pumped back to the lungs to pick up oxygen and get rid of carbon dioxide.

Elimination of carbon dioxide is just as important as getting oxygen. A buildup of carbon dioxide leads to headaches, drowsiness, and even death.

Fast Facts

- Chronic obstructive pulmonary disease (COPD) accounts for more than 100,000 deaths every year. It is the fourth most common cause of death in the United States.

- People with asthma are almost 60% more likely to develop lung cancer.

- Each year, over 25,000 people in the United States get tuberculosis (TB).

Problems that develop in the respiratory tract

There are many disorders and infections of the respiratory system. Infections occur more frequently in the respiratory tract than in any other organ in the body. Examples of upper respiratory infections include the common cold, sinusitis, and influenza (flu). Lower respiratory problems include infections such as bronchitis and pneumonia and disorders like emphysema and asthma. Some of the more serious ones are described in the following pages.

Upper respiratory infections

Influenza (flu)

Influenza is a highly contagious infection of the upper respiratory tract. It is caused by a virus and spreads easily through coughing and sneezing. Influenza can lead to pneumonia and death and is responsible for epidemics that occur almost every winter. Flu vaccine can prevent influenza.

Influenza virus is generally passed from person to person by airborne transmission. However, the virus can live for a short time on objects, such as pens, pencils, keyboards, and telephone receivers. Touching those objects can transmit the virus.

Symptoms of influenza include high fever, headache, sneezing, coughing, sore throat, severe aches and pain, and fatigue. The most common complications of flu are respiratory disorders, especially bronchitis. Pneumonia is the most serious complication.

Treatment includes bed rest and increased fluids, antiviral drugs, and medication to relieve aches and fever. Most people recover in a week, but many flu victims feel exhausted for 3 to 4 weeks. Taking the annual flu shot, washing hands frequently, and avoiding contact with infected persons can prevent influenza.

Lower respiratory infections

Pneumonia

Pneumonia is the most common and most serious type of lung infection. It can be caused by a virus that is inhaled or by bacteria that gets in through the mouth. Pneumonia causes the alveoli to fill with liquid that blocks the exchange of oxygen in the lungs. The lack of oxygen combined with the spread of infection can cause death.

Pneumonia caused by bacteria is spread from person to person through secretions from the nose, mouth, and throat. Symptoms may include high fever, chills, severe chest pain, and a cough that produces mucus. Bacterial pneumonia can come on gradually or suddenly. It often follows what appears to be an ordinary respiratory infection.

Bacterial pneumonia can develop 4–14 days after an apparent recovery from the flu, especially in people with heart disease. Fever returns, along with a cough that produces mucus. This disease can progress rapidly from flu to serious pneumonia, and it often causes death.

Pneumococcal pneumonia is the most common type of bacterial pneumonia. It can be prevented with immunization and hand washing.

Pneumonia caused by a virus resembles the flu at first, with fever, dry cough, headache, muscle pain, weakness, and shortness of breath. Careful hand washing can help prevent its spread.

Tuberculosis (TB)

Tuberculosis is a chronic bacterial infection that affects the lungs. TB germs are airborne, causing illness when they are inhaled.

TB is usually passed to those who share breathing space for a prolonged time with someone with contagious TB disease. The most common places for becoming infected are the home and workplace. TB usually does not result from brief casual contact. Adequate ventilation is the best way to prevent transmission. Those who care for people with TB may have to wear special masks to protect themselves by filtering out the TB bacteria from the air they breathe.

A skin test called a PPD is recommended for people who are at risk for TB. This includes healthcare workers, the elderly, people in group settings such as long-term care facilities, people who work or live with a person with active TB disease, people with AIDS or impaired immune systems, the homeless, and those who abuse alcohol or drugs.

A positive PPD means that the immune system is reacting to TB germs located somewhere in the body, so that person is at increased risk for developing TB disease unless preventive treatment is given. A positive PPD does not mean that one has TB disease or is contagious to others. Most people who become infected never develop active TB. A person with TB usually is not contagious once treatment has begun. To treat the disease, medications are given for 6 to 9 months. The entire treatment must be given or the person can become ill again.

A cough that won't go away is usually the first symptom of TB. Table 35.1 shows what happens with exposure to tuberculosis, TB infection, and active disease.

Table 35.1 Stages of TB

	PPD	Chest X-Ray	Symptoms	Contagious	Medication for Treatment
Stage 1: Exposure	Negative	Normal	None	No	No
Stage 2: TB Infection	Positive	Normal	None	No	Special antibiotic might be given for prevention of active TB
Stage 3: Active Disease	Positive	Abnormal	Cough, weight loss, fever, fatigue, loss of appetite, night sweats, coughing up blood	Yes	Curable in most cases by treatment with several medications taken by mouth for 6–9 months

Lung disorders

Asthma

Asthma is a long-term chronic breathing problem that can affect people of any age. It may be inherited or may be caused by allergies to pollen, pets, dust, or medications. Smoking increases the risk of developing asthma, and stress may make it worse. Persons with asthma can live normal lives with medication and proper care.

A person with asthma has sensitive bronchi that react to triggers such as smoke, air pollution, cold weather, exercise, or allergies. The bronchi may tighten or narrow, becoming inflamed and swollen, making it harder to breathe fresh air in and exhale the stale air. Sometimes it is harder to exhale than inhale. Symptoms of asthma are wheezing, dry cough, or sometimes a cough with mucus, shortness of breath, and chest tightness.

Medications may include an inhaler, puffer, or pills. Some medicines reduce the swelling and in-flammation in the bronchi, helping to prevent asthma attacks from starting, but they do not stop an attack once it has started. Inhalers work quickly, opening the narrowed airways. They help stop an attack once it has begun and are used as needed. Some asthma drugs may cause irregular heartbeats.

Blood pressure medicines, sleeping pills, tranquilizers, sedatives, or aspirin may cause a problem in older people with asthma. These drugs make one breathe more slowly and less deeply, which can be dangerous if one has asthma.

Common Symptoms of Respiratory Problems

The following symptoms should be reported to your supervisor:

- Cough—varies with type of problem. Take notice of these things:

  - Is the cough dry, without sputum?

  - If there is sputum with the cough, what color is it? Is there any blood in the sputum? Is the sputum thick or thin?

  - What factors affect the cough, such as walking, talking, eating, etc.?

Two kinds of medicines are used to treat coughs. Antitussives suppress the cough, and expectorants help loosen mucus so it can be coughed up.

- Shortness of breath (SOB; dyspnea) is the unpleasant sensation of breathlessness or diffi-culty in breathing. Shortness of breath may happen mostly during activity, when it is often called distress on exertion, or DOE. Some people feel short of breath all the time because of narrowed airways. Sometimes shortness of breath occurs when lying down. This is usually due to heart failure and is relieved by sitting up.

- Breathing that is abnormal—too fast, too slow, irregular, shallow, or gasping.

- Pleurisy is a sharp pain caused by an irritation in the lining of the lungs. It is made worse by deep breathing and coughing. Sometimes the area is sore to the touch.

- Cyanosis is a bluish color of the lips, nails, and skin caused by lack of oxygen.

Chronic Obstructive Pulmonary Disease

COPD is the name for reduced airflow in and out of the lungs. It is associated with diseases such as emphysema and chronic bronchitis. Smoking is the cause of 80–90% of COPD. Other causes include heredity, second-hand smoke, and air pollution. There is no cure.

Bronchitis is an inflammation of the bronchi. In chronic bronchitis, the airways become narrow, scarred, and partly clogged with mucus, making it difficult to breathe. There may be a cough that lasts for months and returns often, lasting longer each time.

Emphysema occurs when some of the air sacs deep in the lungs are damaged, often because of long-term infection and irritation. When lung tissue is damaged, the airways collapse, trapping stale air and blocking intake of fresh air. The lungs try to take in more air and become overinflated and stretched out, gradually getting so big they completely fill the chest cavity. Many with severe emphysema develop a barrel-shaped chest because of this.

The stretched-out lungs cannot effectively exhale, creating the feeling that something is blocking the airway. Stale air is never completely replaced with fresh air, and less oxygen gets into the blood. Emphysema makes the heart work harder, eventually leading to heart failure.

Many people with emphysema lose 50–70% of their lung tissue before they are aware of symptoms. A daily morning cough with clear sputum is the earliest symptom. Gradually, the morning cough becomes an all-day cough. Sometimes the first symptom people notice is breathlessness, especially with activity. Other symptoms of COPD include chest tightness and increased mucus.

Care measures for COPD:

- Medications.

- Oxygen therapy.

- Good nutrition and correct body weight.

- Good ventilation. People with COPD often like to have a fan blowing air toward them.

- Rooms should be at a comfortable, moderate temperature, not too hot, too cold, or too humid. Showers and baths should be quick if moisture in the air makes breathing difficult.

- Loose-fitting clothes are best.

- Avoid dust, allergens, air pollution, smoke, and other irritants. Animal hair, scented soaps, colognes, perfumes, powders, cleaners, aerosol sprays, glues, and paints can all cause problems with breathing.

- Exercise can strengthen the body, improve well-being, and reduce shortness of breath.

- Drinking lots of water will keep secretions thin and easy to bring up.

- Tasks should be broken into short segments with frequent rest periods of at least 5–15 minutes.

- Sit when performing tasks if possible.

- Relaxation exercises and special breathing techniques can help the COPD resident feel better (p. 8).

- Caregivers must give frequent support, encouragement, and reassurance.

- Be complimentary, and keep a positive attitude with COPD residents. They often feel anxious and irritable. Lack of oxygen in the blood can cause fatigue, forgetfulness, depression, confusion, poor appetite, moodiness, agitation, frustration, and sleeplessness.

Breathing Techniques and Relaxation Exercises That Help Those Who Feel Breathless

Pursed-lip breathing is helpful in many cases of shortness of breath. It improves ventilation, reduces air trapped in the lungs, relaxes the resident, and eases the effort of breathing. This is especially good to do while exercising or performing any physical activity. Care plan interventions may include assisting the resident to practice breathing exercises. You may be asked to assist the nurse in teaching or demonstrating these steps:

- An erect, upright posture is best for full lung and chest expansion.

- Breathe in slowly through the nose for 1 count. Feel lungs fill with air.

- Purse lips slightly as if to whistle.

- Breathe out gently and slowly through pursed lips for 2 slow counts.

- Do not force the air out; let it escape naturally.

- Keep doing this until breathing eases.

Residents can learn **controlled coughing** techniques to help clear the breathing passages:

- Take a slow, deep breath and hold for 2 seconds.

- Cough twice, with mouth slightly open. The first cough should loosen mucus, and the second should push it out of the lungs.

- Pause. Sniff gently. Do not take a deep breath, as this may push mucus back to the lungs.

The **orthopneic position** can help residents with enlarged lungs breathe better by stabilizing the chest and shoulders and helping the resident use other muscles to support breathing:

- Sit leaning forward. Support the arms on a surface in front. An overbed table provides good support and can be adjusted to the right height. Arms can also be supported on the knees.

Relaxation and visualization exercises can calm anxiety and agitation:

- Sit in a chair with eyes closed and do pursed-lip breathing for a minute or two.

- Frown, tightening the muscles in the forehead. Hold for 3 seconds and then relax.

- Clench jaw by tightening the muscles in the lower jaw. Hold for 3 seconds and relax.

- Tighten and relax arms and hands, then buttocks, and then legs and feet.

- Let the body go limp.

- Imagine the most peaceful scene you can think of.

- Visualize the scene with you in it. Think of as much detail as possible.

- Think about how relaxing it is to be in that place and how easily you can breathe there.

Energy conservation measures can help residents accomplish tasks with less effort:

- Push or slide objects instead of lifting them. Wheeled carts are helpful.

- To stand, take several slow, deep breaths, and then stand while breathing out through pursed lips.

- Always exhale when lifting or pushing heavy objects or when doing an action or exercise.

- When climbing stairs, use pursed-lip breathing, stop often to rest, and use the rail for support.

Respiratory Disorders

Test

Name _____ Date _____ Score _____

Directions: Fill in or circle the correct answer.

1. The normal rate of respiration is _____ to _____ breaths per minute.

2. The main function of the respiratory system is to inhale oxygen into the lungs, transfer the oxygen to the blood, and exhale carbon dioxide.   True   or   False

3. Asthma can affect people of any age.   True   or   False

4. A positive tuberculin test (PPD) means a person has TB disease and is contagious.
   True   or   False

5. Two things that will help prevent the spread of pneumonia and flu are _____ and immunization.

6. Residents with COPD should not exercise.   True   or   False

7. Which of the following symptoms should be reported to a supervisor?

   a. Cough, shortness of breath, cyanosis

   b. Respiratory rate of 16 and regular

   c. Relaxing and visualizing

8. A resident who has difficulty with activities of daily living because of shortness of breath might be advised to _____.

    a. drink less water

    b. use pursed-lip breathing and take frequent breaks

    c. let someone else do everything for them

9. Which of the following can cause breathing problems for a resident with a lung disorder?

    a. Perfume

    b. Dust

    c. Humidity

    d. All of the above

10. Residents with COPD often suffer from depression, anxiety, or forgetfulness due to _____.

    a. old age

    b. personality disorder

    c. lack of oxygen

CERTIFICATE OF COMPLETION

I hereby certify that

has successfully completed the in-Service

Respiratory Disorders

Signature

Seizures and Strokes

Teaching Plan

To use this lesson for self-study, the learner should read the material, do the activity, and take the test. For group study, the leader may give each learner a copy of the learning guide and follow this teaching plan to conduct the lesson. Certificates may be copied for everyone who completes the lesson.

Learning objectives

After this lesson, participants should be able to:

- Define seizure, seizure disorder, and epilepsy

- Recognize when someone is having a seizure and respond appropriately

- List care measures for people on anticonvulsant medications

- List risk factors for strokes

- State the most common symptoms of stroke

- Recognize the symptoms of stroke and respond appropriately

Lesson activities

Introductory activity

Distribute a copy of the learning activity in Figure 36.1 of this course to each participant. Ask participants to read the stories and write or say how they would respond. This can be done as a group discussion or as an individual activity. It is likely that many of the learners will not know the answers. Reassure them that they will learn how to respond to these important situations in today's lesson.

1. Give a copy of the learning guide to each participant. Instruct participants to listen to your lecture and follow along in the learning guide. Ask them to especially listen for the correct

way to respond to the scenarios given to them in the learning activity and to write down answers they didn't know before.

2. Use lecture and discussion to cover the content in the learning guide. Participants can take turns reading and discussing different sections in the guide.

3. Encourage participants to memorize the five most common symptoms of stroke. Allow time for practice if possible.

4. At the conclusion of the lesson, look at the learning activity again and determine whether the participants are able to write or say the correct way to respond in each case.

Rapid response to both seizures and strokes is essential, so each participant should leave the session knowing exactly what to do in both situations.

Conclusion

Have participants take the test. Review the answers together. Award certificates to those who answer 70% of the test questions correctly.

Test answers

1. c			2. True	3. True	4. b and d	5. d
6. numbness/weakness, confusion/trouble speaking, trouble seeing, dizziness/trouble walking, severe headache			7. b	8. False	9. False	10. a

Seizures and Strokes

Learning Guide

Contents:

- Seizure Disorder

  - What is a seizure?

  - What is epilepsy?

  - When is a seizure not epilepsy?

  - Why are seizures harmful?

  - What causes seizures/epilepsy?

  - What are some types of seizures?

  - How is epilepsy treated?

- Stroke

  - What is a stroke?

  - What are the symptoms of stroke?

  - What is transient ischemic attack?

  - Who is at risk for stroke?

  - What should you do if you see someone having a stroke?

Seizure Disorder

About 2.7 million people in the United States have some form of epilepsy, also called seizure disorder. For the vast majority of cases, no single cause has been determined. People with epilepsy often struggle to overcome low self-esteem and the stigma that is attached to having seizures. Some people mistakenly believe that epilepsy is a form of mental illness or disability. The truth is that many people with seizure disorders lead productive and outwardly normal lives.

What is a seizure?

A seizure is rhythmic jerking of the body, or an involuntary change in body movement, sensation, awareness, or behavior. It can last from a few seconds to a few minutes. Seizures are sometimes called convulsions. Seizures are generally described in two major groups of seizures, primary generalized seizures and partial seizures. The difference between these types is in how and where they begin.

What is epilepsy?

The word epilepsy is used when more than one seizure has occurred. If someone has a single seizure, they are not usually said to have epilepsy. The terms epilepsy and seizure disorder are often used interchangeably. The onset of epilepsy is most common in children and the elderly. Epilepsy is the fourth most common neurological disorder in the United States after migraine, stroke, and Alzheimer's disease.

When is a seizure not epilepsy?

Seizures that are first seizures, that are febrile (caused by high fever), or caused by eclampsia (in pregnancy) are not considered epilepsy. Symptoms experienced by a person during a seizure depend on where in the brain the disturbance in electrical activity occurs.

Why are seizures harmful?

A person can be injured during a convulsion, since the body is moving uncontrollably. Also, the brain can be starved of oxygen during long seizures. This can lead to brain damage. Repeated seizures or seizures that last longer than 20–30 minutes can damage the brain's neurons (nerve cells).

What causes seizures/epilepsy?

A seizure occurs when neurons generate uncoordinated electrical discharges that spread throughout the brain. Anything that disturbs the normal pattern of nerve cell activity can lead to seizures. Neurons are very sensitive to abnormal electrical impulses. Illness, injury, an imbalance of the chemicals in the brain that carry messages between nerve cells, and brain abnormalities can be responsible for seizure. Some examples are as follows:

- Heart attacks and strokes, or any condition that deprives the brain of oxygen. Proper treatment of heart disease and high blood pressure can prevent some cases of epilepsy.

- Metabolic disturbances: alcohol withdrawal, severe liver disease, kidney disease.

- Infections such as meningitis and AIDS. Good treatment may prevent seizures.

- Brain tumors or head injury. Wearing seat belts and cycle helmets and using child car seats can prevent brain injury and therefore prevent this type of seizure.

- Presence of certain drugs or stopping certain drugs suddenly (such as narcotics).

- Illicit drug use, like cocaine, heroin, or PCP.

- Alzheimer's disease.

- Neurodegenerative disorders, such as multiple sclerosis.

- Inherited disorders and genetic factors.

What are some types of seizures?

There are many different kinds of seizures. Following are six main types of seizures:

- Grand mal, or tonic-clonic seizures, involve the entire body in a convulsion. When a person has this type of seizure, he or she may cry out, fall to the floor unconscious, twitch or move uncontrollably, drool, or even lose bladder control. It usually lasts for 5–20 minutes. When the seizure is over and the person regains consciousness, he or she feels exhausted and dazed. This is the image most people have when they hear the word epilepsy. Sometimes people experience warning signs beforehand, such as unusual smells, visual changes, or feelings. This warning is called an aura.

- Complex partial seizures causes a person to appear confused or dazed. He will not be able to respond to questions or direction.

- Petit mal (pet-ee mal), or absence seizure, causes a brief loss of consciousness without other symptoms. There is no warning. This type of seizure is not noticeable in some people. The person may briefly stop what he or she is doing, stare for 5–10 seconds or blink rapidly, and then continue his or her activity. The person becomes unresponsive, appears to be daydreaming, and cannot be aroused during this time.

- Status epilepticus is prolonged, repetitive seizure activity that lasts more than 20–30 minutes while the person is unconscious. It is a medical emergency and can result in death if not treated aggressively. It is caused by certain medications, stroke, infection, trauma, cardiac arrest, drug overdose, and brain tumor.

- A drop seizure causes the muscles to go limp. The eyelids may droop, the head may nod, and the person may drop things and often fall to the ground.

- Myoclonic seizure causes muscles to tense. This type of seizure is characterized by rapid, jerk-like movements that can affect the face, limbs, or axial musculature. They are like being jolted by a mild electric shock and may occur frequently through the day.

- There are several other types of seizures as well: simple partial, complex partial, secondarily generalized, and febrile seizures.

How is epilepsy treated?

There are several ways to treat epilepsy. Treatments can control seizures some of the time in about 80% of people with epilepsy. Once epilepsy is diagnosed, it is crucial that treatment begins as soon as possible.

There are many different medications and a variety of surgical procedures that may provide good control of seizures. Some people are helped with special diets.

People with seizure disorders should carry an identification card or wear a bracelet that tells about their condition, their medications, and their doctor's name and phone number.

Medications to control seizures are called anticonvulsants. These must be taken regularly as directed, without missing doses. Missed doses may cause a single seizure, several seizures, or death.

People with severe seizures who don't take their medications have a shorter life expectancy and more risk of cognitive impairment.

Common anticonvulsants are Dilantin (phenytoin), Tegretol (carbamazepine), Depakene (valproate), and phenobarbital. These medications should be taken with food or milk to prevent stomach problems.

Anticonvulsant medications can cause changes in a person's mental status, including mood and behavior. They can also affect speech, balance, the eyes, the stomach, and the gum tissue in the mouth. Changes in any of these areas must be reported. Good oral hygiene will help prevent gum problems.

What should you do if you see someone having a seizure?

1. Alert you supervisor. Follow the directions of the clinical staff. They may ask you to assist with the following:

    a. Roll the person on his or her side to prevent choking on any fluids or vomit.

    b. Loosen any tight clothing around the neck.

    c. Keep the person's airway open. If necessary, grip the person's jaw gently and tilt his or her head back.

    d. DO NOT restrict the person from moving unless he or she is in danger.

    e. DO NOT put anything into the person's mouth, not even medicine or liquid. These can cause choking or damage to the person's jaw, tongue, or teeth. Contrary to widespread belief, people cannot swallow their tongues during a seizure or at any other time.

    f. Remove any sharp or solid objects that the person might hit during the seizure.

    g. Note how long the seizure lasts and what symptoms occurred so you can report it as soon as possible to your supervisor and/or to emergency personnel.

Stay with the person until the seizure ends. After a seizure ends, the person may be sleepy and tired. He or she may have a headache and be confused or embarrassed. Be patient with the person. You may need to help him or her clean up. A seizure is an emergency situation. Call for help as soon as possible. After the seizure has ended, watch for follow-up concerns, including:

- The person does not begin breathing again and return to consciousness after the seizure stops

- Another seizure begins before the person regains consciousness

- The person had injured himself/herself during the seizure

Stroke

About 600,000 Americans will have a stroke this year. Over 160,000 will die from it. Two-thirds of all strokes happen to people over age 65. Stroke risk doubles every 10 years past age 55. Many of the causes of stroke can be controlled, and rapid treatment when stroke occurs can save lives and prevent permanent damage. May is American Stroke Month.

What is a stroke?

A stroke is a "brain attack," meaning it occurs in the same way a heart attack does, only it affects the brain instead of the heart. A stroke occurs when the blood supply to part of the brain is suddenly cut off. This can happen when a blood clot blocks a blood vessel or when a blood vessel breaks and spills blood into the brain. As a result, brain cells in the affected area die. The cells usually die within minutes to a few hours after the attack starts. When brain cells die, they release chemicals that start a chain reaction, killing even more brain cells in a bigger area.

When brain cells die, the abilities that are controlled by that area of the brain are lost. This can include speech, movement, and memory, depending on where in the brain the stroke occurs and how many brain cells are killed. A small stroke might cause weakness of an arm or leg. A large stroke might cause paralysis on one side of the body or loss of the ability to speak and understand language. People can sometimes recover completely from minor strokes, but a severe stroke can be fatal. Rapid treatment is the key to preventing death and paralysis. Stroke is an emergency!

What are the symptoms of stroke?

The five most common stroke symptoms include sudden:

1. Numbness or weakness of face, arm, or leg, especially on one side of the body

2. Confusion, trouble speaking, or trouble understanding

3. Trouble seeing in one or both eyes

4. Dizziness, trouble walking, loss of balance or coordination

5. Severe headache with no known cause

Alert the nurse or your supervisor if you see any of these symptoms in someone.

Treatment is much more effective if given soon after the attack. Every minute can make a difference in preventing serious damage or death. Get help even if the symptoms are painless or go away quickly.

Some other less common stroke symptoms include:

*   Sudden nausea, fever, and vomiting. This is different from a viral illness because it comes on very quickly, in minutes or hours instead of over several days.

*   Brief loss of consciousness or a period of decreased consciousness, such as fainting, confusion, convulsions, or coma.

These symptoms should be reported to your nurse or supervisor immediately.

What is transient ischemic attack?

A transient ischemic attack (TIA) is a stroke that lasts only a few minutes and goes away quickly. A TIA occurs when the blood supply to part of the brain is briefly interrupted. The symptoms are similar to those of stroke, but they usually disappear within an hour.

Only a doctor can tell whether stroke symptoms are from a TIA or a serious stroke. You should assume that all stroke-like symptoms require emergency help. Don't wait to determine whether they go away. TIAs are often warning signs that a person is at risk for a more serious stroke.

Who is at risk for stroke?

People over age 65, African-Americans, people with diabetes, men, and people with a family history of stroke are at greater risk of brain attack than the rest of the population. These things cannot be controlled. People with diabetes can lower their risk of stroke with treatment.

Many things that increase the risk of stroke can be controlled or treated, such as:

- High blood pressure—untreated high blood pressure increases stroke risk four to six times. Blood pressure is too high if it is usually more than 140/90.

- Heart disease—some heart conditions increase stroke risk by up to six times.

- High cholesterol—this increases the risk of stroke by clogging blood vessels.

- Personal history of stroke or TIA—people who have had a stroke or TIA are at risk for having another stroke. Thirty-five percent of those who experience TIAs have a stroke within 5 years.

- Sleep apnea—people who do not breathe for periods of time while they are sleeping develop low levels of oxygen in the blood, possibly leading to blood clots and stroke.

- Smoking—cigarette or cigar use doubles the risk of stroke by damaging blood vessels.

- Alcohol—excessive alcohol consumption is associated with stroke in some studies.

- Weight—excess weight puts a strain on the blood vessels and is often linked to high blood pressure, high cholesterol, and diabetes.

What should you do if you see someone having a stroke?

Fifty-two percent of the stroke residents in one study were not aware they were experiencing a stroke. Most strokes are recognized by someone other than the victim. If you see the symptoms, alert the nurse or your supervisor. If you are at home or out in the community and see a person with these symptoms, call 911.

Figure 36.1 Seizure and Stroke Learning Activity

Seizures and Strokes Learning Activity

Read the stories below, and then decide how you would respond in each situation.

You find a resident on the floor. Her arms and legs are jerking and thrashing around, and it appears that she has wet herself. She does not respond when you call her name. What is the first thing you should do? List five or six things you should do to respond to this resident's seizure.

a. _____

b. _____

c. _____

d. _____

e. _____

f. _____

2. After the resident in the first scenario has stopped convulsing, she does not open her eyes or respond when you call her name. After a minute or two she begins convulsing again. How should you respond now?

   _____

3. You are helping a resident with a shower. Suddenly the resident begins acting strangely.
   He doesn't seem to understand what you are saying to him, and he appears confused.
   This is not normal behavior for this resident.
   What is this a possible symptom of? _____
   How should you respond to this problem? _____

4. You notice that your resident is not using his right arm like he usually does. He is letting the arm hang at his side while he uses his left hand to do things. When you ask him about it, he says his arm is feeling weak today, but he's sure it will pass. What, if anything, should you do about this?

   _____

Seizures and Strokes Learning Activity Answer Key

Read the stories below, and then decide how you would respond in each situation.

1. You find a resident on the floor. Her arms and legs are jerking and thrashing around, and it appears that she has wet herself. She does not respond when you call her name. What is the first thing you should do? List five or six things you should do to respond to this resident's seizure.

    1. Alert the nurse, follow nurses instructions.

    2. Roll her on her side to prevent choking.

    3. Loosen any tight clothing around her neck.

    4. Keep her airway open.

    5. Remove anything sharp or solid that she might hit.

    6. Stay with the resident until she is fully conscious and calm.

2. After the resident in the first scenario has stopped convulsing, she does not open her eyes or respond when you call her name. After a minute or two she begins convulsing again. How should you respond now?

    ### Alert the nurse
    ### Status epilepticus, or repetitive seizure activity, is life-threatening.

3. You are helping a resident with a shower. Suddenly the resident begins acting strangely. He doesn't seem to understand what you are saying to him, and he appears confused. This is not normal behavior for this resident.

    What is this a possible symptom of? It could be a stroke.

    How should you respond to this problem? Alert the nurse.

4. You notice that your resident is not using his right arm like he usually does. He is letting the arm hang at his side while he uses his left hand to do things. When you ask him about it, he says his arm is feeling weak today, but he's sure it will pass. What, if anything, should you do about this?

    ### This is a symptom of possible stroke. Alert the nurse.

Seizures and Strokes

Test

Name _____ Date _____ Score _____

Directions: Fill in or circle the correct answer(s).

1. A seizure is _____.

   a. a heart attack

   b. a voluntary change in body movement, sensation, awareness, or behavior

   c. an involuntary change in body movement, sensation, awareness, or behavior

   d. the same thing as epilepsy

2. There are many different types of seizures.   True   or   False

3. People who take anticonvulsant medications may be prone to gum problems and need good oral hygiene.   True   or   False

4. The nurse may ask you to assist when a resident is having a seizure. You may be asked to? (More than one answer.)

   a. put a tongue blade in their mouth to keep them from swallowing their tongue

   b. remove any sharp or solid objects they might hit during the seizure

   c. try to hold their body still

   d. stay with them until the seizure ends

5. When is a seizure a medical emergency?

   a. Another seizure begins before the person regains consciousness

   b. The person injures himself/herself during the seizure

   c. The person does not return to consciousness after the seizure stops

   d. All of the above

6. List the five most common symptoms of stroke (five points).

   a. _____

   b. _____

   c. _____

   d. _____

   e. _____

7. Some risk factors for stroke that can be controlled include _____.

   a. age, gender, race, diabetes

   b. high blood pressure, heart disease, high cholesterol, smoking, weight

   c. occupation, allergies, finances, education

   d. there is nothing anyone can do to lower their risk of having a stroke

8. Stroke cannot be treated. True   or   False

9. There is no hurry in getting treatment for stroke, because the damage is already done.
   True   or   False

10. Which of the following is a true statement about stroke?

    a. 52% of stroke occurrences were identified by someone other than the victim

    b. Stroke and seizures occur together

    c. Exercise cannot help prevent stroke

    d. All of the above

CERTIFICATE OF COMPLETION

I hereby certify that

_____

has successfully completed the in-Service

Seizures and Strokes

_____
Signature

37

Skin Care

Teaching Plan

To use this lesson for self-study, the learner should read the material, do the activity, and take the test. For group study, the leader may give each learner a copy of the learning guide and follow this teaching plan to conduct the lesson. Certificates may be copied for everyone who completes the lesson.

Learning objectives

After this lesson, participants should be able to:

- Understand the structure and functions of the skin

- Understand what happens to the skin as people age

- Understand how to care for residents' skin and how to prevent skin problems

- Be able to recognize and report skin problems

Lesson activities

Skin Care Jeopardy Game (Figure 37.1):

1. Review the game answers and the learning guide so you are knowledgeable about the lesson content.

2. The game answers may be read to the learners, or if you have time you can write each one on a separate sheet of paper and tack them to the wall behind cover sheets with the point values. Tack the answers and cover sheets in columns, and place a paper with the category name at the head of each column. The cover sheet can be removed when a learner chooses that category and point value, revealing the answer underneath.

3. If you are reading the game answers, mark the numbers off the game categories chart as they are chosen.

4. Prepare several small gift certificates or other inexpensive prizes, as it is possible that there will be more than one game winner. If prizes are not an option, use the award certificate included with this packet.

5. If possible, enlist the help of another worker to keep score during the game.

6. Remember that the point of the exercise is to learn the material in an interesting way, not to cause conflict. Keep the game fun and educational.

Introduction:

1. Begin by explaining that this lesson will be taught in the form of a game similar to the television game show Jeopardy. The learners will be given answers, and they must come up with the correct questions to match the answers.

2. Review the learning goals for the session.

3. Give everyone a copy of the learning guide, and allow the learners to spend a few minutes reading the material to prepare for the game.

The game

Explain the rules of the game:

1. Each learner will take a turn as a "contestant."

2. By turns, each contestant will choose a category and a value. For example, "Skin Functions for 30."

3. The answer to the question will be read, and the first person to call out the correct question to match the answer given will receive the assigned point value. If preferred, ask learners to raise their hands and be recognized. Learners may refer to their learning guide for help in formulating the correct question.

4. The learner with the most points at the end of the session will receive an award.

Use the game as an opportunity for teaching. Expand upon the information presented in the game as needed, giving illustrations that are specific to your agency.

Make sure everyone understands both the answers and the questions and is able to find the appropriate material in the learning guide.

Conclusion

Have participants take the test. Review the answers together. Award certificates to those who answer 70% of the test questions correctly.

Test answers

1. False	2. d	3. d	4. b	5. c
6. True	7. False	8. a	9. True	10. True

Skin Care

Learning Guide

Contents:

- The Structure of Skin: What Skin Is

- Functions of Skin: What Skin Does

- The Aging of Skin: What Happens

- Caring for Older Skin: What to Do

- Skin Problems

    - What to report to the nurse or supervisor

    - Preventing skin problems

The Structure of Skin: What Skin Is

Epidermis: The thin, top layer of skin surface.

Dermis: The thicker layer underneath the surface. The dermis contains:

- Blood vessels: Tubes that carry blood through the body, with oxygen and food

- Nerves: Fibers that carry sensations to and from the brain

- Oil glands: Organs that secrete an oily lubricating fluid

- Sweat glands: Organs that separate waste products from the blood and secrete them as sweat

- Hair follicles: Organs that create hair

Fatty tissue: Layer of fat under the skin. While not part of the skin, the fatty tissue provides a protective layer of padding (to prevent injury to underlying bones and muscles) and insulation (to keep heat in).

Functions of Skin: What Skin Does

1. Controls body temperature:

   - Releases heat through sweat

   - Constricts and expands surface blood vessels to insulate or cool the body

2. Protects against injury and disease:

   - Covers and pads muscles and bones, preventing damage

   - Forms a barrier against harmful organisms and infection

3. Provides sensations:

   - Nerve endings sense danger

   - Sensitive to pressure, pleasure, pain, and temperature

4. Creates vitamin D:

   - Produced by sunlight on the skin

5. Cares for itself:

   - Self-lubricating with oil glands

6. Warns of disease:

   - Changes in color, temperature, or moistness may signal illness

The Aging of Skin: What Happens

- The skin and fatty tissue layer get thinner

- The skin becomes less elastic

- Oil glands produce less oil, so skin is dry

- Blood vessel walls get thinner and more delicate, so they break easily

- Circulation of the blood slows down, so the skin is not getting as much oxygen and nutrition from the blood, causing the skin to become poorly nourished and fragile

Because of these changes in the skin, older people:

- Tend to feel cold

- Suffer from skin tears

- Heal slowly

- Become wrinkled

- Develop pressure sores

Caring for Older Skin: What to Do

- Keep skin clean:

    – Pat skin, don't rub, when washing or drying

    – Use powder sparingly—excess powder can cause irritation

- Keep skin lubricated:

    – Use lotions liberally

    – Frequent bathing with soap will dry the skin—use lotion cleansers

- Keep skin creases and folds dry

- Keep clothes and bedding dry

- Eat nutritious food and drink lots of water

- Change position often to improve circulation and prevent pressure sores

- Don't disturb moles

- Massage the skin, but avoid bony projections and irritated areas: Massage around but not directly on them

- Use chair cushions and good beds

- Inspect skin daily for redness, tears, blisters, scrapes, or irritated areas

- Report concerns to a nurse

Skin Problems

Decubitus ulcers (bed sores or pressure sores)

Causes:

- Sustained pressure on the skin compresses the blood vessels and prevents nutrition and oxygen from getting to the skin cells. Over time, the skin tissue dies and decubitus ulcers develop.

- The skin is under pressure where the bones press against the skin tissue, especially when the weight of the body or a body part is pushing down on a pressure point.

- Body fluids such as urine and feces contain damaging chemicals. When they remain on the skin, they cause moist areas that become irritated and develop sores.

- Friction from clothing or bedding can injure the skin and lead to skin ulcers.

What to report to the nurse or supervisor

- A red pressure area that does not become normal after 20 minutes without pressure

- A reddened area of the skin that does not turn white when you push on it

- A skin area that is warm or hot to the touch

- Any swelling

- Any opening in the skin

- Blisters, tears, craters, rashes, or holes

- Scrapes or abrasions

- Drainage or weeping from the skin

Be especially alert when you are caring for residents that are frail, don't move around much, or have poor nutrition. *Residents with little or no feeling in parts of the body, such as stroke victims, must be watched because they don't feel pressure spots and change position when they should.*

Preventing skin problems

- Encourage or assist residents to walk or exercise several times per day

- Encourage or assist residents to keep their skin clean, dry, and lubricated

- Encourage or assist residents to keep their bedding free of wrinkles

- Encourage or assist residents to eat well and drink plenty of liquid

For residents that are in chairs most of the time:

- Encourage or assist them to stand, walk, or shift their weight every 15 minutes.

- Teach them how to do chair pushups with their arms.

- Teach them to sit with their knees at the same level as their hips, with their thighs horizontal to the chair. This will distribute their weight along their thighs and away from pressure points.

- If a resident cannot do these things, he or she should return to bed after an hour in a chair.

For residents that are in bed most of the time:

- Teach them how to use side rails and the trapeze to change position frequently, at least every two hours. Be available to assist them if necessary. Even small shifts in body weight are helpful.

- When you are assisting a resident to change position, move him or her carefully so you do not create friction and shearing between the skin and the bedding or clothes.

- The head of the bed should be raised as little as possible, no more than 30 degrees, to prevent sliding and pressure on the bony areas. If it must be raised higher for eating, it should be lowered an hour later.

- Massage the skin when possible, but avoid massaging pressure points or irritated areas.

- For residents that use special chair cushions or mattress overlay pads, check to be sure that the pads are thick enough to do the job. Place your hand under the pad while the patient is on top of it—if you can feel their body through the cushion, the pad is too thin.

For residents with pressure sores:

- Keep weight and pressure off any reddened areas and wounds.

- Use pillows to elevate or separate body parts and keep pressure off an area, such as a pillow under the calf to raise the heel off the bed, or a pillow between the legs to keep the knees from touching.

Skin Care

Test

Name _____ Date _____ Score _____

Directions: Circle the correct answer.

1. A little blister on a resident's skin is normal and nothing to be concerned about.
   True   or   False

2. You should report a reddened area on the skin to the nurse or your supervisor if _____.

   a. it has a dark black or brown center

   b. it doesn't turn white under your thumb when you press on it

   c. you remove all pressure from it and it still doesn't return to a normal skin color after
       20 minutes

   d. b and c

3. You should encourage residents to have healthy skin by _____.

   a. bathing frequently with soap and water

   b. only bathing occasionally

   c. using lots of powder in all the skin folds and creases

   d. staying clean, using lotion, eating well, drinking water, and exercising

4. When sitting in a chair for long periods, your resident should _____.

   a. sit with knees higher than hips

   b. get up or shift their weight every 15 minutes

   c. stay there as long as possible

   d. avoid shifting their weight in the chair too much

5. Older people are at risk for pressure sores because _____.

    a. they eat too much

    b. they bathe too often

    c. the skin, the fatty tissue layer, and the blood vessel walls are thinner and more fragile

    d. their bones get sharper as they age

6. Changes in a person's skin color could be a sign of illness.   True   or   False

7. People who are in bed most of the time should keep the head of their bed raised as high as possible, because a sitting position is better for circulation than a lying position.
   True   or   False

8. Older people tend to feel cold because _____.

    a. the fatty tissue layer is thinner and the blood vessels don't expand and contract as well

    b. they don't wear enough clothes

    c. their internal thermostat doesn't work anymore

    d. none of the above

9. Older people heal slowly because the skin is not getting enough oxygen and nutrition.
   True   or   False

10. People who have had strokes or are paralyzed must be watched closely for skin ulcers.
    True or   False

CERTIFICATE OF COMPLETION

I hereby certify that

_____

has successfully completed the in-Service

Skin Care

_____

Signature _____

38

Feeding Tubes and Oral Care

Teaching Plan

To use this lesson for self-study, the learner should read the material, do the activity, and take the test. For group study, the leader may give each learner a copy of the learning guide and follow this teaching plan to conduct the lesson. Certificates may be copied for everyone who completes the lesson.

Learning objectives

After this lesson, participants should be able to:

- Care for residents who have feeding tubes

- Provide effective oral care

> Note: Parts of this lesson may not be appropriate for every type of worker; it might be beyond your scope of practice. Be sure to know the rules in your state and organization regarding the level of worker allowed to give food, fluids, or medication through feeding tubes. Be ready to explain these rules to your workers.

Lesson activities

If available, bring the equipment used in your facility for tube feeding. Have participants handle the equipment to become familiar with it. Discuss the content of the learning guide with participants. You may wish to ask some of the participants to read the material in advance and present part of the lesson.

If needed, have participants practice oral care by brushing each other's teeth. Prepare for this by asking them in advance to bring toothbrushes and toothpaste to the session. Emphasize the importance of handling and storing dentures correctly to avoid breakage, chipping, warping, and loss.

Conclusion

After participants take the test, review it together. Award certificates to those who answer 70% of the test questions correctly.

Test answers

1. liquid	2. water	3. b	4.b	5. True
6. comfort, prevent bad breath, mouth dryness, infections, and irritations, reduce heart disease	7. 30 minutes to an hour	8. flush with water, avoid acidic liquids, do not mix medicine with formulas, crush tablets completely	9. soft	10. stomach juices

Feeding Tubes and Oral Care

Learning Guide

Contents:

- Feeding Tubes

    - Types of tubes

    - Nourishment

    - Medications

    - Daily care of a gastronomy tube

    - Nasogastric (NG) tube care

- Oral Care

    - Assisting with mouth care

    - Denture care

Feeding Tubes

Sometimes people with certain conditions become unable to eat or drink enough to have adequate nutrition. When this happens, a doctor might put a tube into the patient's stomach to enable the patient to receive nutrition, medicines, or fluids. These tubes come in various sizes and are usually called feeding tubes or enteral tubes. Enteral means "within the digestive tract." Feeding a patient through a tube placed in the digestive tract is known as tube feeding or enteral feeding.

Types of tubes

Occasionally, temporary tubes called nasogastric (NG) tubes are inserted through the nose and into the stomach. These are often used after surgery or when the tube will be needed for only a short time.

Some people have a more permanent feeding tube inserted into the digestive tract through a surgical incision called a stoma.

There are two main types of permanent feeding tubes. One type goes directly into the stomach and is called a gastrostomy tube or G-tube. Sometimes these are called percutaneous endoscopic gastrostomy tubes (**PEG tubes**) because a doctor inserts them with a special instrument called an endoscope. Not all feeding tubes are PEG tubes. Anyone caring for a tube should learn what kind of tube it is.

The second type is a **J-tube** or jejunostomy tube. J-tubes go directly into the small intestine (the upper part of the bowels). These are used when there is a need to bypass the stomach.

Most feeding tubes have an anchoring device inside and outside the digestive tract. The internal anchor, or bumper, keeps the tube from falling out. The external bumper is a disc that keeps the tube from going too far into the stomach.

There is usually a plug at the end of the feeding tube. Adapters on the end of the tube can connect it to a feeding device. Some have a side port for medication administration. Tubes range from size 8 to size 30 and are made of soft, flexible materials such as silicone, rubber, or polyurethane.

Figure 38.1 Feeding Tube

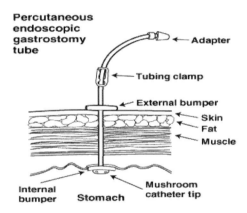

Nourishment

There are many different formulas used to feed people through feeding tubes. Commercially prepared formulas contain all the basic nutrients needed to maintain health.

A resident might have continuous feeding, with a machine that pumps a specific amount of formula per hour into the tube. Follow your facility policy and state's regulations on scope of practice for who can administer tube feedings. It is important for CNAs, who care for residents who have feeding tubes, to understand nourishment is fed through a feeding tube. Some residents receive bolus feedings, also called intermittent feedings, which means they get a certain amount of formula all at one time, usually several times per day.

Once opened, formulas need to be refrigerated at a specific temperature and used within a certain amount of time. If a formula is supposed to be mixed with water, it is important to follow the directions about how much water to use and whether to use sterile water or tap water. Usually, liquid formula should not be diluted with water, because it increases the risk of contamination.

Sometimes formula is given through a food container that is washed after every use. Food containers and tubings used to give the formula must be kept clean. If the feeding is continuous, the tubings and feeding containers should be changed regularly, usually at least every 24 hours. In this case, the container should be marked to show when it was started and how long it should be used.

Medications

The nurse may give residents with feeding tubes their medications through the feeding tube. The doctor orders and pharmacist who dispenses the medicines can give advice about which medications need to be given on a full or empty stomach. This will help determine the timing of feedings and medications.

Not all medicine can be given safely through a feeding tube. The pharmacist will let the facility know if tablets may be crushed and whether time-release capsules may be opened. Liquid forms of medication should be used when available. Liquid medications may usually be diluted with water. Soft gelatin capsules filled with liquid can be given by pricking a hole in the capsule and squeezing out the contents.

Medications should normally not be mixed with formula because of possible interactions between the drug and the formula. Medications should not be mixed together for the same reason. To avoid drug interactions, give 30 cc of water between medications. After giving medicine through a feeding tube, flush the tube with at least 20 to 30 cc of water.

Feeding Tubes and Medication Types

Medications easily given via tube:

- Liquids (best alternative)

- Immediate-release oral tabs

- Soft gelatin capsules

Avoid or ask pharmacist about:

- Crushed enteric-coated tabs

- Sublingual or buccal meds

- Sustained-release caps/tabs

- Syrups

Usually these are **not** given via tubes.

Daily care of a gastrostomy tube

- Always wash your hands and wear gloves when caring for the tube.

- Check the tube site daily for redness, bleeding, drainage, or tenderness.

- Note the length of the tube every day. Use the external marks on the tube if available, or measure the length of the tube from the stoma site to the end of the feeding tube. If the length of the tube changes, it might not be at the right place in the digestive tract. Changes in tube length must be reported to your nurse supervisor.

- Be sure the tube is secured and that there is a small amount of space between the disc or bumper and the skin.

- If there is a button, it should be rotated daily during routine skin cleansing.

- Gently clean the skin around the tube site with soap and water or according to your organization's protocols. Dry the site thoroughly.

Nasogastric (NG) tube care

- Brush teeth twice daily.

- Clean the area where the NG tube goes into the nostrils every day. Use a cotton-tip applicator moistened with warm water. If the patient's nose is sore, apply water-soluble lubricant such as Surgilube or KY jelly.

- Change the nasal tape when it is loose or dirty, or as needed. Make sure the nasal tape is secure at all times.

- A nasogastric tube may irritate the nasal passages. Be gentle when feeding or cleaning around the tube.

Oral Care

Keeping the mouth moist and clean is important for comfort. Good mouth care may help prevent bad breath, mouth dryness, infections, and irritations. Encourage the resident to do his own oral care. If he is unable, staff may assist.

Good nutrition is another way to improve oral health. Acidic juices such as orange juice help reduce the buildup of plaque deposits on the teeth. Encourage residents to floss daily. Research shows that good oral hygiene is linked to a reduced risk of heart disease, probably because good oral cleanliness reduces the bacteria in the body.

Assisting with mouth care

- Gather supplies:

    - Soft toothbrush

    - Toothpaste

    - Emesis basin

    - Washcloth

    - Water or alcohol-free mouth wash

    - Moisturizer or lubricant for lips

- Raise head of bed or assist the resident to sit or stand at the sink

- Place a towel under the resident's head or around the shoulders

- Apply gloves

- Use the toothbrush and a small amount of toothpaste to brush gently the teeth, gums, and tongue

- Do not put the toothbrush too far in the back of the mouth, as this can cause gagging

- Ask the resident to rinse mouth

- Apply lubricant, such as KY jelly, to lips

Denture care

- Dentures should be removed and cleaned at least once per day.

- Apply gloves.

- Use a piece of gauze to handle the dentures. Dentures are slippery and easily dropped.

- Place a washcloth in the bottom of the sink to provide a cushion in case you accidentally drop the dentures in the sink.

- Take dentures from resident. If dentures are difficult to remove, instruct the resident to puff out his cheeks with air. This usually breaks the suction and allows the dentures to be removed.

- Clean dentures over a basin filled with water to avoid chipping them.

- Use only cool water. Hot water can warp dentures.

- Use a denture brush or soft toothbrush and cleaning agent. If there is no denture cleaning agent, use baking soda and water.

- Have the resident rinse his mouth before reinserting dentures.

- Apply denture cream or adhesive as needed and have the resident reinsert dentures in mouth.

- If storing dentures, store in a clearly labeled container filled with cool water. Storing dentures dry can cause them to warp. Keep the container in a safe place.

Feeding Tubes and Oral Care

Test

Name _____ Date _____ Score _____

Directions: Circle or fill in the correct answer.

1. It is best to use _____ medications when giving medications through a feeding tube.

2. It is best to use _____ to flush feeding tubes.

3. All tablets may be crushed in order to administer them through a feeding tube.

   a. True

   b. False

4. When a feeding tube is being used, it is not necessary to consider whether a medication should be given on a full or empty stomach.

   a. True

   b. False

5. Denture warp may occur if dentures are not stored in water. True or False

6. Keeping the mouth moist and clean is important for several reasons. List three reasons:

   a. _____

   b. _____

   c. _____

7. It is important to keep the resident's head higher than the stomach during a tube feeding and for how long afterward?

   a. _____

8. List two ways to prevent clogging of a feeding tube:

    a. _____

    b. _____

9. When assisting with oral care, use a _____ toothbrush.

10. You know that a feeding tube is in the stomach when you see _____ _____ in your syringe.

CERTIFICATE OF COMPLETION

I hereby certify that

_____

has successfully completed the in-Service

_____

Feeding Tubes and Oral Care

_____
Signature

39

Urinary Catheter Care

Teaching Plan

To use this lesson for self-study, the learner should read the material, do the activity, and take the test. For group study, the leader may give each learner a copy of the learning guide and follow this teaching plan to conduct the lesson. Certificates may be copied for everyone who completes the lesson.

Learning objectives

After this lesson, participants should be able to:

- Identify three types of urinary catheters

- Describe three signs and symptoms of a catheter-associated urinary tract infection (UTI)

- List three things that should be considered when performing catheter care

- Understand the importance of proper care of patients with indwelling urinary catheters

Lesson activities

1. Show your team how various types of urinary catheters function

2. Invite an infection-control nurse to talk with your team about catheter-associated infections, the prevalence in skilled nursing and measures to prevent infections

3. Visit the following websites:

    – National Association for Continence (NAFC) at *www.nafc.org*

    – The American Urological Association (AUA) Foundation at *www.urologyhealth.org*

    – Wound, Ostomy, and Continence Nurses Society at *www.wocn.org*

4. Have participants use Figure 39.1 to match types of catheters with their descriptions

Conclusion

Have participants take the test. Review the answers together. Award certificates to those who answer 70% of the test questions correctly.

Test answers

1. c	2. True	3. d	4. d	5. d
6. False	7. b	8. True	9. c	10. d

Urinary Catheter Care

Learning Guide

Contents:

- Introduction

- How the Bladder Works

  - Why a resident needs a urinary catheter

- Types of Urinary Catheters

  - Indwelling catheters

  - External catheters

- Common Problems With Catheter Use

- The CNA's Role

  - Reinforce proper fluid intake education

  - Perform catheter care and maintenance

  - Empty the collection bag

  - Offer comfort and support

  - Observe and report

Introduction

The use of urinary catheters in skilled nursing is not uncommon. For residents with urinary retention, the use of intermittent catheterization or an indwelling catheter is an appropriate treatment option. In some cases, residents with urinary incontinence may benefit from short-term use of a catheter if they have a stage III or stage IV pressure ulcer in an area that would be exposed to urine if the incontinence were managed with another modality. Other indications for catheter use include monitoring urinary output in postoperative or severely ill residents and managing incontinence in terminally or severely ill residents that experience pain with movement.

Staff members are in a position to observe and report potential catheter-related problems early and hopefully prevent the resident from experiencing significant complications.

How the Bladder Works

The kidneys are responsible for filtering waste products from the blood and producing urine for elimination from the body. Ureters (small tube-like structures) take the urine form the kidneys to the bladder. The bladder is a balloon-shaped organ that is made of muscle that can stretch and contract. The bladder is responsible for storing urine (muscle stretches to hold urine) and eliminating urine (muscle contracts to force urine out of the body).

The urine travels from the bladder through the urethra, a tube-like structure, to exit the body. Muscle fibers called a sphincter wrap around the urethra to keep urine in the bladder until nerves carry messages from the bladder to the brain to tell it when the bladder is beginning to feel full. The brain will alert the person that it is time to empty his or her bladder, and, at the same time, it will tell the sphincter muscles to remain closed until the person is able to get to the toilet. A normal bladder empties about four to seven times in 24 hours and does not leak urine.

Key Terms to Aid Your Understanding

- **Alkaline:** a term used to describe substances that rate above 7 on the pH scale.

- **Catheterization:** passage of a catheter into a body channel or cavity (e.g., the bladder).

- **Pressure ulcer:** an inflammation, sore, or injury to the skin and/or underlying tissue over a bony prominence, as a result of prolonged pressure. A stage III and stage IV pressure ulcer refers to the level of tissue damage that has occurred.

- **Sphincter:** the muscles surrounding the urethra that are used to control the flow of urine from the bladder. The muscles relax and contract; when they contract, the urethra is closed.

Why a resident needs a urinary catheter

In skilled nursing facilities, the two most common problems causing a resident to need a urinary catheter are urinary incontinence (when the urine leaks and can't be controlled) and urinary retention (when the bladder doesn't empty completely). In some cases, the resident needs a urinary catheter to capture all urine output for measurement. For some conditions, the physician may need to know exactly how much fluid is going into the resident and how much urine is coming out. In all cases, a urinary catheter is used when there is not a more suitable treatment of the resident's condition, despite problems and risks that can occur with catheter use.

The urinary tract is a common source of bacteremia in residents with urinary catheters. UTI is one of the most common infections and is often related to an indwelling urinary catheter. This lesson will explain the proper way to care for resident with an indwelling urinary catheter.

Types of Urinary Catheters

There are various types of catheters available. The type utilized is based on the reason the resident needs catheterization and the resident's ability to self-manage his or her catheterization. A catheter can be placed in the bladder through the urethra and removed immediately following bladder emptying (in-and-out catheterization), placed into the bladder through the urethra and left in place for a period of time (indwelling catheter), or placed directly into the bladder through a surgical opening in the lower abdomen (suprapubic catheter). External or condom catheters are sometimes options for male residents.

Intermittent catheters are used with residents that cannot completely empty their bladder. The inability to empty the bladder completely is called urinary retention. The nurse briefly inserts the catheter into the bladder to drain the urine. Once the bladder is empty, the catheter is removed. A routine bladder-emptying schedule is determined based on the amount of fluid the patient typically drinks but usually no less than three to four times per day. Intermittent catheters are left in the bladder short term, which lowers the chance of infection.

Indwelling catheters

An **indwelling catheter** is often called a Foley catheter. The indwelling catheter is inserted by the nurse based on the physician's order. The catheter is inserted through the urethra into the bladder. The tip of the catheter is held in place with a water-filled balloon. The catheter is connected to drainage tubing and a collection bag. This type of catheter is used for residents with uncontrollable urine leakage (urinary incontinence) that is caused by a blockage in the urethra or urinary retention that cannot be treated with other methods. Residents with urinary incontinence who develop skin irritation or pressure ulcers (stage III or stage IV) may also benefit from the use of an indwelling catheter to prevent prolonged exposure to urine and promote healing. It is also used when the physicians and nurses need to measure urine output and the incontinence prevents accurate measurement. Terminally ill or severely impaired residents also may use a catheter when moving about is painful.

A **suprapubic catheter** is a type of indwelling catheter. Instead of inserting the catheter through the urethra, it is inserted into the bladder through an incision made in the abdomen just above the pubic bone. A suprapubic catheter may be used because it tends to be more comfortable for residents who need to have a catheter for an extended period of time. They create less risk for UTI than standard catheters. Some problems unique to suprapubic catheters are uncontrolled urine leakage and skin irritation around the insertion site.

External catheters

External catheters, also called condom catheters, are available for men with urinary incontinence (unexpected urine leakage). Condom catheters are used to collect urine leakage. This catheter fits over the penis like a condom. External condom catheters attach to the penis with either a double-sided adhesive, a latex inflatable cuff, or a foam strap. In addition, adhesive-free catheters are held in place by a belt or special underwear. Once the external catheter is applied, it is attached to a urine collection bag by a tube. Residents who are in a chair and/or are otherwise mobile often prefer a smaller collection bag that can be attached to their leg. External catheters are typically disposable and need to be changed every 24 to 72 hours.

External collection devices exist for women. The devices are pouches or form-fitting cups that fit over the perineal area and are attached to the skin by adhesive or straps. The devices are seldom used, because they are uncomfortable for the patient and difficult to keep in place if the patient has any ability to move.

Common Problems With Catheter Use

Infection is the most common problem associated with the use of indwelling catheters. Bacteria (germs) grow in the urine. This is called bacteriuria (bacteria in the urine). As the number of bacteria increases, infection within the bladder and/or other parts of the urinary tract can occur. In the homecare setting, about 8% of residents with an indwelling catheter will develop a UTI.

Bacteriuria develops in most residents within two to four weeks after the catheter is inserted. Even with proper technique for catheter insertion and meticulous hygiene, bacteria may enter the bladder and contaminate the urine. Bacteria can enter from the point the urethra opens to the outside of the body and travel up the catheter or can travel up from the bag to the bladder from inside the catheter system or outside on the surface of the system.

Bladder spasms sometimes occur with indwelling catheters. The balloon that holds the catheter tip inside the bladder may cause the bladder to become irritable and spasm. The risk of spasm increases when the catheter is not properly secured and there is unnecessary movement of the catheter and balloon. The spasms may cause some urine to leak out, which could cause skin irritation due to exposure to urine. Bladder spasms resulting in a small amount of urine leakage are not a reason
to worry unless the catheter leaks continuously or if there is little or no urine in the bag.

Indwelling catheters can become dislodged and/or be pulled out while the balloon at the end of the catheter is still inflated. If this occurs, the balloon can cause damage to the bladder and urethra as it passes out of the body. This can occur when the catheter is secured with too much tension placed on the tubing or can be accidentally pulled out by a confused or ambulatory patient.

External (condom) catheters can also fall off or be pulled off by mistake, resulting in potential skin damage due to prolonged contact with urine. The stripping of the catheter off the penis may also cause skin damage or irritation.

Catheter blockage or obstruction is a serious problem that must be corrected immediately. Occasionally, the catheter gets clogged with **encrustations** (e.g., buildup of bacteria, protein debris, uric acid, or other particles in the urine) or a mucous plug. This causes a blockage of urine flow out of the bladder. The flow of urine can be partially or completely blocked. The blockage could cause increased pressure in the urinary tract, which can cause the bladder, ureters, and kidneys to distend (to swell out or expand). The increase in pressure and distention of the urinary tract can lead to permanent damage to the organs; therefore, it is important that diminished urinary output or absence of output be reported immediately to the home health nurse for further assessment and follow-up. Residents that tend to have encrustation often require more frequent catheter changes to avoid catheter obstruction.

Always Report the Signs and Symptoms of UTIs to the Nurse

- Fever greater than 100.4 degrees F

- Pain or burning in the area of the bladder

- Offensive urine odor

- Change in the appearance of the urine (e.g., cloudy, hematuria [blood in the urine], sediment particles)

- Change in mental status (e.g., confusion, especially in older adults)

A catheter is inserted into the bladder for the purpose of continuous urine drainage. This includes catheters inserted through the urethra or by suprapubic incision. It is a strong risk factor for infection; infection can lead to sepsis and even death.

Special Precautions

- Check the drainage bag to make sure the urine is flowing into the tubing and then into the drainage bag

- Check the area around the urethra for inflammation or signs of infection, such as irritated, swollen, red, or tender skin at the insertion site or drainage around the catheter

- Keep the urinary drainage bag below the level of the bladder

- Make sure the urinary drainage bag does not drag and pull on the catheter

- Report to the nurse any concerns

Figure 39.1 Match the Catheter Description with Catheter Type

1. Used with patients that cannot completely empty their bladder.	a. suprapubic catheter
2. Often called a Foley catheter; inserted through the urethra into the bladder.	b. external catheters
3. A type of indwelling catheter. Instead of inserting the catheter through the urethra, it is inserted into the bladder through an incision made in the abdomen just above the pubic bone.	c. intermittent catheters
4. Also called condom catheters, are available for male patients with urinary incontinence (unexpected urine leakage).	d. indwelling catheter

Answer key

1. c	2. d	3. a	4. b

The CNA's Role

When caring for a patient with a catheter, your role is to follow the plan of care and provide comfort and support, promote dignity, and assist with personal hygiene. You play an important role in preventing problems associated with catheter use and can identify and report signs of potential problems, such as infection, for further assessment.

Reinforce proper fluid intake education

Ideally, your resident's urine should be clear and transparent and not cloudy or dark yellow. The best way to see these results is for the resident to drink at least 8–12 eight-oz. glasses of liquid per day. It is important to know if your patient has any fluid or diet restrictions (e.g., limit fluid to 1,000 cc per day, limit caffeine intake) prior to encouraging the resident to drink more.

Water is the preferred fluid. Tea and juice are also good choices for your residents to have some variety. Carbonated drinks should be avoided or taken in moderation because they make the pH of urine more alkaline, which can cause encrustation, stone formation, and bacterial growth. It is also important to remind patients that foods such as Jell-O, ice cream, and soup are considered fluids and should be counted in their daily consumption.

Tips for fluid intake

Some suggestions to assist residents maintaining needed fluid intake include, but are not limited to:

- Keep a water pitcher or glass of water close at hand to the resident. Easy access to the glass of water will encourage your residents to drink throughout the day.

- For residents who do not typically drink water because they don't like the taste, encourage them to try adding lemon juice or other flavoring to water, use a water filter to get rid of some of the unpleasant taste, and keeping the water cold (cold water tastes better than room-temperature water). Residents with dementia may need frequent reminders to maintain hydration.

Perform catheter care and maintenance

It is important to follow your facility's policy and clinical procedure for performing routine catheter care. Regular catheter care is very important to prevent infection and other complications. The most important factor is keeping the insertion site clean; therefore, residents with catheters will need assistance to maintain their daily hygiene. If your resident is able to shower, he or she may do so without harm. Clean the body with soap and warm water as usual. You will not harm the catheter. The following are steps to consider when providing basic catheter care:

- Before cleaning the catheter, you should tell the resident what you are going to do. Explain that you are going to take care of the catheter to prevent infection and make sure it's working properly.

- Always provide privacy for dignity..

- Make sure you have good lighting so you can clearly see the catheter insertion site, the catheter, the drainage tubing, and the collection bag.

- Hand washing is the top defense against infection. You must always perform hand hygiene according to your agency's policy (wash with soap and water or use an alcohol-based hand sanitizer) before applying your gloves and after glove removal. If the resident performs any self-care, he or she must wash his or her hands before handling the catheter, tubing, or drainage bag.

- It is very important to keep the general perineal area clean. Wash the entire perineal area with warm soapy water. Rinse well and dry thoroughly. Reminder, for women, always clean from front to back, and for men, you may have to retract (pull back) the foreskin on the penis to see the urethra and clean thoroughly.

- Following perineal care, obtain fresh water and a clean washcloth to wash the catheter tubing. Firmly grasp the catheter to prevent tugging on it and gently wash the tubing with soap and water. Begin at the point the catheter enters the body and wash the first 2 to 3 inches of the tube, moving away from the body toward the drainage bag. Do not wash toward the body because this may push bacteria into the catheter insertion site. Gently remove any drainage or crusting that may be present on the tube. Gently dry the tubing.

- Do not apply powder or lotion around the catheter insertion site. The powder can become moist and cause irritation to the surrounding area and/or can provide an environment that enables bacteria to grow.

- Always inspect the catheter insertion site and report any redness, rash, swelling, irritation, or drainage.

- Always inspect the drainage system to ensure there are no leaks, kinks in the tubing, encrustations forming inside the tubing, or anything else that may seem unusual for the resident. It is important that urine can always flow freely from the bladder.

- Inspect the urine drainage. Look for any mucus, blood clots, or other sediment in the tubing. If you notice any of these things, you should notify the care team and follow up as warranted.

- Properly position the collection bag to make certain the urine is always flowing downhill. This can be accomplished by positioned the collection bag below the level of your resident's bladder at all times. This is important whether the resident is sitting, standing, lying down, or walking. Do not place the bag on the floor because of the risk of bacteria getting on the bag and moving up the tubing onto the body.

- Never pull or tug on the catheter. It is important to stabilize the catheter to avoid any tensions or pulling that could cause the catheter to come out of the bladder and/or cause bladder irritation or spasms. For women, the catheter is typically secured to the inner thigh. For men, the catheter can be secured to the lower abdomen when lying in bed or the thigh when sitting in a chair or walking.

Empty the collection bag

The collection bag should be emptied as often as needed but at least every 8 to 12 hours. If using a leg bag, it should be emptied more often, about every 3 to 4 hours. For some residents, you may be required to measure and record the amount of urine collected. Normally, adults make 1 to 2 quarts of clear, yellow urine per day.

To empty the bag, you will need disposable gloves, a container to collect the urine, and alcohol swabs. Because you will be opening a port on a closed drainage system, it is important to follow these guidelines to minimize the risk of bacteria entering the system:

1. Wash your hands with soap and water or use alcohol-based hand sanitizer according to your facility's policy.

2. Put on disposable gloves.

3. Remove the drainage tube from the holder on the collection bag. Point the drainage tube into the container.

4. Unclamp (open) the drainage tube.

5. Drain the urine into the collection container. Do not allow the end of the tube to touch any surface.

6. Reclamp (close) the drainage tube.

7. Clean the tip of the drainage tube with the alcohol swab.

8. Reinsert the drainage tube into the holder on the collection bag.

9. If specified, document the amount of urine as output.

10. Discard the urine into the toilet.

11. Rinse the container that contained the urine, or dispose of it according to your agency's policy.

12. Remove and discard gloves.

13. Wash your hands with soap and water or use an alcohol-based sanitizer according to policy.

Offer comfort and support

You play an important role in helping the resident feel comfortable and accepted. Residents often feel a sense of loss when they require a catheter (long-term or short-term) for elimination of urine instead of going to the toilet as they have done in the past. Provide comfort and support and aid them in maintaining their dignity. You may want to inquire how to obtain a decorative or discreet cover bag for the collection bag to maintain dignity if the person is going in public.

Observe and report

Residents with a urinary catheter are at risk for a number of complications that can cause long-term damage to the urinary tract unless they are quickly recognized and corrected. If you notice any of the following, you should notify your care team:

- Signs and symptoms of a possible UTI.

- Change in urine characteristics (e.g., change in color, cloudy, presence of sediment, hematuria).

- Decrease in the amount of urine output could indicate the resident is not drinking enough or there may be something in the catheter blocking urine flow.

- Absence of urine output must be reported immediately. It could indicate a complete blockage of urine flow, which can be life-threatening.

- Changes around the catheter insertion site (e.g., skin irritation, redness, rash, swelling, drainage).

- Changes in the amount of mucus or sediment buildup on the inside of the drainage tubing.

Urinary Catheter Care

Test

Name _____ Date _____ Score _____

Directions: Circle the correct answer.

1. In skilled nursing, what is one of the most common problems causing a patient to need a urinary catheter?

    a. Excessive urine output

    b. Damaged kidneys

    c. Incomplete bladder emptying

    d. Lack of caregiver

2. Indwelling and external catheters are two types of urinary catheters. True or False

3. What is the most common problem associated with indwelling catheter use?

    a. Encrustation in the catheter

    b. Leaking from the insertion site

    c. Tripping over the tubing

    d. UTI

4. What frequency should the resident with an indwelling catheter perform perineal care?

    a. At least daily and when experiencing discomfort

    b. Following every shower or sponge bath

    c. The same frequency to prior to receiving the catheter

    d. Twice daily and after each bowel movement

5. Which of the following is part of routine catheter care?

    a. Avoid using soap near the catheter insertion site.

    b. Clean the catheter tubing with an up-and-down motion 2 to 3 inches from the insertion site

    c. Gently pull or tug on the catheter to be sure it is securely in the bladder

    d. Secure the catheter tubing to the female patient's thigh

6. When applying an external catheter, you should gently retract the foreskin to completely expose the urethral opening in the penis. True or False

7. What are the signs and symptoms of urinary tract infection?

    a. Excessive urine output, burning, and clear, yellow urine

    b. Fever greater than 100.4°F, blood in the urine, and offensive urine odor

    c. Change in mental status, decreased urine output, and bladder spasms

    d. Sediment in the urine, redness around the insertion site, and urine leakage

8. Adequate fluid intake is an important consideration for residents with a urinary catheter. True or False

9. What should staff do while emptying the collection bag to minimize the risk of infection?

    a. Hold the bag higher than the level of the bladder to ensure proper drainage

    b. Clamp the tubing and remove the collection bag to drain contents into the toilet

    c. Clean the drainage tube with an alcohol swab prior to placing it back in the sleeve (holder)

    d. Place the end of the drainage tube against the bottom of the collection container

10. Which of the following is an area in which staff can have a positive effect while caring for a resident with a urinary catheter?

    a. Observing for signs and symptoms of a UTI

    b. Encouraging fluid intake of at least 8–12 glasses per day

    c. Providing assistance with personal care

    d. All of the above

CERTIFICATE OF COMPLETION

I hereby certify that

has successfully completed the in-Service

Urinary Catheter Care

Signature

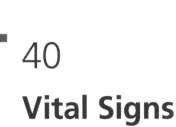

40

Vital Signs

Teaching Plan

To use this lesson for self-study, the learner should read the material, do the activity, and take the test. For group study, the leader may give each learner a copy of the learning guide and follow this teaching plan to conduct the lesson. Certificates may be copied for everyone who completes the lesson.

Learning objectives

After this lesson, participants should be able to:

- State how to measure pulse, respiration, body temperature, and blood pressure

- State the importance of weight measurement

Lesson activities

Preparation:

Gather the following equipment: blood-pressure cuff, stethoscope, thermometer, scale, and forms for documentation. Use the same equipment that is used in your agency for measuring vital signs and weight. Provide a copy of your documentation procedures, or an example of the correct way to document vital signs in your facility, to every learner.

Self-study:

If your workers are using this lesson plan for self-study, have them work with at least one other employee (two others is better) so they can check each other's performance of the required skills according to the skills checklist. The learners will need to read all the material, including this teaching plan, take and check the pretest (Figure 40.1), and perform the skills on the checklists before they receive the certificate. They should also review the correct way to document vital signs in your facility.

Introduction:

1. Give all learners a copy of the learning guide, and ask them to complete Figure 40.1, the pretest, by following the instructions in each section.

2. Go over the pretest with the learners, being sure they understand the correct answers, using the answer key. Allow for questions and explanations.

What's normal?

Point out to your learners that older adults tend to have slightly lower temperatures than younger people, as well as slightly higher blood pressure, pulse, and respirations. Although older people may be in a lower or higher part of the "normal" range, this may still be normal for the individual and the age. Some people may have conditions that mean their "normal" vital signs are different from the ranges given. When a resident can be expected to operate outside the normal range most of the time, the physician should be contacted to establish a normal and acceptable range for the resident. Otherwise, all vital signs outside normal ranges should be reported to the nurse.

Testing vital sign measurements

1. Give the learners time to review the vital sign measurement techniques in the learning guide. Allow for questions.

2. Give each learner a copy of the approved documentation used in your facility for recording vital signs. Review the correct procedure in your facility for documenting vital signs and weight.

3. Explain that each learner will demonstrate his or her ability to correctly measure vital signs and weight as the test for this session.

4. Arrange learners into groups of three. Ask one learner in each group to be the "resident," while the other two learners measure his or her vital signs and weight. Each learner should document the vital signs they obtain. The vital signs obtained by two different people on the same resident should be very close to the same measurement. Variations should be checked by the teacher to determine whether there is a problem with the technique used by one of the learners.

5. Have the resident change places with other learners so that everyone has an opportunity to demonstrate their ability to measure vital signs correctly. Use the check-off boxes under each section of the lesson to document that each learner has demonstrated the abilities on the checklists, and keep these in your training files.

Conclusion

Have participants take the test. Review the answers together. Award certificates to those who answer 70% of the test questions correctly.

Test answers

1. c	2. a	3. a	4. a	5. b
6. b	7. a	8. b	9. c	10. False

Vital Signs

Learning Guide

Contents:

- Measuring Pulse and Respirations

- Measuring Body Temperature

  - Oral temperature

  - Axillary temperature (under the arm)

  - Rectal temperature

- Measuring Blood Pressure

- Weight Measurement

Measuring Pulse and Respirations

☐ Wash your hands

☐ Place the resident's hand in a resting position on a surface, palm up.

☐ Feel along the inside of the wrist with your fingertips, locating the pulse below the patient's thumb and just below the bend of the wrist. Do not use your thumb, as it has a strong pulse of its own.

☐ Look at your watch and find a starting point. Count the beats you feel for 30 seconds, and then multiply that number by two. If the pulse is irregular, count for a full minute and don't multiply.

☐ When you have finished counting the pulse, stay in the same position and watch the patient's chest. It is best if the resident is not aware that you are counting his breathing, because he may alter his breathing rate if he is conscious of being watched.

☐ Look at your watch and find a starting point. Count each time the resident's chest rises and falls as one single respiration.

☐ Count respirations for 30 seconds and multiply by two. If breathing is irregular, count for a full minute and don't multiply.

☐ Wash hands

☐ Document both the pulse and the respirations, writing down the number of heartbeats and the number of breaths you counted per minute.

☐ Notify your supervisor of irregularities or measurements outside the normal range.

Measuring Body Temperature

Oral temperature

☐ Wait at least 15 minutes after the resident has eaten, smoked, or had a drink.

☐ Place a disposable cover on the thermometer, or follow your agency's policy for disinfecting thermometers before reusing them. Be sure the thermometer is not broken, chipped, or cracked.

☐ Ask the resident to wet his lips, and then insert the tip of the thermometer under the patient's tongue and slightly to the side. You may have to push a button on an electronic thermometer to activate it.

☐ Ask the resident to close his lips over the thermometer. An electronic thermometer should stay in place until it beeps.

☐ When finished, remove the thermometer from the resident's mouth and dispose of the cover.

☐ Electronic thermometers will tell you the temperature with a digital reading.

☐ Document the reading. Disinfect and store the thermometer according to policy.

Axillary temperature (under the arm)

☐ Hold the thermometer in the center of the resident's armpit for at least nine minutes or until it beeps.

Rectal temperature

Follow direction from the nurse and your facility's policy on rectal temperatures.

☐ Assist the resident to lie on his or her side with the upper leg pulled up toward the chest as much as possible.

☐ Lubricate the covered rectal thermometer or rectal electronic probe and gently insert it no further than one inch into the resident's rectum. Keep the resident covered during this procedure to protect privacy.

☐ Hold in place for at least 3 minutes, while supporting the resident to prevent any movement that could cause injury. Be careful to avoid trauma to the rectum. Use gloves and standard precautions.

Measuring Blood Pressure

☐ The resident should be relaxed and comfortable, either sitting or lying down. Be sure there is no tight clothing restricting circulation on the arm. The arm should be bare. Loose sleeves can be pushed up.

☐ Rest the resident's arm on a surface such as a table or chair arm, with the palm up and the arm out straight. The resident should not hold the arm up, as using muscles could raise the pressure.

☐ Use a blood pressure cuff that is the right size for the resident. The cuff should fit easily around the arm and overlap but not be so large that it overlaps itself too far. A cuff that is the wrong size will give an incorrect reading.

☐ Wrap the fully deflated cuff snugly (not too tight) around the resident's arm about an inch above the bend in the elbow. The cuff contains a sensor, usually marked with an arrow, which should be placed over the brachial artery. The brachial artery runs along the inside of the arm, on the side next to the body.

☐ Place the gauge where you can easily see it. Put your stethoscope earpieces in your ears.

☐ Close the valve on the sphygmomanometer bulb. This usually means turning the valve clockwise.

☐ Find the brachial pulse by placing your fingers just above the bend in the elbow along the side of the arm closest to the body. Keeping your fingers on the brachial artery, inflate the cuff until you can no longer feel the pulse and then continue inflating for an additional 30 mm on the gauge. Usually you will inflate the cuff until the gauge reads between 170 and 200.

☐ Place the flat disk part of your stethoscope (the diaphragm) on the brachial artery just below the cuff and just above the bend in the elbow.

☐ Open the valve on the bulb slowly and steadily, turning it counterclockwise. The cuff will begin to deflate.

☐ Listen closely to the sounds coming through the stethoscope. At the first pulse sound you hear, note the gauge reading. This is the systolic pressure reading.

☐ Note the gauge reading again when the pulse sound disappears. This is the diastolic pressure.

☐ Deflate the cuff and remove it. Record the blood pressure according to your agency's policy.

Weight Measurement

☐ Weight is not a vital sign, but changes in weight can be important symptoms of illness.

☐ Weigh the resident at about the same time of day each time, using the same scale. Periodically check the scale's accuracy by weighing yourself and comparing this weight with your weight on other scales.

☐ Place the scale on a stable, solid surface, preferably a hard floor without carpeting.

☐ Assist the resident to remove shoes and unneeded clothing. Put a paper towel on the scale.

☐ Be sure the scale is set at zero before having the resident step on it (or sit if it is a chair scale).

☐ Make sure the resident is able to stand safely, and be prepared to provide support.

☐ Wait until the scale stops moving before reading the measurement.

☐ Document the weight measurement.

☐ If using a wheelchair scale or a mechanical lift scale, follow equipment user guide instructions.

Vital Signs

Test

Name _____ Date _____ Score _____

Directions: Circle the correct answer.

1. What is a sphygmomanometer used for?

    a. Temperature

    b. All vital signs

    c. Blood pressure

    d. None of the above

2. Which term refers to how much force is being put on the arteries when the heart is contracting?

    a. Systolic

    b. Diastolic

    c. Respiration

    d. Radial

3. Where is a apical pulse taken?

    a. Chest

    b. Carotid

    c. Wrist

    d. Leg

4. When measuring pulse, you should _____.

    a. place the resident's hand in a resting position on a surface, palm up

    b. use your thumb

    c. count beats for 30 seconds even if the beat is irregular

    d. none of the above

5. When measuring body temperature, you should wait how long after a resident has eaten, smoked, or had a drink?

    a. 1 minute

    b. 15 minutes

    c. A day

    d. An hour

6. When taking blood pressure, the resident's arm should be _____.

    a. flexed, with the hand in a fist

    b. out straight with the palm of the hand up

    c. higher than his chest

    d. none of the above

7. When taking blood pressure, you need to find what type of pulse?

    a. Brachial

    b. Chest

    c. Radial

    d. Carotid

8. Normal values for diastolic blood pressure is between _____.

    a. 20 and 70

    b. 60 and 90

    c. 100 and 140

    d. 150 and 200

9. Normal respirations are between how many per minute?

    a. 70 and 75

    b. 10 and 25

    c. 14 and 25

    d. 14 and 35

10. Weight is a vital sign. True   or   False

CERTIFICATE OF COMPLETION

I hereby certify that

_____

has successfully completed the in-Service

Vital Signs

_____

Signature